Liver imaging: MRI with CT correlation

Current Clinical Imaging Series
Series Editor – Richard C. Semelka

Vascular Imaging of the Central Nervous System: Physical Principles, Clinical Applications and Emerging Techniques;
Joana Ramalho, Mauricio Castillo, 2014

Other books in the Series
Imaging MSK Trauma; Andrea Donovan, Mark E. Schweitzer, 2012

Health Care Reform in Radiology; Richard C. Semelka, Jorge Elias, 2013

Text Atlas of Skeletal Age Determination; Ernesto Tomei, Richard C. Semelka, Daniel Nissman, 2014

Women's Imaging; Michele A. Brown, Haydee Ojeda-Fournier, Dragana Djilas, Mohamed El-Azzazi, Richard C. Semelka, 2014

Liver imaging: MRI with CT correlation

Editors

Ersan Altun MD

Associate Professor of Radiology,
Attending Radiologist,
Abdominal Imaging, Department of Radiology,
The University of North Carolina at Chapel Hill, NC, USA

Mohamed El-Azzazi MD, PhD

Associate Professor of Radiology
University of Dammam, Department of Radiology, Saudi Arabia;
Consultant in the Department of Radiology
King Fahd Hospital of the University, Saudi Arabia;
Assistant Professor of Radiology
University of Al Azhar, Cairo, Egypt,
Clinical Research Scholar
Department of Radiology, University of North Carolina, Chapel Hill, NC, USA

Richard C. Semelka MD

Professor of Radiology
Abdominal Imaging, Department of Radiology
Director of MRI Services
Vice Chair of Quality and Safety
The University of North Carolina at Chapel Hill, NC, USA

WILEY Blackwell

Library of Congress Cataloging-in-Publication Data

Liver imaging : MRI with CT correlation / editors, Ersan Altun, Mohamed El-Azzazi, Richard C. Semelka.
    p. ; cm.
  Includes bibliographical references and index.
    ISBN 978-0-470-90625-5 (hardback)
  I. Altun, Ersan, 1975-, editor. II. El-Azzazi, Mohamed, editor. III. Semelka, Richard C., editor.
  [DNLM: 1. Liver Diseases–diagnosis. 2. Diagnosis, Differential. 3. Imaging, Three-Dimensional. 4. Magnetic Resonance Imaging. 5. Tomography, X-Ray Computed. WI 700]
  RC847
  616.3′620757–dc23

                                                                              2014049427

A catalogue record for this book is available from the British Library.

Wiley also publishes its books in a variety of electronic formats. Some content that appears in print may not be available in electronic books.

Typeset in 9.5/12pt MinionPro by Laserwords Private Limited, Chennai, India

Printed in Singapore by C.O.S. Printers Pte Ltd

1   2015

Contents

List of Contributors

Mamdoh AlObaidy

The University of North Carolina at Chapel Hill, Department of Radiology, Chapel Hill, NC, USA

King Faisal Specialist Hospital & Research Center, Department of Radiology, Riyadh, Saudi Arabia

Ersan Altun

The University of North Carolina at Chapel Hill, Department of Radiology, Chapel Hill, NC, USA

Mohamed El-Azzazi

The University of North Carolina at Chapel Hill, Department of Radiology, Chapel Hill, NC, USA

University of Dammam, Department of Radiology, Dammam, Saudi Arabia

King Fahd Hospital of the University, Department of Radiology, Khobar, Saudi Arabia

University of Al Azhar, Department of Radiology, Cairo, Egypt

Miguel Ramalho

The University of North Carolina at Chapel Hill, Department of Radiology, Chapel Hill, NC, USA

Hospital Garcia de Orta, Department of Radiology, Almada, Portugal

Richard C. Semelka

The University of North Carolina at Chapel Hill, Department of Radiology, Chapel Hill, NC, USA

Preface

In this text we describe the techniques used in modern liver imaging with MRI and CT. Although the breadth of information may be greater on MRI, it is critical to also appreciate all available information that CT conveys. This is essential as CT remains a common tool to evaluate the liver in general practice.

We have striven to show a full range of disease processes, illustrated with comparative examples for both CT and MRI. We have also drawn to the readers' attention examples and settings where MRI findings may be more informative.

CHAPTER 1

The cross-sectional anatomy of the liver and normal variations

Ersan Altun[1], Mohamed El-Azzazi[1,2,3,4], and Richard C. Semelka[1]

[1] The University of North Carolina at Chapel Hill, Department of Radiology, Chapel Hill, NC, USA
[2] University of Dammam, Department of Radiology, Dammam, Saudi Arabia
[3] King Fahd Hospital of the University, Department of Radiology, Khobar, Saudi Arabia
[4] University of Al Azhar, Department of Radiology, Cairo, Egypt

Knowledge of cross-sectional anatomy of the liver is essential for the determination of localization of disease processes and for their management. To have a good knowledge and sense of the cross-sectional anatomy of the liver on computerized tomography (CT) and magnetic resonance imaging (MRI) studies, the segmental anatomy of the hepatic parenchyma and the anatomy of hepatic fissures, hepatic vessels, and bile ducts should be understood.

Liver anatomy can be described using two different approaches, including morphological anatomy and functional anatomy (1).

Morphological anatomy of the liver describes the liver anatomy depending on external appearance of the liver (1). Four lobes of the liver including the right, left, caudate and quadrate can be identified on the basis of the fissures of the liver surface (1). Morphological anatomy is not sufficient for the needs of modern radiology, hepatology, and hepatobiliary surgery.

Functional anatomy of the liver describes the functional segments of the liver on the basis of the anatomy of hepatic vessels and bile ducts (1). Functional anatomy is necessary to meet the needs of modern radiology, hepatology, and hepatobiliary surgery. Functional anatomy of the liver has been described by a number of different nomenclature systems for the determination of anatomic segments of the liver. A single, universally accepted classification system for the functional segmental anatomy of the liver does not exist. The Goldsmith and Woodburne system (1957), the Couinaud system (1957) and the Bismuth system (1982) are the most commonly used nomenclaturel systems (1).

Functional anatomy

The segments of the liver

The Bismuth system, which is a modified version of the Couinaud system, is the most commonly used anatomic nomenclature system, particularly in the United States. This hepatic segmental nomenclature system meets the needs of modern surgical techniques (Table 1.1) (1–5) and allows hepatobiliary surgeons, hepatologists, and radiologists to use a common nomenclature that meets their needs and enables them to understand each other.

The three vertical planes (scissurae) hosting the hepatic veins, and a transverse plane passing through the right and left portal vein branches are used to describe the segments of the liver (1,5).

The three vertical scissurae hosting the hepatic veins divide the liver into four sectors and a transverse plane passing through the right and left portal vein branches divides these sectors into the eight segments, which are numbered clockwise on the frontal view. These segments can be described in a straightforward approach by combining the definitions of two systems including the Bismuth, and Goldsmith and Woodburne systems (Table 1.1). These liver segments, including the caudate lobe, can be described on the basis of this approach as follows: caudate lobe (I), left lateral superior (II), left lateral inferior (III), left medial superior (IVa), left medial inferior (IVb), right anterior inferior (V), right posterior inferior (VI), right posterior superior (VII), and right anterior superior (VIII) (Figures 1.1 and 1.2).

In the Bismuth system, each segment has an independent vascular supply, including arterial, portal, and venous supplies, as well as independent lymphatic and biliary drainage (1–5).

Liver Imaging: MRI with CT Correlation, First Edition. Edited by Ersan Altun, Mohamed El-Azzazi and Richard C. Semelka.
© 2015 John Wiley & Sons, Inc. Published 2015 by John Wiley & Sons, Inc.

Table 1.1 Description of the liver segments according to the three most commonly used nomenclature systems.

Part	N. Goldsmith and R. Woodburne (1957)		C. Couinaud (1957)		H. Bismuth (1982)	
	Segment	Subsegment	Sector	Segment	Sector	Segment
Dorsal	Caudate L.		Caudate L.	I	Caudate L.	I
Left	Lateral	Superior	Lateral	II	Posterior	II
		Inferior	Paramedian	III	Anterior	III
Left	Medial	Superior		IV		IVa
		Inferior				IVb
Right	Anterior	Inferior	Paramedian	V	Anteromedial	V
		Superior		VIII		VIII
Right	Posterior	Inferior	Lateral	VI	Posterolateral	VI
		Superior		VII		VII

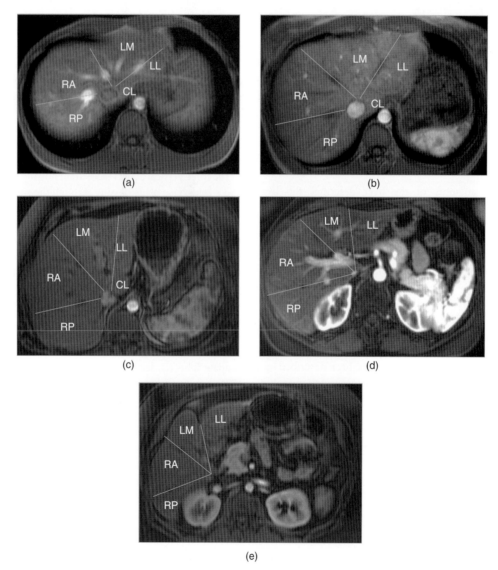

(a)

(b)

(c)

(d)

(e)

Figure 1.1 *Segments of the Liver.* T1-weighted axial hepatic venous (a) and hepatic arterial dominant (b–e) phase 3D-GE images acquired at different levels demonstrate the segments of liver, which are determined based on the distribution of diagonal planes (lines) hosting hepatic veins according to Goldsmith and Woodburne classification. RP, Right lobe posterior segment; RA, Right lobe anterior segment; LM, Left lobe medial segment; LL, Left lobe lateral segment; CL, Caudate lobe.

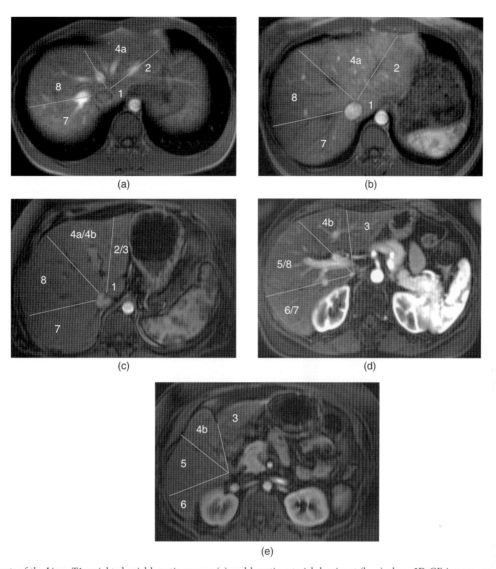

Figure 1.2 *Segments of the Liver.* T1-weighted axial hepatic venous (a) and hepatic arterial dominant (b–e) phase 3D-GE images acquired at different levels demonstrate the segments of liver, which are determined based on the distribution of diagonal planes hosting hepatic veins (lines) and transverse planes hosting portal veins according to Bismuth classification. 1: Caudate lobe. 2: Left Lateral inferior segment. 3: Left lateral superior segment. 4a: Left medial superior segment. 4b: Left medial inferior segment. 5: Right anterior inferior segment. 6: Right posterior inferior segment. 7: Right posterior superior segment. 8: Right anterior superior segment.

The caudate lobe has been described as a separate sector in the Bismuth system (1,5). The caudate lob or segment I is located posteriorly, and positioned between the fissure for ligamentum venosum, the inferior vena cava (IVC), and porta hepatis (Figure 1.2) (1,5). It is anatomically different from other segments as it may often have direct connections to the IVC through hepatic veins, which are different from the main hepatic veins (1,5). The caudate lobe may also be supplied by both branches of the right and left hepatic arteries, and both branches of right and left portal veins (1,5). Because of its different blood supply, the caudate lobe may be spared and/or may be hypertrophied to compensate for the loss of normal liver parenchyma in some liver disorders such as the Budd–Chiari syndrome or cirrhosis.

The corresponding branches of the hepatic arteries, portal veins, and tributaries of the bile ducts are intra-segmental and serve the corresponding segments of the liver by traveling together, while the hepatic veins run independently and are located inter-segmental (1,5). The hepatic arteries, hepatic veins, portal veins, and bile ducts demonstrate frequent variations which may affect surgical procedures in liver transplantations and liver resections.

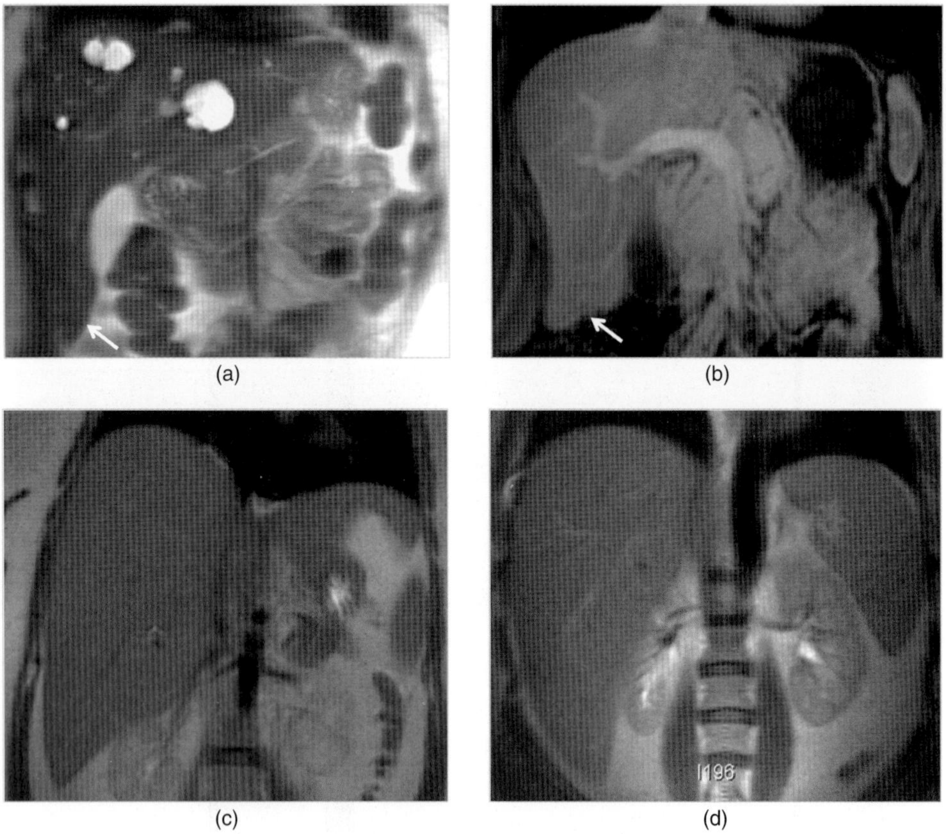

Figure 1.3 *Riedel Lobe.* Coronal T2-weighted single shot echo train spin echo (a) and T1-weighted post-gadolinium fat-suppressed hepatic venous phase (b) images acquired at 3.0 T demonstrate the Riedel lobe as a downward tongue-like vertical elongation of the right lobe with tapered inferior margin with narrow angles (arrows; a, b) in two different patients. Note the cysts in the liver in the first patient (a). Coronal T2-weighted single shot echo train spin echo images acquired at 1.5 T (c, d) demonstrate enlarged liver, with blunt and obtuse angles except the inferior tip of the right lobe, in two different patients with acute hepatitis (c) and fatty liver (d).

Normal variations of the liver segments

One of the most common normal variations of the segments of the liver is Riedel's lobe, which is characterized by the vertical elongation of the right lobe and it appears as a downward tongue-like projection of segment V and VI (Figure 1.3). It is more frequent in women. The Riedel's lobe has frequently a tapered inferior margin with narrow angles on all imaging planes, best appreciated on the coronal plane; however, hepatomegaly often results in a rounded inferior contour with blunt and obtuse angles (Figure 1.3).

Another common normal variation of the liver is the horizontal elongation of the lateral segment of the liver which wraps around the anterior aspect of the upper abdomen and extends laterally to the spleen (Figure 1.4). Focal lesions located in the horizontally elongated left lateral segment, particularly when they are exophytic, may be overlooked or misinterpreted as lesions arising from the adjacent organs such as the stomach or spleen.

Another common variation is the hypoplasia or aplasia of segments of the liver (Figure 1.5). It is more common in the segments VII–VIII–IV. When these segments are hypoplastic, the colonic segments are frequently inter-posed between the normal segments of the liver.

Another common variation is the interposition of the colon between the morphologically normal liver and the chest wall. Rarely, the colon, particularly hepatic flexura, may be interposed between the liver and right hemidiaphragm. The interposition of the colon between the hypoplastic / aplastic liver segments, between the chest wall and the normal liver or between the diaphragm and the liver may require critical technical modifications for the performance of the interventional procedures such as percutaneous biopsies, percutaneous biliary drainage, or transjugular intrahepatic portosystemic shunt creation.

Another variation of the liver segments is the presence of contour undulation resulting from the diaphragmatic insertions along the lateral aspect of the liver. These contour undulations tend to be multiple and closely related to overlying ribs and usually appear as wedge shaped capsular margins (Figure 1.6). They may occasionally appear as longitudinal striations of decreased signal due to the presence of diaphragmatic muscular tissue on T1- and T2-weighted sequences. They may also occasionally appear as rounded pseudolesions along the

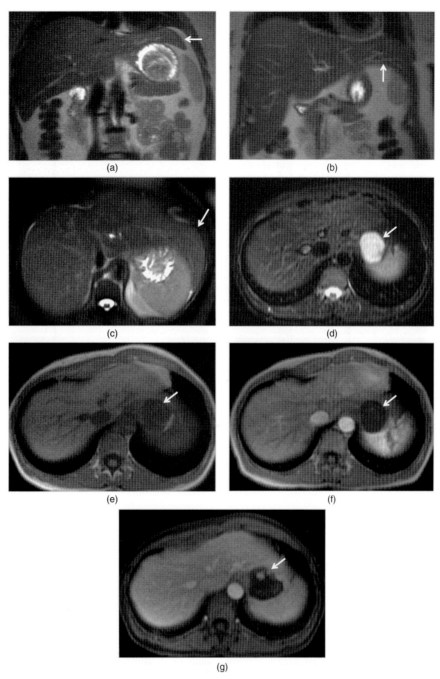

Figure 1.4 *Horizontal Elongation of the Lateral Segment of the Liver.* Coronal (a, b) and transverse fat-suppressed (c) T2-weighted single shot echo train spin echo images show elongated left lateral segment of the liver (arrows, a–c) which wraps around the anterior aspect of the upper abdomen and spleen in three different patients. Transverse T2-weighted fat-suppressed echo train spin echo (d), T1-weighted in-phase SGE (e), T1-weighted postgadolinium hepatic arterial dominant phase SGE (f) and hepatic venous phase fat-suppressed 3D-GE (g) images acquired at 1.5 T show an exophytic hemangioma (arrows, d–g) taking origin from the elongated left lateral segment. The hemangioma, which is adjacent to the spleen, demonstrates markedly high signal on T2-weighted image (d) and peripheral nodular enhancement on post-gadolinium images (f, g). Coronal T2-weighted single shot echo train spin echo (h), transverse T1-weighted pre-contrast SGE (i), T1-weighted post-gadolinium fatsuppressed hepatic arterial dominant phase (j) and hepatic venous phase (k) 3D-GE images acquired at 1.5 T show an exophytic focal nodular hyperplasia (FNH) (arrows, j, k) located in the left lateral segment adjacent to the spleen. The FNH is isointense to the liver on precontrast images (h, i), and demonstrates higher enhancement on the hepatic arterial dominant phase (j) and becomes isointense on the hepatic venous phase (k); compared to the liver parencyhma. Transverse T2-weighted fat-suppressed single shot echo train spin echo (l), T1-weighted pre-contrast SGE (m), post-gadolinium fat-suppressed hepatic arterial dominant phase (n) and hepatic venous phase (o) 3D-GE images demonstrate an exophytic hepatocellular carcinoma (HCC) (arrows, l, m) located in the left lateral segment of the liver. Heterogenous signal consistent with hemorrhage is detected within the tumor on pre-contrast images (l, m). The tumor showed heterogeneous enhancement on the hepatic arterial dominant phase (n) and washout with capsular enhancement on the hepatic venous phase (o).

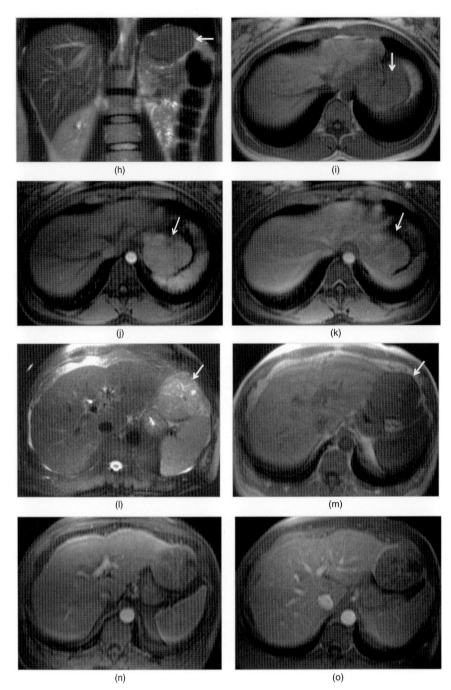

Figure 1.4 (*Continued*)

liver edge (Figure 1.6). These pseudolesions form due to the prominent diaphragmatic insertions and contain perihepatic fat tissue, which shows high signal on both T1- and T2-weighted sequences.

The hepatic vessels and bile ducts
The hepatic arteries
The celiac axis has three branches typically, including the common hepatic artery, splenic artery, and left gastric artery (3,6).

The common hepatic artery has three branches typically, including the proper hepatic artery, right gastric artery, and gastroduodenal artery (Figure 1.7) (3,6). The proper hepatic artery is the artery feeding the liver. This classical hepatic arterial anatomy is seen in 60% of the population and the proper hepatic artery classically divides into right and left hepatic arteries feeding the right and left lobes of the liver, respectively (Figure 1.7) (3,6). However, the right and left hepatic arteries demonstrate significant amount of variations (3,6).

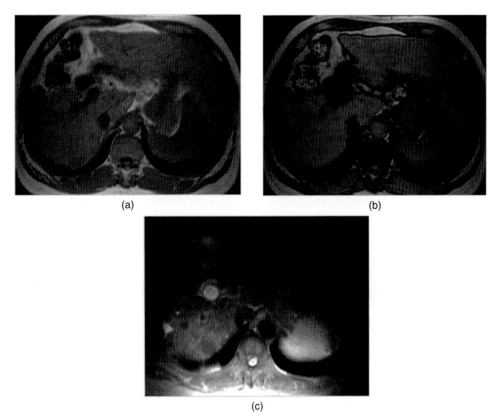

(a)

(b)

(c)

Figure 1.5 *Hypoplasia or Aplasia of the Segments of the Liver.* Segments 8 and 4 are hypoplastic, and the hepatic flexura is interposed between the liver segments. Note that the liver is cirrhotic, and the left lateral segment of the liver is elongated and enlarged.

The right hepatic artery arises from the proper hepatic artery in 55–60% of the population. The right hepatic artery may arise from the common hepatic artery, superior mesenteric artery, celiac artery, gastroduodenal artery, or right gastric artery in 9–11%. The left hepatic artery arises from the proper hepatic artery in 55–60% of the population, but may arise from the common hepatic artery, left gastric artery, the celiac artery, or splenic artery in 4–10% of the population. Both right and left hepatic arteries may arise from the arteries other than the proper hepatic artery in 0.5–1%. The entire hepatic artery proper arises from the superior mesenteric artery in 2–4.5% of the population and from the left gastric artery in 0.5%. The accessory left or right hepatic arteries or both may also be present in 13–16% of the population. The accessory left or right hepatic arteries may arise from the common hepatic artery, left or right hepatic arteries, gastroduodenal artery, superior mesenteric artery, splenic artery, celiac artery, or left or right gastric artery. The hepatic arteries may arise from the arteries other than the proper hepatic artery in the presence of additional accessory hepatic arteries in 2–3% of the population. The middle hepatic artery which is an extrahepatic branch of the proper hepatic artery may also exist in 40% of the population (Figure 1.7). The cystic artery arises from the right hepatic artery in 75% of the population, from the middle hepatic artery

in 13%, from the gastroduodenal artery in 7%, and from the left hepatic artery in 4.5% (3,6).

The portal veins

The main portal vein is classically formed by the confluence of the superior mesenteric vein and splenic vein behind the neck of the pancreas (Figure 1.8) (2,5). It drains the blood from the gastrointestinal tract and spleen (2). It also receives blood from the inferior mesenteric, gastric, and cystic veins. The main portal vein and the right and left portal veins are in the hilar fissure (Figure 1.8). The portal bifurcation may be extrahepatic (48% of cases), intrahepatic (26%), or located at the entrance of the liver (26%) (2). The right portal vein has two sectoral portal branches including the anterior and posterior branches which supply segments V, VIII and VI, and VII, respectively (Figure 1.8) (2). The left portal vein consists of two parts, including the horizontal (extrahepatic) and vertical (intrahepatic) parts (Figure 1.8) (2). The vertical part supplies segments IV, III, and II (2). One segmental branch usually supplies segments II, VI, and VII and more rarely segment III (2). Segments IV, V, and VIII are generally supplied by more than one segmental branch (2).

Anatomic variants of the portal vein are uncommon and seen in only 10–20% of the population (2,3). Normal classic branching pattern, which is characterized by the bifurcation

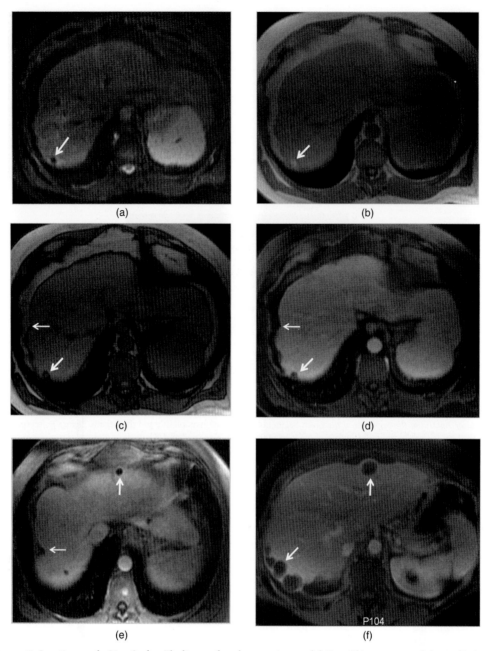

(a)

(b)

(c)

(d)

(e)

(f)

Figure 1.6 *Diaphragmatic Insertions on the Liver Surface.* The liver surface shows contour undulations (thin arrows, c–e) due to diaphragmatic insertions. Note that a round pseudolesion (thick arrows, a–d), which forms due to a prominent diaphragmatic insertion, shows fat signal and no enhancement. These pseudolesions should not be confused with capsular and subcapsular lesions such as metastases. Cystic metastases (thick arrows, e, f) in another patient show peripheral wall enhancement in addition to their contour bulging and high fluid content (not shown).

of the main portal vein into right and left portal veins, is seen in 78.5% (2,3,5). Trifurcation of the main portal vein into right anterior portal vein, right posterior portal vein and left portal vein is seen in 11% of the population (Figure 1.8) (2,3,5). The right anterior segment branch may arise from the left portal vein in 4% of the population (2,3,5). The left portal vein may arise from the right anterior segment branch. The right posterior branch may arise from the main portal vein as the first and separate branch, while the right anterior branch

forms a bifurcation with the left portal vein in 5–10% of the population (2,3,5). Quadrification of the portal vein consisting of the branches for segment VII and VI, the right anterior sector branch, and the left portal vein may also be present in a few (2,3,5). Branches for subsegments or segments may directly arise from the portal bifurcation very rarely (2). Another very rare variation is the absence of portal vein bifurcation, and in this case, the solitary portal vein passes through the entire liver (2).

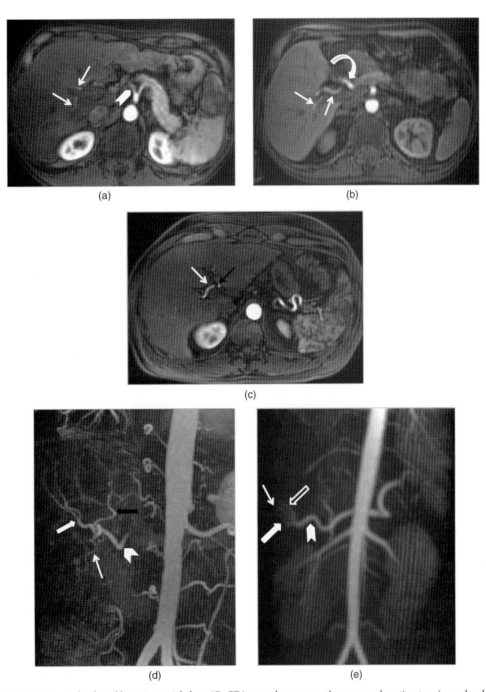

Figure 1.7 *Hepatic Arteries.* T1-weighted axial hepatic arterial phase 3D-GE images demonstrate the common hepatic artery (arrowhead, a), proper hepatic artery (curved arrow, b), right hepatic artery and its branches (white arrows, a – c) and left hepatic artery (black arrow, c) at different levels. Maximum intensity projection images reconstructed from 3D-GE MR angiography coronal source images can also demonstrate the common hepatic artery (arrowhead, d), proper hepatic artery (arrowhead, e), right hepatic artery (white thick arrow, d; white thick arrow, e), left hepatic artery (black arrow, d; white hollow arrow, e), middle hepatic artery (white thin arrow, e), and gastroduodenal artery (white thin arrow, d).

The hepatic veins

The hepatic veins drain into the IVC at the dome of the liver (Figure 1.9) (1). The right hepatic vein drains the segments V – VII and part of VIII (1). The middle hepatic vein drains the segments IV, V, and VIII, although it mainly drains segment IV (1). The left hepatic vein drains the segments II – III and part of IV (1). Variations of the hepatic veins are common. The middle and left hepatic veins form a single trunk before draining into the IVC in 60% of the population (3). Right inferior accessory hepatic veins draining the segment V – VII

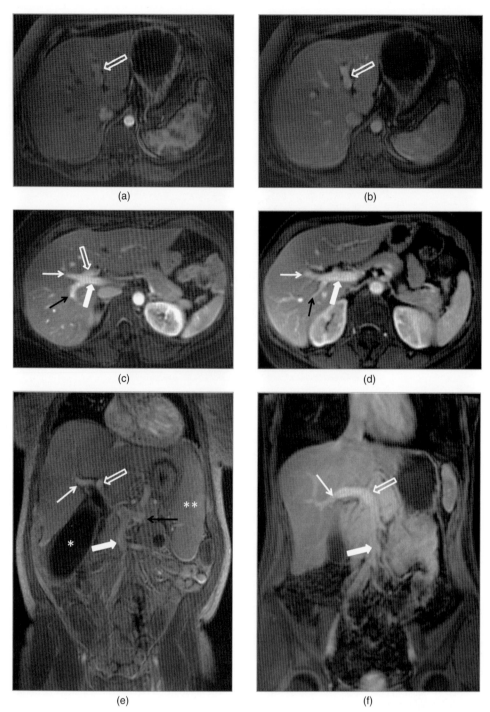

(a)

(b)

(c)

(d)

(e)

(f)

Figure 1.8 *Portal Vein.* T1-weighted axial hepatic arterial dominant (a), hepatic venous (b–d) 3D-GE images demonstrate horizontal part of left portal vein (white hollow arrows, a–c), right portal vein (white thick arrows, c–d), anterior (white thin arrows, c–d), and posterior (black arrows, c, d) branches of right portal vein. Note the trifurcation of the main portal vein (white thick arrow, c) into the right anterior (white thin arrow, c), right posterior (black arrow, c) and left portal vein (white hollow arrow, c) which is the most frequent variation of the main portal vein and its branches. T1- weighted coronal hepatic venous phase magnetization prepared rapid gradient echo (e) and 3D-GE (f) images demonstrate the main portal vein (hollow arrow, e, f), right portal vein (thin arrow, e, f), superior mesenteric vein (thick arrow, e, f) and splenic vein (black arrow, e). Note that the gall bladder (single asteriks, e) is hydropic and the spleen (double asteriks, e) is enlarged. Maximum intensity projection images reconstructed from 3D-GE MR angiography coronal source images can also demonstrate the portal vein (arrow, g) and its branches on the venous phase.

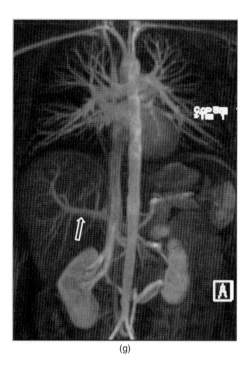

(g)

Figure 1.8 (*Continued*)

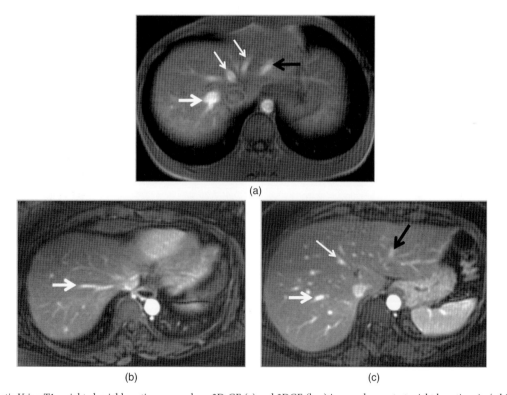

(a)

(b)   (c)

Figure 1.9 *Hepatic Veins*. T1-weighted axial hepatic venous phase 2D-GE (a) and 3DGE (b, c) images demonstrate right hepatic vein (white thick arrow, a–c), middle hepatic vein and its tributaries (white thin arrows, a–c) and left hepatic vein (black arrow, a–c) at different levels. T1-weighted coronal hepatic venous phase 3D-GE image demonstrates the accessory right hepatic vein (thick arrow, d) draining the segment 6. Note the small hemangioma (thin arrow, d) which shows prominent and continuous enhancement on the hepatic venous phase.

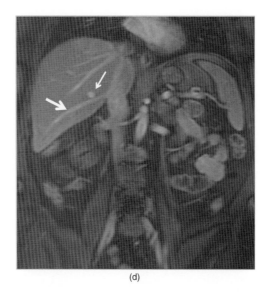

(d)

Figure 1.9 (*Continued*)

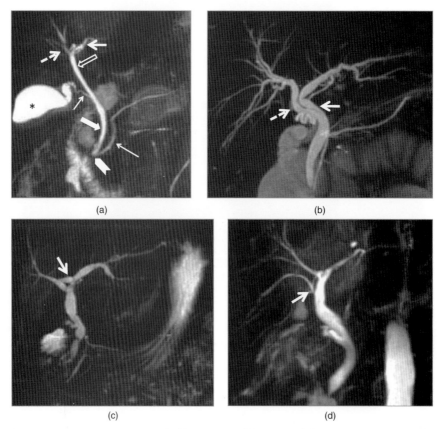

(a) (b)

(c) (d)

Figure 1.10 *Bile Ducts*. Maximum intensity projection images (a–b) reconstructed from coronal thin section source images demonstrate normal (a) and mildly dilated biliary ducts (b) in two different patients. In a patient with normal biliary system (a); intrahepatic bile ducts, right (white thick dashed arrow, a) and left (white thick arrow, a) hepatic ducts, common hepatic duct (white hollow arrow, a), cystic duct (white thin short arrow, a), gall bladder (asteriks, a), common bile duct (white filled arrow, a), and pancreatic duct (white thin long arrow, a). Note that ampulla of Vater (arrowhead, a) which is located at the second portion of the duodenum is visualized well. In another patient with mildly dilated biliary system (b); right (dashed arrow, b) and left (arrow, b) hepatic ducts demonstrate low insertion to the common hepatic duct. Note that fourth order branches of intrahepatic bile ducts can be visualized if they are dilated. Maximum intensity projection images (c, d) reconstructed from coronal thin section source images demonstrate mildly dilated (c) and normal biliary ducts (d) in two different patients. In another patient with mildly dilated biliary system, the right posterior duct directly drains into the left hepatic duct (arrow, c), which is the most common variation of the biliary system. In another patient with normal biliary system, the right posterior duct (arrow, d) drains directly into the common hepatic duct, which is not an uncommon variation. Source: Semelka 2010. Reproduced with permission of Wiley.

may also be commonly seen (Figure 1.9) (3). Right inferior accessory hepatic veins and the drainage of segment V and VIII veins into the middle hepatic vein affect surgical procedures (3).

The bile ducts

Peripheral bile ducts drain into the right and left hepatic ducts, which unite to form the common hepatic duct (Figure 1.10) (3,5). The cystic duct drains into the common hepatic duct, and they together form the common bile duct (Figure 1.10). The common bile duct and main pancreatic duct (duct of Wirsung) unite and form the ampulla of Vater which opens into the second portion of the duodenum at the major papilla (Figure 1.10). The right hepatic duct drains the segments of the right liver lobe [V–VIII] and has two major branches: the right posterior duct draining the posterior segments [VI, VII], and the right anterior duct draining the anterior segments [V, VIII]. The right posterior duct usually runs posterior to the right anterior duct and fuses it from a medial approach to form the right hepatic duct (1). The left hepatic duct is formed by segmental branches draining the segments of the left liver lobe [II–IV] (1). The bile duct draining the caudate lobe usually joins the right and left hepatic ducts at their bifurcation. This normal biliary anatomy is seen in approximately 58% of the population (Figure 1.10) (3).

The most frequent anatomic variation is the drainage of the right posterior hepatic duct into the left hepatic duct in 13–19% of the population (Figure 1.10) (3,5). Simultaneous drainage of the right anterior hepatic duct, right posterior hepatic duct, and left hepatic duct into the common hepatic duct is seen in 11% of the population (3,5). The drainage of the right posterior hepatic duct into the common hepatic duct is seen in 5% of the population (Figure 1.10), and the drainage of the left hepatic duct into the right hepatic anterior duct in 4% of the population (3,5). Accessory hepatic ducts are seen in 2% of the population (3).

The cystic duct also demonstrates three common types of variations as follows: (i) cystic duct's insertion from a lower level, (ii) medial cystic duct insertion and (iii) parallel extension of the cystic duct and common hepatic duct.

References

1 Skandalakis, J.E., Skandalakis, L.J., Skandalakis, P.N., and Mirilas, P. (2004) Hepatic surgical anatomy. Surg Clin N Am, 84, 413–435.

2 Madoff, D., Hicks, M.E., Vauthey, J.-N. *et al.* (2002) Transhepatic portal vein embolization: anatomy, indications, technical considerations. Radiographics, 22, 1063–1067.

3 Catalano, O.A., Singh, A.H., Uppot, R.N. *et al.* (2008) Vascular and biliary variants in the liver: implications for liver surgery. Radiographics, 28, 359–378.

4 Rutkauskas, S., Gedrimas, V., Pundzius, J. *et al.* (2006) Clinical and anatomical basis for the classification of the structural parts of liver. Medicina, 42, 98–106.

5 Macdonald, D.B., Haider, M.A., Khalili, K. *et al.* (2005) Relationship between vascular and biliary anatomy in living liver donors. AJR Am J Roentgenol, 185, 247–252.

6 Covey, A.M., Brody, L.A., Maluccio, M.A. *et al.* (2002) Variant hepatic arterial anatomy revisited: digital subtraction angiography performed in 600 patients. Radiology, 224, 542–547.

CHAPTER 2

The cross-sectional imaging techniques and diagnostic approach

Ersan Altun and Richard C. Semelka

The University of North Carolina at Chapel Hill, Department of Radiology, Chapel Hill, NC, USA

The main cross-sectional imaging techniques of the liver include MRI and CT imaging. MR imaging is the best technique for the imaging of the liver and has higher sensitivity and specificity and resultant diagnostic accuracy for the detection and differentiation of hepatic disease processes compared to CT, mainly due to its higher soft tissue contrast resolution despite the fact that the spatial and temporal resolution of MRI is still lower compared to CT (1). However, the gap between MRI and CT in terms of spatial and temporal resolution has been decreasing dramatically in the last 10 years.

The main focus of this book is to summarize the most common disease process of the liver briefly, to define the MR imaging features with characteristic examples and to correlate MR imaging features and examples with their CT counterparts.

Good image quality is crucial for the evaluation of patients in all modalities in modern radiology. Therefore, imaging techniques which will result in good diagnostic image quality should be applied for liver imaging on both MR and CT.

MR imaging techniques

Diagnostic high image quality, reproducibility of this image quality in each sequence and in each patient, and good conspicuity of disease processes require the use of sequences that are fast and consistent and avoid artifacts (2–4). Maximizing these principles to achieve high-quality diagnostic MR images requires the use of fast scanning techniques which result in consistent high diagnostic image quality with the consistent display of disease processes without any artifacts in all patient groups (2–4).

Motion is still the most common and important obstacle for the acquisition of high quality images. Respiration, bowel peristalsis, and vascular pulsations are the major motion artifacts that have lessened the reproducibility of MRI. However, the use of very fast breathing-independent sequences and breath-hold sequences has decreased, and will decrease more with the help of new faster hardware and sequence designs in the future, these artifacts significantly and form the foundation of high-quality and reproducible MRI studies of the abdomen, including the liver.

Disease conspicuity depends on the principle of maximizing the difference in signal intensities between diseased tissues and the background tissue in the abdomen. For disease processes situated within or adjacent to fat in the abdomen including the liver, such as capsular/subcapsular liver lesions or portal hilar lesions, this is readily performed by manipulating the signal intensity of fat, which can range from low to high in signal intensity on both T1-weighted and T2-weighted images, depending on the use of fat-suppressed or non-fat-suppressed techniques. For example, diseases that are low in signal intensity on T1-weighted images, such as peritoneal fluid or portal hilar lymph nodes, are more conspicuous on T1-weighted sequences in which fat is high in signal intensity (i.e., sequences without fat suppression) (Figure 2.1). Conversely, diseases which are high in signal intensity on T1-weighted images, such as subacute blood as in subcapsular hematoma, hemorrhage in the gallbladder wall or high protein content, are more conspicuous if fat is rendered low in signal intensity with the use of fat-suppression techniques (Figure 2.2). Additionally, lesions containing abundant amount of fat which show high signal intensity on T1-weighted images also can be differentiated from the subacute blood or protein content with the help of fat-suppressed imaging techniques in which fat containing lesions become hypointense due to fat-suppression (Figure 2.3) in contrast to subacute blood or protein content (Figure 2.2). On T2-weighted images, diseases which are low in signal intensity, such as siderotic or some regenerative liver nodules, lesions with subacute blood or high protein, chronic fibrosis or lesions with fibrosis, are more conspicuous on sequences in which background fat is

Liver Imaging: MRI with CT Correlation, First Edition. Edited by Ersan Altun, Mohamed El-Azzazi and Richard C. Semelka.
© 2015 John Wiley & Sons, Inc. Published 2015 by John Wiley & Sons, Inc.

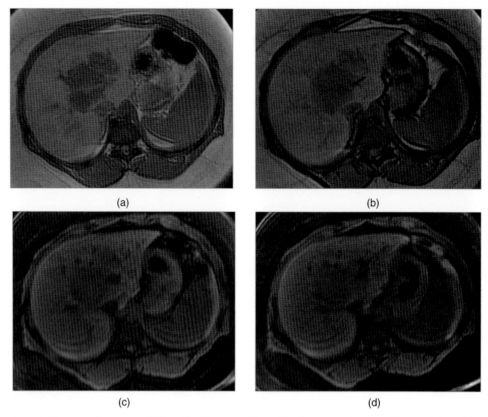

(a)
(b)
(c)
(d)

Figure 2.1 *Increased conspicuity on non-fat-suppressed T1-weighted Sequences.* T1-weighted transverse in-phase (a), out-of-phase (b) 2D-GE, fat-saturated (c, d) 3D-GE images at 3.0 T demonstrate a lesion which invades portal hilus and infiltrates the liver parenchyma in a patient with lymphoma. The lesion is detectable on all sequences; however, it is more conspicuous on in-phase (a) and out-of-phase (b) images. Since the lesion does not contain fat, it does not show any decrease in signal on out-of-phase image (b) compared to in-phase image (a), and on fat-suppressed images (c, d) compared to in-phase image (a).

high in signal intensity, such as non-fat-suppressed sequences (Figure 2.4). Disease processes which demonstrate mild to high signal intensity on T2-weighted sequences, such as focal liver lesions, lymphadenopathy, or mild ascites are most conspicuous using sequences in which fat signal intensity is low, such as fat-suppressed sequences (Figure 2.5).

Gadolinium-enhanced imaging (Figure 2.6) is routinely performed on three phases, including the hepatic arterial dominant, early hepatic venous, and interstitial phases, respectively. An additional hepatocyte phase may also be acquired as a fourth and delayed phase, depending on employed contrast media, protocol, or specific medical condition of the patient.

Gadolinium-enhanced imaging (Figure 2.6) provides at least three further imaging properties that facilitate detection and characterization of disease, specifically, the pattern of blood delivery (i.e., capillary enhancement which is evaluated on the hepatic arterial dominant phase), the patency of hepatic venous and portal venous systems (i.e., venous enhancement which is detected on the hepatic venous phase), and the size and/or rapidity of drainage of the interstitial space (i.e., interstitial enhancement which is evaluated on the interstitial phase) (5). Additionally, hepatocyte specific gadolinium-enhanced imaging phase demonstrates the intracellular distribution of

hepatocyte specific gadolinium agents within the liver and their resultant excretion within the bile ducts (6).

The great majority of diseases can be characterized by defining their appearance on T1-, T2-weighted and different phases of postgadolinium T1-weighted images.

T1-weighted sequences

T1-weighted sequences are routinely useful for investigating diseases of the abdomen and pelvis, including the liver. The primary information that precontrast T1-weighted images provide includes (i) information on abnormally increased fluid content or fibrous tissue content that appears low in signal intensity on T1-weighted images (Figure 2.1), and (ii) information on the presence of subacute blood or concentrated protein, which are both high in signal intensity on T1-weighted images (Figure 2.2). T1-weighted sequences obtained without fat suppression also demonstrate the presence of fat as high signal intensity tissue (Figure 2.3). The routine use of an additional fat attenuating technique permits reliable characterization of fatty lesions (Figure 2.3). In the abdomen and pelvis, gradient echo (GE) sequences including spoiled gradient echo (SGE) or three dimensional gradient echo (3D-GE) sequences are preferred to spin-echo sequence. GE sequences have a number

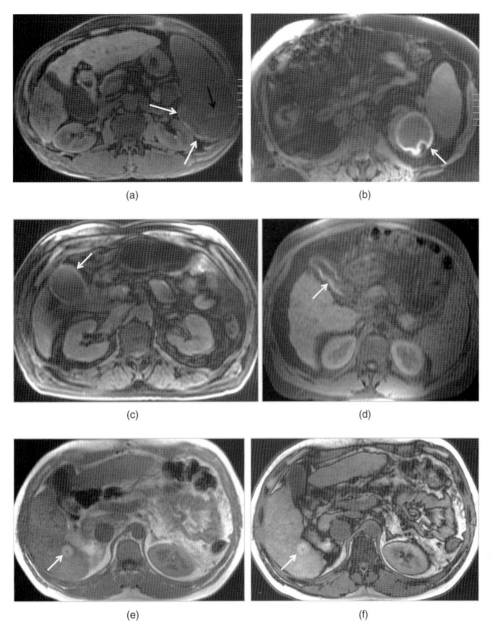

Figure 2.2 *Increased conspicuity on fat-suppressed T1-weighted Sequences.* T1-weighted transverse fat-saturated 3D-GE images demonstrate early subcapsular hematoma (white arrows; a, b) located in the spleen and the left kidney in two different patients. The subcapsular hematoma located in the spleen shows a capsular high signal intensity linear signal at 3.0 T (a). The subcapsular hematoma located in the left kidney shows peripheral high signal intensity surrounding a low signal core (b). Note the lacerations (black arrow, a) as linear high signal intensity tracks in the spleen as well. T1-weighted transverse fat-saturated 3D-GE image (c) at 3.0 T and 2D-GE (d) image at 1.5 T demonstrate thickened gallbladder walls with high signal (arrows; c, d) in two different patients. High signal intensity of the gallbladder walls is consistent with hemorrhage. The diagnosis in both cases is acute hemorrhagic cholecystitis. T1-weighted transverse 2D-GE in-phase (e) and out-of-phase (f) images at 3.0 T demonstrated a small lesion (arrows; e, f) with high signal which does not demonstrate any signal drop on out-of-phase image (f) compared to in-phase image in another patient. The lesion which is diagnosed as hepatocellular carcinoma did not show any change in the signal intensity of lesion in months. Therefore, the high signal intensity of the lesion in this case is due to its high protein content but not due to hemorrhage. Note the central scar of the tumor as well.

of advantages over spin-echo sequences: (i) Similar T1 tissue contrast can be generated with GE sequences as spin-echo sequences in much shorter acquisition times. The two most important implications of this advantage include the use of breath-hold imaging to minimize motion artifacts and the ability to perform contrast-enhanced dynamic exams of the abdomen, including the liver with distinct arterial, venous, and interstitial phases in breath-hold times. (ii) GE sequences enable the use of chemical shift imaging for the detection of small amounts of fat in organs or lesions such as fatty infiltration of

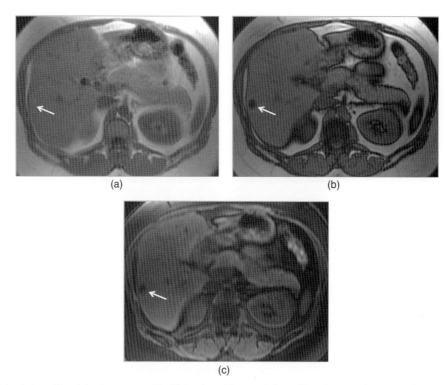

Figure 2.3 *Fat containing lesions.* T1 weighted transverse 2D-GE in-phase (a), out-of-phase (b) and 3D-GE fat-saturated 3D-GE images demonstrate a hepatic adenoma (arrows, a–c). The lesion shows high signal on in-phase image (a), and prominent signal drop on out-of-phase image (b) and fat-saturated image (c). These findings reveal that the lesion contains large amount of fat.

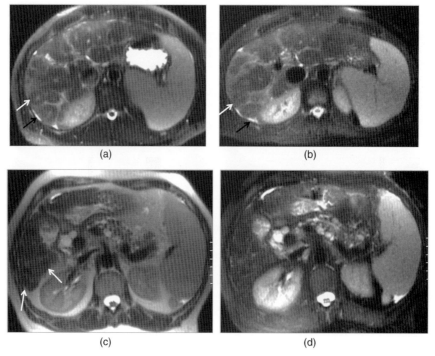

Figure 2.4 *Increased conspicuity of regenerative and siderotic nodules on non-fat-suppressed T2-weighted sequences.* T2-weighted transverse non-fat-suppressed (a) and fat-suppressed (b) single shot echo train spin echo sequences demonstrate macronodular regenerative nodules in a cirrhotic patient. Macronodular regenerative nodules (white arrows; a, b) which demonstrate low signal with central focal high signal on both images, are slightly better appreciated on non-fat-suppressed image. Note the mild ascites (black arrows; a, b) located in the perihepatic space and enlarged spleen developing secondary to portal hypertension. T2-weighted transverse non-fat-suppressed (c) and fat-suppressed (d) single shot echo train spin echo sequences demonstrate siderotic nodules and micronodular regenerative nodules in a cirrhotic patient with common bile duct dilation and multiple cysts located in the pancreas secondary to chronic pancreatitis. The nodules (arrows, c) in the cirrhotic liver demonstrate low signal on both images; however, these nodules are slightly better appreciated on non-fat-suppressed T2-weighted image (c).

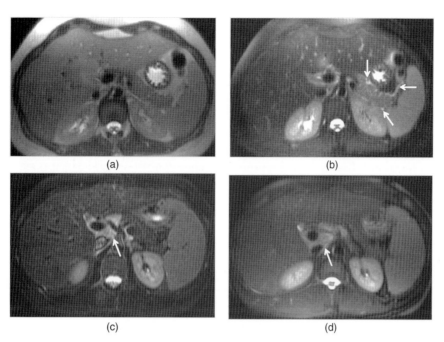

Figure 2.5 *Increased conspicuity on fat-suppressed T2-weighted sequences.* T2-weighted transverse non-fat-suppressed (a) image does no and fat-suppressed (b) single shot echo train spin echo images in a patient with mild acute pancreatitis. The presence of mild peripancreatic free fluid (arrows, b) is not appreciated on non-fat-suppressed image (a) but is seen on fat-suppressed image (b). T2 weighted fat-suppressed single shot echo train spin echo (c) and short tau inversion recovery (d) sequences demonstrate multiple lymph nodes (arrows; c, d) showing high signal at the porta hepatis in another patient with Hepatitis C.

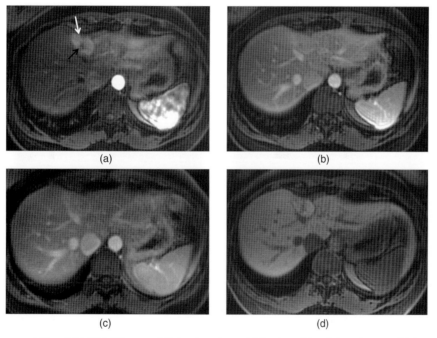

Figure 2.6 *Phases of enhancement.* T1-weighted 3D-GE post-gadolinium hepatic arterial dominant (a), early hepatic venous (b), interstitial (c) and hepatocyte (d) phase images at 3.0 T obtained with the use of gadobenate dimeglumine (Multihance) which is a hepatocyte specific gadolinium based contrast agent demonstrate a focal nodular hyperplasia (white arrow, a). The capillary enhancement of the lesion is evaluated on the hepatic arterial dominant phase (a), and is characterized by the prominent homogeneous enhancement. The drainage of the interstitial space is evaluated on the interstitial phase (c). The interstitial space of the lesion is drained more rapidly compared to the interstitial space of the remaining liver parenchyma so that the lesion becomes isointense to the remaining liver parenchyma on this phase. The central scar of the lesion (black arrow, a) contains fibrosis; therefore, it shows enhancement on the interstitial phase (c) but not on the hepatic arterial dominant phase. Note the capsular enhancement of the lesion as well on the interstitial phase (c). On the early hepatic venous phase (b), the lesion tends to become isointense to the remaining liver parenchyma. The hepatic veins are patent on the early hepatic venous and interstitial phases. On the hepatocyte phase (d), the lesion shows enhancement and becomes isointense to the remaining liver parenchyma due to the presence of hepatocytes and biliary canaliculi.

the liver or hepatocellular adenomas, hepatocellular carcinomas (HCCs), and angiomyolipomas (7).

Gradient echo sequences

The most commonly used GE sequences for routine abdominal imaging are SGE and 3D-GE sequences.

SGE sequences (Figure 2.7) are two dimensional sequences and can also be used as a single (breathing independent) or multi acquisition (breath hold) technique. Image parameters for breath-hold SGE sequences involve (1) relatively long repetition time (TR) (approximately 150 ms) and (2) the shortest in-phase

echo time (TE) (approximately 4.4 ms at 1.5 T, 2.2 ms at 3.0 T), both to maximize signal-to-noise ratio (SNR) and the number of sections that can be acquired in one multisection acquisition (7,8). For routine T1-weighted images, in-phase TE are preferable to the shorter out-of-phase echo times (2.2 ms at 1.5 T, 1.1 ms at 3.0 T), to avoid both phase-cancellation artifact around the borders of organs and fat-water phase cancellation in tissues containing both fat and water protons. Flip angle should be approximately 70° to 90° to maximize T1-weighted information. Using the body coil, the SNR of 2D SGE sequences is usually suboptimal with section thickness less than 8 mm,

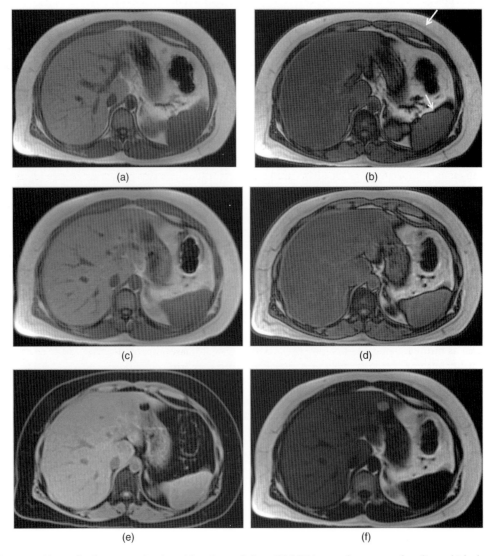

Figure 2.7 *GE Sequences.* T1-weighted transverse in-phase (a) and out-of-phase (b) SGE images demonstrate fatty liver which shows signal drop on out-of-phase image (b). Note the phase cancellation artifact (chemical shift artifact or Indian ink artifact) (arrows, b) as linear hypointense band around the borders of organs on out-of-phase image (b). Fat-water phase cancellation is present in the fatty liver tissue containing both fat and water protons resulting in signal drop on out-of-phase image (b) compared to in-phase image (a). T1-weighted transverse 3D-GE in-phase (c), out-of-phase (d), water-only (e) and fat-only (f) images demonstrate fatty liver in the same patient. The image quality of in-phase and out-of-phase 3D-GE images (c, d) are almost equal to the image quality of SGE images (a, b). Water-only 3D-GE image (e) only demonstrates the water signal of the tissues; therefore, the fat signal is attenuated. Fat-only 3D-GE image (f) only demonstrates the fat signal of the tissues. Since the liver is fatty, increased signal coming from the fat content of the liver is detected on the fat-only image (f).

whereas with the phased-array multicoil, section thickness of 5 mm results in diagnostically adequate images. On new MRI machines more than 22 sections may be acquired in a 20-s breath hold (7,8).

In single-shot techniques, all of the k-space lines for one slice are acquired before acquiring the lines for another slice, that is, in sequential rather than interleaved fashion. SGE may be modified to a single-shot technique by minimizing TR, to achieve breathing-independent images for noncooperative patients (7,8).

GE sequences can be performed as a 3D acquisition, which can be used both for volumetric imaging of organs such as the liver and for pre- and postgadolinium administration.

A 3D-GE sequence is typically performed with minimum TR and TE and a flip angle between 10° and 15°. The flip angle is related to the TR to maximize T1 signal. With a minimum TR, flip angle can also be relatively low and still achieve good T1 contrast. As TR and TE of these sequences have minimum values (TR < 5 ms and TE < 2.5 ms), the flip angle will mainly determine the contrast in the images. In 3D-GE, a volume of data is obtained rather than individual slices. There are several advantages of 3D versus 2D GE sequences: (i) higher inherent SNR than 2D GE sequences, (ii) higher in-plane resolution with larger matrices, (iii) contiguous, thinner sections for higher through plane resolution which facilitates reformats in other planes, (iv) homogenous and fast fat-suppression, which allows scan times that are still short enough to perform breath-hold imaging with fat suppression, (v) the enhancement of vessels and tissues with gadolinium is more obvious because of the fat suppressed nature of the sequence, (vi) gadolinium-enhanced 3D-GE sequences also are the most clinically effective techniques for MR angiography (MRA) of the body (7,8).

3D-GE sequences, in combination with or without robust segmented fat-suppression techniques, overlapping reconstruction, and in-plane as well as through-plane interpolation of the MR data, allow high quality imaging with larger volume coverage in breath-hold times. 3D-GE sequences can be obtained with sufficient anatomic coverage, very thin sections, and high spatial resolution matrices in scan times of only 15–20 s.

Precontrast in-phase and out-of-phase 3D-GE sequences (Figure 2.7) can be acquired with high image quality, although the image quality is slightly below the image quality of 2D SGE. However, their higher spatial resolution is their main advantage. Additionally, the four-point Dixon method allows the acquisition of water-only and fat-only images (Figure 2.7).

3D-GE is particularly suitable for dynamic contrast-enhanced MR imaging because of its excellent inherent fat suppression and sensitivity to enhanced tissues and abnormalities. Currently, most of the 3D-GE sequences used for dynamic gadolinium-enhanced MR exams employ sequential k-space filling as opposed to the sequences with centric or elliptic-centric k-space filling used in MRA in most centers. These beneficial features, in combination with clinically viable acquisition breath hold times, make 3D-GE the primary technique over 2D SGE

for dynamic contrast enhanced imaging of the abdomen and pelvis, including the liver (Figure 2.6) (7,8).

Additionally, 3D-GE sequences with radial acquisition have recently been used in noncooperative patients who cannot hold their breaths. In noncooperative patients, pre and postgadolinium fat-suppressed T1-weighted imaging can be performed with 3D-GE sequences acquired with radial acquisition without breath holding.

Fat-suppressed gradient echo sequences

Fat-suppressed SGE or 3D-GE sequences are routinely used as precontrast images (Figure 2.8). They are important for the detection of subacute blood, high protein content, and fat containing lesions, and particularly for the evaluation of pancreas (Figure 2.8). Image parameters are similar to those for standard SGE or 3D-GE; however, it is advantageous to employ a lower out-of-phase echo time (2.2 to 2.5 ms at 1.5 T) for SGE, which benefits from additional fat-attenuating effects, and also increases SNR and the number of sections per acquisition. Fat-suppressed 3D-GE sequences are now routinely used for the acquisition of fat-suppressed precontrast T1-weighted images. Although the contrast resolution of fat-suppressed 3D-GE is mildly lower compared to fat-suppressed SGE, the acquisition of thin sections with higher matrices is advantageous (7,8).

Fat-suppressed-SGE and 3D-GE images are often used to acquire postgadolinium images (Figure 2.6). Fat-suppression is particularly essential for interstitial-phase gadolinium-enhanced images. The complementary roles of gadolinium enhancement, which generally increases the signal intensity of disease tissue, and fat suppression, which diminishes the competing high signal intensity of background fat, are particularly effective at maximizing conspicuity of diseased tissue (7,8).

Out-of-phase gradient echo sequences

Out-of-phase (opposed-phase) SGE images are useful for demonstrating diseased tissue in which fat and water protons are present within the same voxel. A TE = 2.2 ms is advisable at 1.5 T. A TE = 6.6 ms is also out-of-phase at 1.5 T but the shorter TE of 2.2 ms is preferable as more sections can be acquired per sequence acquisition, the signal is higher, the sequence is more T1-weighted, and in combination with a T2-weighted sequence, it is easier to distinguish fat and iron in the liver. At TE = 6.6 ms both fat and iron in the liver result in signal loss relative to the TE = 4.4 ms in-phase sequence; while on TE = 2.2 ms out-of-phase sequences fat is darker and iron is brighter relative to TE = 4.4 ms, facilitating their distinction (Figure 2.9). At 3.0 T, the shortest in-phase and out-of-phase values are 2.2 and 1.1 ms, respectively. It is not possible to acquire the first echoes at these optimal in-phase and out-of-phase TE times due to gradient capabilities, unless separate in-phase and out-of-phase acquisitions are used or highly asymmetric echoes are utilized in a single scan. Therefore, asymmetric TE values can be preferred for in-phase (2.5 ms) and out-of-phase (1.58 ms) echoes and these values vary depending on the vendor. When

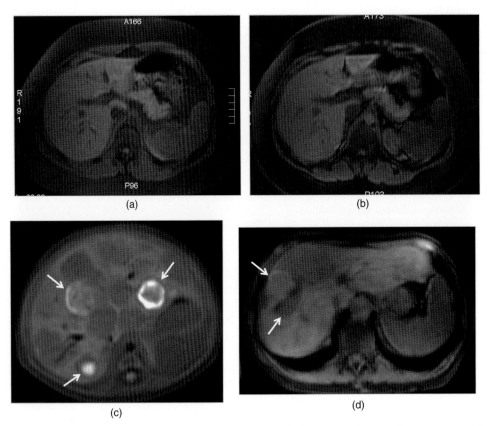

Figure 2.8 *Fat-suppressed GE sequences.* T1-weighted transverse SGE (a) and 3D-GE (b) fat-suppressed images demonstrate normal pancreas with high signal intensity in the same patient. This sequence is particularly essential for the detection of focal lesions such as pancreatic adenocarcinoma, and diffuse disease processes such as pancreatitis and pancreatic fibrosis. Note that the image quality of SGE is slightly better compared to 3D-GE image while the fat-suppression of 3D-GE is better compared to SGE. T1-weighted transverse fat-suppressed SGE image (c) demonstrate multiple hypointense nodular lesions containing hemorrhage which shows high signal in an infant with infantile hemangioendothelioma. T1-weighted transverse fat-suppressed 3D-GE image (d) demonstrate hemorrhagic metastasis in another patient carcinoid tumor.

acquiring in-phase/out-of-phase GE sequences, it is essential to use an opposed-phase TE which is less than the in-phase TE. Additionally, it is also possible to acquire in-phase and out-of-phase images with high in-plane and through-plane spatial resolution with the help of 3D-GE sequences; however, the image quality of this technique is still developing (7,8).

The most common indication for an out-of-phase sequence is the presence of fat in the organs or lesions such as fatty infiltration of the liver, or hepatic adenoma, or HCCs (Figures 2.3, 2.9, and 2.10). Another useful feature is that the generation of a phase-cancellation artifact around high signal intensity masses, located in water-based tissues, confirms that these lesions are fatty. An example of this is angiomyolipoma of the liver (Figure 2.10). In addition to out-of-phase effects, the different TE, for the out-of-phase sequence compared to the in-phase sequence, provides information on magnetic susceptibility effects that increase with increase in TE. This can be used to distinguish iron-containing structures (e.g., surgical clips, iron deposition in the liver, gamna gandy bodies in the spleen) from nonmagnetic signal void structures (e.g., calcium) (Figures 2.9 and 2.11). To illustrate this point, the signal void

susceptibility artifact from surgical clips increases in size, from a shorter TE (e.g., 2.2 ms) out-of-phase sequence to a longer TE (e.g., 4.4 ms) in-phase sequence, whereas the signal void from calcium remains unchanged (7,8). Therefore, 3D-GE or SGE with out-of-phase TE can be used for pre- and postcontrast imaging in patients with prominent susceptibility artifacts which arise from metallic implants, clips, prostheses, or air (free air or bowel gas) and impair the evaluation of adjacent structures, because short TE times decrease the size of those artifacts compared to long TE times as on in-phase images.

Magnetization-prepared rapid-acquisition gradient echo (MP-RAGE) sequences

One limitation of GE sequences, both SGE and 3D-GE, is relative motion sensitivity, and requirement for cooperation by the patient in following breathing instructions. Despite using relatively short breath-hold times, motion artifacts are still the most common and important obstacle for the acquisition of good image quality (Figure 2.12). Therefore, the development of extremely fast breath-hold and/or breathing-independent

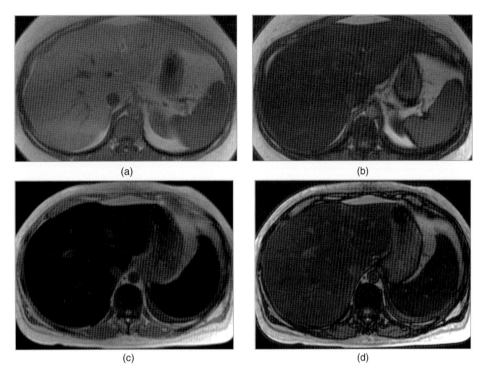

Figure 2.9 *Detection of fatty liver and transfusional hemosiderosis on SGE sequences.* T1-weighted transverse in-phase (a) and out-of-phase (b) SGE images demonstrate diffuse fatty infiltration of the liver which is characterized by the signal drop on out-of-phase image (TE = 2.2 ms) compared to in-phase image (TE = 4.4 ms). This is due to phase cancellation of fat and water signal located in the same tissue. T1-weighted transverse in-phase (c) and out-of-phase (d) images demonstrate diffuse iron deposition in the liver and spleen. Iron deposition is characterized by low signal of the hepatic and splenic parenchyma on in-phase image (TE = 4.4 ms) and by relatively increased signal of the hepatic and splenic parenchyma on out-of-phase image (TE = 2.2 ms) compared to in-phase image. This is due to the effect of shorter TE times used on out-of-phase images.

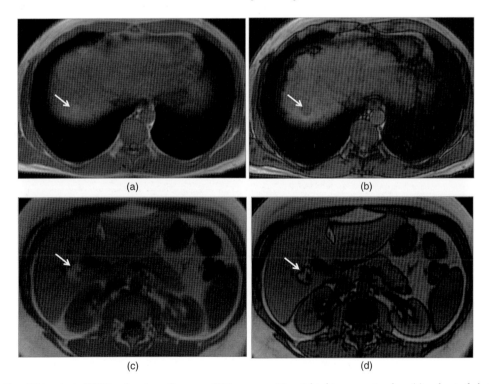

Figure 2.10 *Detection of fat content of HCC and angiomyolipoma on SGE sequences.* T1-weighted transverse in-phase (a) and out-of-phase (b) SGE images demonstrate a small HCC which shows high signal on in-phase image and signal drop on out-of-phase image due to its fat content. T1-weighted transverse in-phase (c) and out-of-phase (d) SGE images demonstrate an angiomyolipoma which shows high signal on both in-phase and out-of-phase images, and phase cancellation artifact around the borders of the lesion. Lesions with abundant fat content do not show signal drop as in angiomyolipomas.

sequences, which would dramatically reduce the motion artifacts, is still in progress.

In uncooperative patients, GE sequences may be modified as a single-shot technique using the minimum TR to achieve breathing-independent images. Such sequences have included so-called magnetization prepared rapid acquisition gradient echo (MP-RAGE). MP-RAGE sequences include turbo fast low-angle shot (turboFLASH) sequence. In 2D multi-section

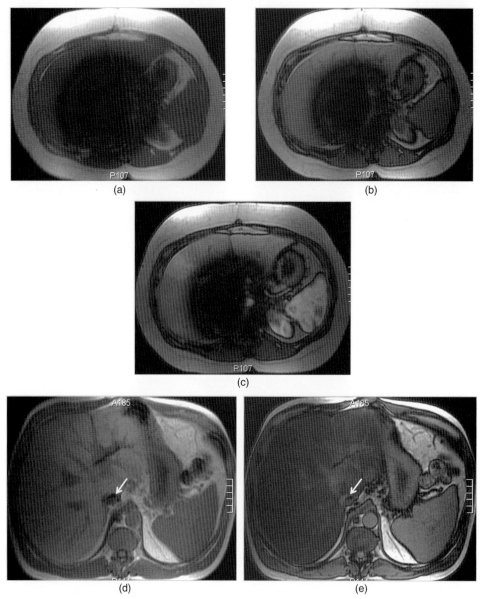

(a)

(b)

(c)

(d)

(e)

Figure 2.11 *Change in the size of susceptibility artifacts on SGE sequences.* T1-weighted transverse in-phase (a), out-of-phase (b) and post-gadolinium hepatic arterial dominant phase (c) SGE images show the decrease in the size of prominent susceptibility artifact arising from IVC filter with short TE times. The artifact is very large and impairs the diagnostic evaluation. However, the artifact decreases in size when shorter TE times (TE = 2.2 ms) are employed on pre-contrast (b) and post-contrast (c) out-of-phase images compared to in-phase (TE = 4.4 ms) image (a). T1-weighted transverse in-phase (d) and out-of-phase (e) SGE images demonstrate the susceptibility artifacts arising from the surgical clips adjacent to the IVC in a patient with liver transplantation. The artifact (arrows; d, e) decreases in size on out-of-phase image compared to in-phase image due to the use of shorter TE times on out-of-phase image. Note that the liver shows signal drop on out-of-phase image compared to in-phase image due to its fat content. T1-weighted transverse in-phase (f) and out-of-phase (g) SGE images in a patient with primary sclerosing cholangitis (PSC). The liver is bizarre shaped and its contours are very irregular due to PSC. Gamna-gandy bodies containing iron are present within the spleen. Since gamna-gandy bodies contain iron, the size and number of these nodules demonstrate decrease on shorter TE sequences including short TE out-of-phase images. T1-weighted transverse in-phase (h) and out-of-phase (i) SGE images demonstrate an angiomyolipoma (thick arrows; h, i) located in the right kidney which shows partial signal decrease and phase cancellation artifact due to its abundant fat content on out-of-phase image. Also note that the susceptibility artifacts (thin arrows; f–i) arising from the bowel gas decreased in size with short TE times employed on out-of-phase imaging.

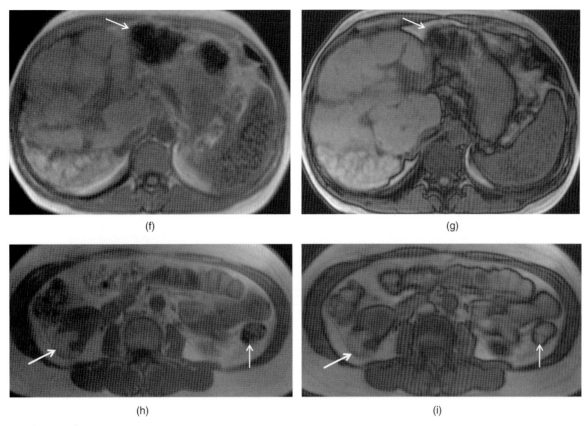

Figure 2.11 (*Continued*)

varieties, these techniques are generally performed as a single shot, with image acquisition duration of 1 to 2 s, which renders them relatively breathing-independent. Magnetization preparation is currently performed with a 180° inversion pulse to impart greater T1-weighted information. The inversion pulse may be either slice or non-slice selective. Slice-selective means that only the tissue section that is being imaged experiences the inverting pulse, while non-slice-selective means that all the tissue in the bore of the magnet experiences the inverting pulse. The advantage of a non-slice-selective inversion pulse is that no time delay is required between acquisition of single sections in multiple single-section acquisition. A stack of single-section images can be acquired in a rapid fashion. This is important for dynamic gadolinium-enhanced studies. A non-slice-selective inversion pulse results in slightly better image quality, particularly because flowing blood is signal-void. Approximately 3 s of tissue relaxation is required between acquisition of individual sections, which limits the usefulness of this sequence for dynamic gadolinium-enhanced acquisitions. Current versions of MP-RAGE are limited because of low signal-to-noise, varying signal intensity and contrast between sections, unpredictable bounce-point boundary artifacts due to signal-nulling effects caused by the inverting 180° pulse, and unpredictable nulling of tissue enhanced with gadolinium (Figure 2.13). Research

is ongoing to solve these problems with MP-RAGE so that it may assume a more important clinical role. Routine use of a high quality MP-RAGE sequence would further increase the reproducibility of MR image quality by obviating the need for breath-holding, particularly in patients unable to suspend respiration (Figure 2.13). 3.0 T MR imaging particularly improves the image quality of MPRAGE sequences due to higher signal to noise ratio and greater spectral separation (Figure 2.13) (7,9,10). Additionally, the use of spatial-spectral selective water excitation (WE), which is a special fat suppression technique compatible with MPRAGE sequence, allows the use of fat suppression with MPRAGE, particularly on postgadolinium sequences (Figure 2.13). Spatial-spectral selective WE is a newer fat-attenuation technique which selectively excites water protons, leaving protons in fat unperturbed, rather than exciting all protons and then spoiling the signal from fat protons (10).

T2-weighted sequences

The predominant information provided by T2-weighted sequences includes (i) the presence of increased fluid in diseased tissue, which results in high signal intensity, (ii) the presence of chronic fibrotic tissue, which results in low signal intensity, and (iii) the presence of iron deposition, which results in very low signal intensity.

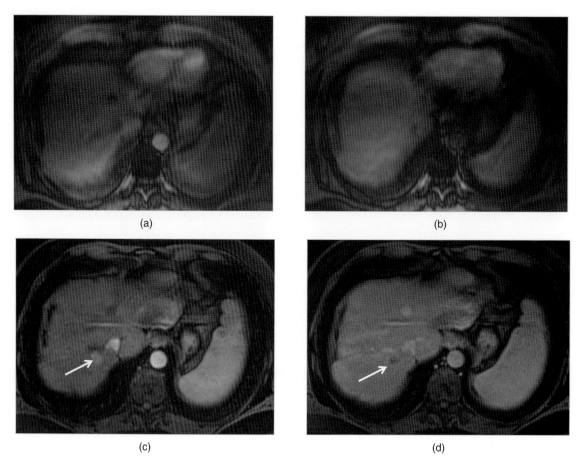

(a) (b)

(c) (d)

Figure 2.12 *Motion artifacts.* Transverse T1-weighted fat-suppressed 3D-GE images acquired at 1.5 T on the early arterial phase (a) and interstitial phase (b) are blurred due to motion artifacts and no lesion is detected. However, transverse T1-weighted fat-suppressed 3D-GE images acquired at 1.5 T one month later shows a lesion with higher enhancement (arrow, c) on the hepatic arterial dominant phase (c) and washout (arrow, d) on the interstitial phase (d). Note that the enhancement of the tumor, which is a hepatocellular carcinoma, could not be demonstrated on the early arterial phase image (a) because of the incorrect timing in addition to the motion artifacts. Furthermore, the washout of the tumor could not be detected on the interstitial phase (b) due to motion artifacts.

Echo-train spin-echo sequences

Echo-train spin-echo (ETSE) sequences are termed *fast spin-echo*, *turbo spin-echo*, or *rapid acquisition with relaxation enhancement* (RARE) sequences. The principle of ETSE sequences is to summate multiple echoes within the same repetition time interval to decrease examination time, increase spatial resolution, or both.

ETSE sequences allows the acquisition of higher matrices with shorter acquisition times and resultant decreased motion artifacts compared to conventional T2-weighted spine echo sequences. Due to this advantage, ETSE sequences are generally used for evaluation of the pancreaticobiliary ductal system.

ETSE sequences, acquired as contiguous thin 2D sections, 3D thin section, or as a thick 3D volume slab, form the basis for MR cholangiography (Figure 2.14). The greatest concern with high resolution 3D ETSE sequences is the significant increase in specific absorption rate (SAR). This is particularly relevant as most 3D implementations must increase the echo-train length compared to 2D varieties because of the added data that needs to be acquired. Recently, newer MR systems, in combination with advances in gradient and software design, have allowed the development of efficient long echo-train 3D ETSE using variable flip angle refocusing pulses. Concerns of SAR are offset by using smaller (constant or variable) flip angles during data acquisition. With this strategy, T2 information can be maintained throughout the echo-train, or used more effectively, for high SNR imaging. Efficiency is further aided by implementing an additional "restore" pulse at the end of data collection to expedite magnetization recovery, allowing shorter TRs (~1200 ms) to be used for T2 imaging. These recent modifications to conventional 3D-ETSE imaging have made high resolution isotropic T2 imaging of the pelvis and biliary system feasible in a relatively short acquisition time (~5 min) (7,11).

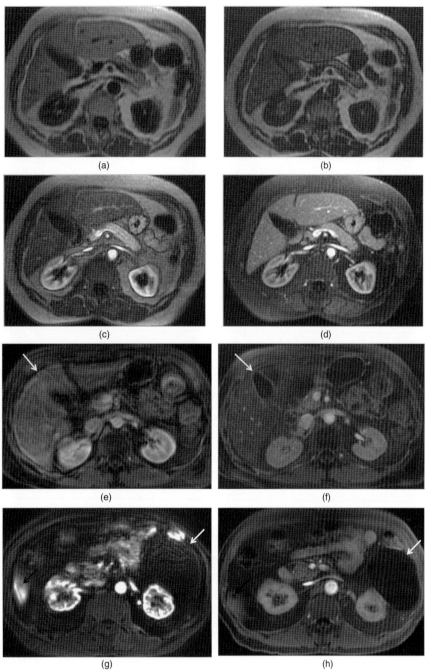

Figure 2.13 *MPRAGE sequences and 3D-GR sequences with radial sampling.* T1-weighted transverse in-phase (a), out-of-phase (b), hepatic arterial dominant phase (c) and early hepatic venous phase water excitation (d) MPRAGE images demonstrate fair but diagnostic image quality in an uncooperative patient with fatty liver. The liver shows mild signal drop on out-of-phase image. Fair image quality of MPRAGE sequences is due to lower signal to noise ratio, higher susceptibility artifacts and signal nulling effects such as varying signal intensity – contrast between sections, unpredictable bounce-point boundary artifacts and unpredictable nulling of tissue with gadolinium. Note that the kidneys show low signal on pre-contrast MPRAGE images due to signal nulling effects. T1-weighted transverse post-gadolinium 3D-GE image (e) acquired in a non-cooperative patient at 1.5 T is not diagnostic due to breathing artifacts; however, post-gadolinium water excitation (WE) MPRAGE image (f) acquired with a breathing independent technique is diagnostic without breathing artifacts with fair image quality. Note that even the gallbladder (arrows; e, f) on 3D-GE image at 1.5 T (e) is not visualized well due to breathing artifacts. However, all organs are visualized well with WE-MRAGE sequence at 1.5 T (f). T1-weighted transverse post-gadolinium 3D-GE image (g) acquired in a non-cooperative patient at 3.0 T is not diagnostic due to breathing artifacts; however, post-gadolinium WE-MPRAGE image (h) acquired with a breathing independent technique is diagnostic without breathing artifacts with good image quality. Note that even the big renal cyst (white arrows; g, h) is not visualized well on 3D-GE at 3.0 T due to breathing artifacts while even the small liver cyst (black arrows; g, h) is visualized well on WE-MPRAGE sequence at 3.0 T. WE-MPRAGE sequence at 3.0 T has superior image quality compared to 1.5 T due to its higher signal to noise ratio. Noncooperative patient protocol including transverse fat-suppressed T2-weighted SS-ETSE (i, j), T1-weighted in-phase MP-RAGE (k, l), precontrast fat-suppressed T1-weighted 3D-GE sequences with radial sampling (m, n), postgadolinium fat-suppressed T1-weighted 3D-GE sequences with radial sampling acquired on the interstitial phase demonstrate infiltrative gallbladder cancer involving the liver. A gallbladder tumor arising from the gallbladder wall is detected (arrows; i, k, m, o). The tumor is large extending into the liver and shows heterogeneous enhancement (asteriks; j, l, n, p). Note the higher image quality of 3D-GE sequences with radial sampling compared to MPRAGE sequences. Source: Semelka 2010. Reproduced with permission of Wiley.

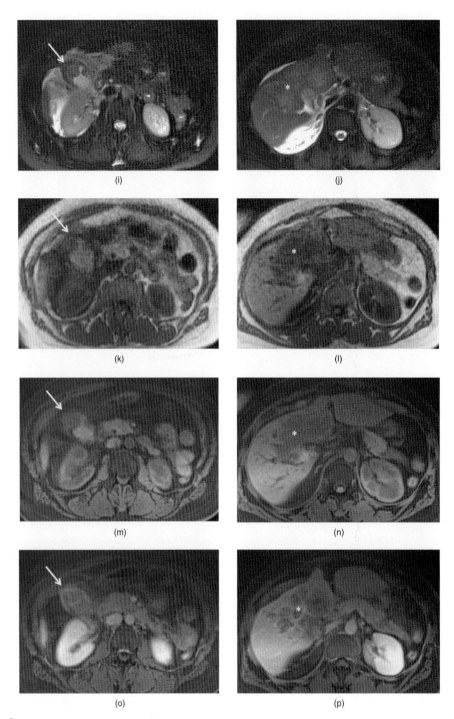

Figure 2.13 (*Continued*)

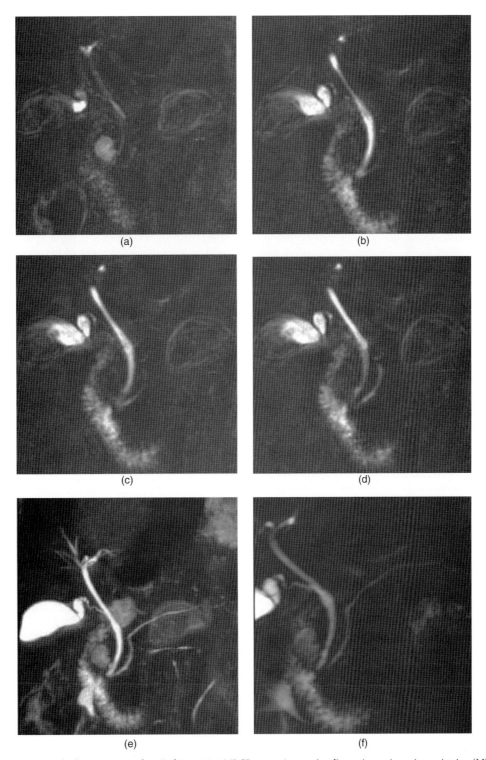

(a)

(b)

(c)

(d)

(e)

(f)

Figure 2.14 *MRCP.* T2-weighted echo train spin echo 3D thin section MRCP source images (a–d), maximum intensity projection (MIP) reconstruction image (e) and thick section MRCP image (f) show normal intra and extrahepatic bile ducts, normal ampulla of vater and normal pancreatic duct. T2-weighted echo train spin echo 3D thin section MRCP source images (a–d), maximum intensity projection (MIP) reconstruction image (e) and thick section MRCP image (f) show normal intra and extrahepatic bile ducts, normal ampulla of vater and normal pancreatic duct. Source: Semelka 2010. Reproduced with permission of Wiley.

Single-shot echo-train spin-echo sequence

Single-shot ETSE sequence (e.g.: half-fourier acquisition single shot turbo spin-echo (HASTE), single shot fast or turbo spin echo (SSFSE or SSTSE) or single shot echo-train spin echo (SS-ETSE) is a breathing independent T2-weighted sequence that has had a substantial impact on abdominal imaging (Figures 2.4 and 2.5). Typical imaging involves a 400 ms image acquisition time, in which k-space is completely filled using half-Fourier reconstruction. Shorter effective echo time (e.g., 60 ms) is recommended for bowel-peritoneal disease, and longer effective echo time (e.g., 100 ms and greater) is recommended for liver-biliary disease. Since the technique is single-shot, the echo train length is typically greater than 100 echoes, while the effective TR for one slice is infinite. A stack of sections should be acquired in single-section mode in one breath-hold to avoid slice misregistration; however, the method lends itself to free-breathing application under uncooperative imaging circumstances. Recently, 3D versions of this technique have been implemented. Motion artifacts from respiration and bowel peristalsis are obviated; chemical-shift artifact is negligible; and susceptibility artifact from air in bowel, lungs, and other locations is minimized, such that the bowel wall is clearly demonstrated (Figure 2.15). Similarly, susceptibility artifact from metallic devices such as surgical clips or hip prostheses is minimal (Figure 2.15). All of these effects render SS-ETSE an attractive sequence for evaluating abdomino-pelvic disease. In patients with implanted metallic devices and extensive surgical clips, SS-ETSE is the sequence least affected by metal susceptibility artifact (7,11).

However, one disadvantage of SS-ETSE sequences is that T2 differences between tissues are reduced in part due to averaging of T2 echoes, which has the greatest effect of diminishing contrast between background organs and focal lesions with minimal T2 differences. This generally is not problematic in the pelvis due to substantial differences in the T2 values between diseased and normal tissue. In the liver, however, the T2 difference between diseased (solid tissue) and background liver may be small and the T2-averaging effects of summated multiple echoes blur this T2 difference. These effects are most commonly observed with HCC. Fortunately, diseases with T2 values similar to those of the liver generally have longer T1 values than the liver, so the lesions poorly visualized on ETSE are generally apparent on precontrast GE as low signal lesions or on postgadolinium GE images as low or high signal lesions, depending on the enhancement features (7,11).

Fat-suppressed (FS) echo-train spin-echo sequences

Fat suppression in spin echo sequences is useful for investigating focal liver disease to attenuate the high signal intensity of fatty infiltration, if present. Fatty liver is high in signal intensity on ETSE, in particular single shot versions, which lessens the conspicuity of high signal intensity liver lesions. Diminishing fat signal intensity with fat suppression accentuates the high signal intensity of focal liver lesions (Figure 2.16). FS SS-ETSE is also

useful for evaluating the biliary tree. Fat suppression appears to diminish the image quality of the bowel due to susceptibility artifact from air–bowel wall interface and is not recommended for bowel studies, although bowel-related extraluminal disease (such as appendicial abscess) may be well shown with this technique.

Fat suppression in ETSE sequences is achieved through either spectrally-selective or non-spectral selective preparation pulses. Non-spectral selective fat suppression, which is termed *short tau inversion recovery* (STIR), is performed with a slice-selective inversion pulse timed to suppress the T1 of fat (TI = 150 ms at 1.5 T) (Figure 2.16). As the pulse is broadband, both water and fat are magnetization-prepared, resulting in suppression of fat signal, alteration of contrast from water signal, and depression of water signal from equilibrium. While fat signal is uniformly suppressed, the remaining soft tissue (water signal) has lower signal as a direct consequence of the inversion pulse. As soft tissue in the abdomen has long T1 relative to fat, adequate SNR is still maintained. Although STIR is sensitive to non-uniform inversion (due to B1 field effects), the method is well-accepted as a robust technique for fat suppression in the abdomen, using spin echo-based sequences. As the sequence is fundamentally different from SS-ETSE, it may be useful to combine both short duration sequences for the liver in place of longer, breathing-averaged ETSE (7,12).

An alternate method of fat suppression involves spectral selection of fat resonances exclusively. Preparation pulses (inversion or saturation) can be spectrally tuned to fat signal, while avoiding undue suppression or alteration of water signal, as seen with STIR techniques. Conceptually, the technique is similar to STIR, in which magnetization (in this case, only fat) is prepared with an inversion pulse timed to suppress fat. Ideally, other soft tissue will remain unaffected, preserving high contrast-to-noise ratio. Since spectral fat suppression is frequency-specific, it is sensitive to spatial susceptibility, which creates an inhomogeneous magnetic field (Figure 2.17). The water and fat resonances are not clearly delineated in this circumstance, causing fat–water frequency "overlap", and potentially a significant number of fat spins to be unsuppressed. This effect is also prevalent at the edges of the FOV, or any regions away from the magnet isocenter (Figure 2.17) (7,12).

Further improvement in uniform fat suppression can be achieved by incorporating adiabatic pulses, which are a specially designed class of RF pulses that provide B1 insensitive spin nutation. Recently, spectral (fat)-selective adiabatic inversion pulses, termed *SPAIR*, have been used in T2-weighted imaging of the abdomen (Figure 2.18). The uniformity of fat suppression is more robust than traditional spectral-selective techniques, making it the method of choice for liver and bowel imaging. Moreover, its inherent high CNR provides important diagnostic advantages over STIR, since soft tissue signal is preserved. The effects of inhomogeneous main magnetic field still pose challenges to SPAIR, due to spectral overlap. But the improved inversion profile and frequency cutoff of SPAIR alleviates the degree

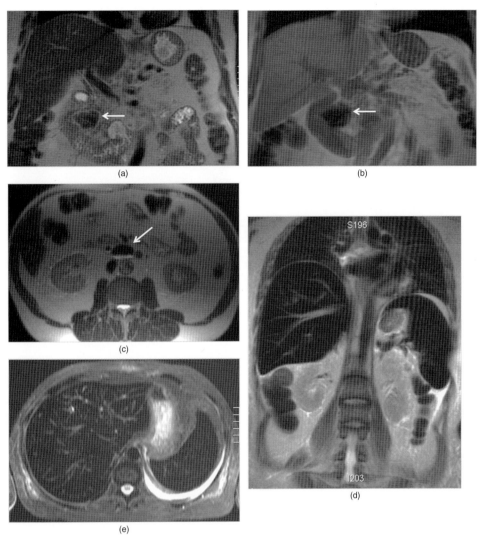

Figure 2.15 *Susceptibility and iron effects on T2-weighted sequences.* Coronal T2-weighted single shot echo train spin echo (a), coronal T1-weighted SGE (b) and transverse T2-weighted single shot echo train spin echo (c) images demonstrate duodenal diverticules (arrows; a–c) detected in two different patients. The liver, common bile duct, and small and large bowel wall and their lumens are visualized with very good image quality on T2-weighted images due to short acquisition time and decreased sensitivity to susceptibility artifacts. Note the smaller size of susceptibility artifact (arrow, a) detected in the diverticule (a) on T2-weighted image compared to the large size of susceptibility artifact (arrow, b) on T1-weighted image (b). Due to smaller sizes of susceptibility artifacts, the bowel wall and lumen can be visualized well on single shot echo train spin echo sequences. T2-weighted coronal non-fat-suppressed (d) and transverse fat-suppressed (e) single shot echo train spin echo sequences demonstrate low signal intensity of the liver and spleen due to iron deposition secondary to transfusional hemosiderosis. The lungs, stomach and large bowel are all well visualized on single shot echo train spin echo sequences due to decreased sensitivity to the susceptibility artifacts. Note the pleural effusion at the left side. T1-weighted in-phase SGE (f) and T2-weighted single shot echo train spin echo (g) images demonstrate a bizarre shaped liver with very irregular contours diagnosed as primary sclerosing cholangitis. Gamna-gandy bodies containing iron are present in the enlarged spleen. Gamna-gandy bodies are seen as hypointense nodules on SGE image due to its susceptibility artifact. However, these nodules are not appreciated on T2-weighted single shot echo train spin echo sequence due to its lesser sensitivity to susceptibility artifacts. T1-weighted in-phase SGE (h) image demonstrate surgical clips (arrows, h) adjacent to the IVC in a patient with liver transplantation with ischemic changes and findings of portal hypertension including enlarged spleen and ascites. However, surgical clips are not visualized on T2-weighted fat-suppressed single shot echo train spin echo due its lesser sensitivity to susceptibility artifacts.

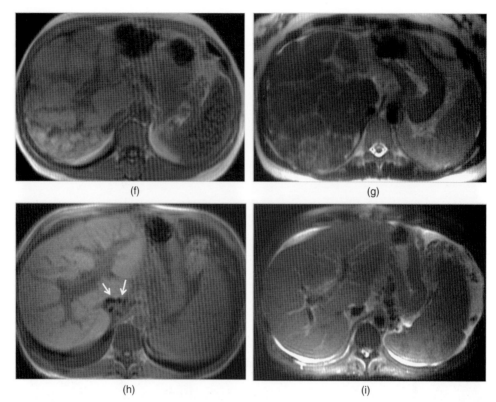

(f)

(g)

(h)

(i)

Figure 2.15 (*Continued*)

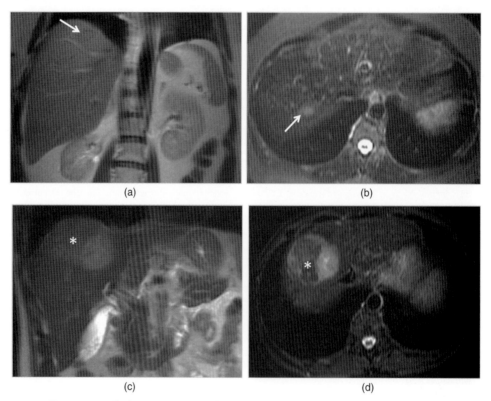

(a)

(b)

(c)

(d)

Figure 2.16 *Fat-suppression effects on T2-weighted sequences.* T2-weighted coronal single shot echo train spin echo image (a) demonstrate a subtle focal lesion (arrow, a) with hypointense signal located in the liver which has higher signal compared to psoas muscle due to its diffuse fatty infiltration. T2-weighted transverse echo train spin echo image (b) acquired with short tau inversion recovery technique (STIR) shows diffuse signal decrease in the liver due to fat suppression. Additionally, the focal lesion (arrow, b) shows mildly higher signal compared to the background fatty liver on fat-suppressed image (b). T2-weighted coronal single shot echo train spin echo image (c) demonstrate a large HCC with abundant fat (asteriks; c, d) which show hypointense signal on STIR image due to signal loss secondary to fat attenuation.

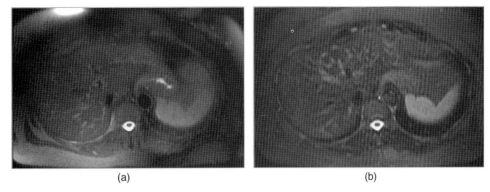

Figure 2.17 *Fat-suppression techniques.* T2-weighted transverse spectrally saturated fat-suppressed single shot echo train spin echo (a) demonstrate inhomogeneous fat-suppression, especially at the periphery, compared to STIR image (b).

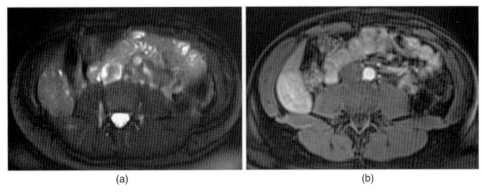

Figure 2.18 *Fat-suppression techniques.* T2-weighted transverse single shot echo train spin echo (a) and T1-weighted 3D-GE post-gadolinium interstitial phase (b) images at 3.0 T acquired with SPAIR technique demonstrate prominent fat-suppression although fat-suppression is inhomogeneous at the periphery of the images due to magnetic field inhomogeneity. Note the adenoma located in the right lobe of the liver.

of poor fat suppression. Implementation of SPAIR fat suppression takes longer than its other counterparts, due to the longer pulse length required for the adiabatic condition. This may increase scan times for segmented T2 and T1 acquisitions (7,12).

Alternative fat-suppressed T2-weighted sequences for the liver, such as echo-planar imaging, have also been employed at some centers.

Focal or diffuse lesions may show mild, moderate, or markedly high signal, depending on fluid content on non-fat-suppressed and fat-suppressed images; high or low signal, depending on fat content on non-fat-suppressed images or fat-suppressed images, respectively; and low signal, depending on iron, fibrosis, or protein content on non-fat-suppressed and fat-suppressed images (Figures 2.15, 2.16, and 2.19).

Postgadolinium sequences

Gadolinium-containing contrast agents are the most useful and most commonly used MR contrast agents. They are most effective when administered as a rapid bolus, with imaging performed using T1-weighted SGE or 3D-GE sequences obtained in a dynamic serial fashion. Dynamic MR imaging is performed on at least three phases consecutively, including (i) hepatic arterial dominant phase, (ii) early hepatic venous phase, and (iii) interstitial phase. An additional hepatocyte-specific phase

may be obtained as a fourth delayed phase if hepatocyte-specific gadolinium-containing agents are employed (7).

A critical aspect of the use of GBCA agents is the recognition of the importance of timing of data acquisition in order to maximize the information available, regarding the dynamic handling of contrast by the vascular and extracellular spaces of various organs, tissues, and disease processes.

Hepatic arterial dominant phase

Appropriate early timing of data acquisition immediately following contrast is the most critical aspect of timing. Three different techniques, including empirical timing, test bolus, and bolus tracking methods are employed in order to acquire the optimal phase of early enhancement in a short time window of early postgadolinium imaging, which is the hepatic arterial dominant phase (13). It has been recently reported that arterial-phase bolus-track liver examination (ABLE) technique is a successful method for the acquisition of hepatic arterial dominant phase (14). A bolus track sequence, which produces an image approximately every second, is used to detect the arrival of GBCAs to the level of celiac axis. After 8 s, the liver is scanned using 3D-GE with centric re-ordered k space in 16–20 s. During the 8-s period, the patient is given breathing

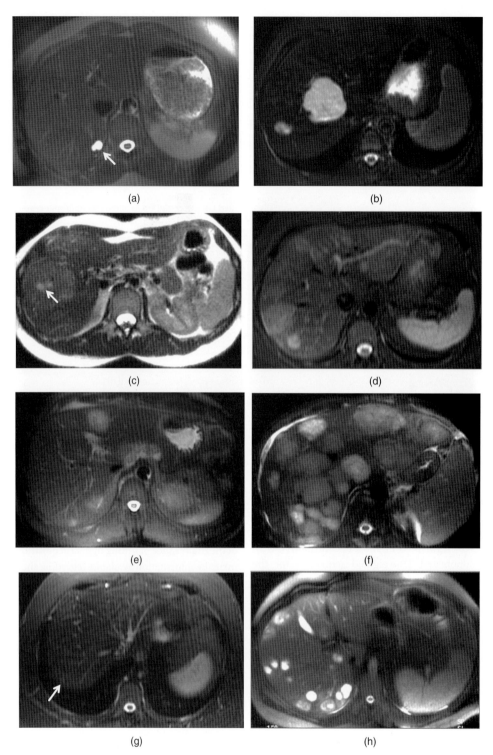

Figure 2.19 *Appearances of common lesions and their signal intensities on T2-weighted echo trains spin echo (ETSE) sequences.* Simple cysts, which are the most common benign lesion seen in the liver, are seen as markedly hyperintense lesions (arrow, a). Hemangiomas, which are the most common benign neoplasm of the liver, are seen as markedly hyperintense lesions (b). Focal nodular hyperplasias (FNHs), which are the second common benign neoplasm of the liver, are seen as mildly hyperintense or isointense lesions (c). The central scar (arrow, c) may exist in FNHs and demonstrate mild to moderate high signal. Hepatocellular adenomas, which are the third common neoplasm of the liver, are seen as mildly hyperintense or isointense lesions (d). Hypovascular liver metastases usually demonstrate mild to moderate high signal as in seen in a patient with colon cancer metastases (e). Hypervascular metastases demonstrate variable high signal intensity although moderate to markedly high signal are seen frequently as seen in a patient with carcinoid metastases (f). Chemotherapy treated liver metastases (arrow, g) usually show low signal intensity or mildly high signal intensity due to its lesser fluid and higher fibrotic content. Abscesses (h) usually demonstrate moderate to markedly high signal intensity. Hepatocellular carcinomas may show low signal intensity (arrow, i) due to its protein or hemorrhagic content, mild to moderate homogeneous high signal intensity (arrows, j) due to its fluid content and heterogeneous signal intensity (arrow, k) due to its necrotic component. Confluent fibrosis at segment 8 (l) and diffuse reticular fibrotic network (m) show mildly high signal.

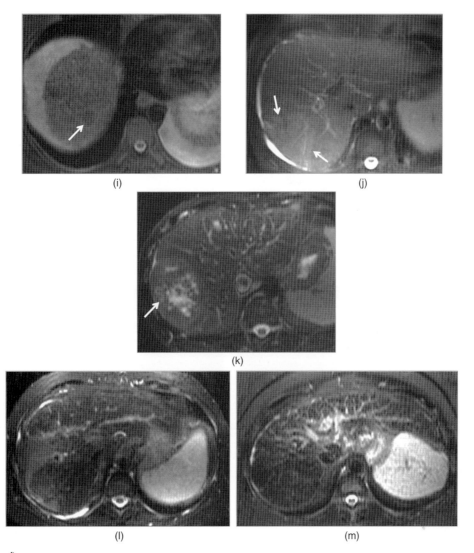

Figure 2.19 (*Continued*)

instructions. This is also the technique that we routinely use now in our institution.

However, all these techniques depend on the estimation of circulation time of the contrast material from the site of injection or abdominal aorta to the liver (13). Because the circulation time of the contrast material to the liver shows variations depending on various factors, different sub-phases of arterial phase enhancement other than the hepatic arterial dominant phase may be detected (13).

These sub-phases can be summarized on the basis of the vessel enhancement patterns and extent of organ enhancements as displayed in Table 2.1. These sub-phases are as follows: (a) early hepatic arterial phase (EHAP), (b) mid hepatic arterial phase (MHAP), (c) late hepatic arterial phase (LHAP), (d) splenic vein only hepatic arterial dominant phase (SVHADP), and (e) hepatic arterial dominant phase (HADP).

(a) EHAP is characterized by the presence of contrast in the arteries including the hepatic arteries; the absence of contrast in any venous structure; and the presence of no or slight enhancement in the renal cortex, pancreas, spleen, and liver (Figure 2.20).

(b) MHAP is characterized by the presence of contrast in the arteries including the hepatic arteries; the absence of contrast in any venous structure; and the presence of mild to moderate enhancement in the renal cortex and the spleen, and slight to mild enhancement in the pancreas and liver (Figure 2.20).

(c) LHAP is characterized by the presence of contrast in the arteries including the hepatic arteries and renal veins; the presence or absence of contrast in the suprarenal IVC and the absence of contrast in the other venous structures; the presence of moderate to intense enhancement in the renal cortex and the spleen; mild to moderate enhancement in the pancreas; and slight to mild enhancement in the liver (Figure 2.21).

Table 2.1 The vessel and organ enhancement patterns according to sub-phases of early enhancement.

	EHAP	MHAP	LHAP	SVHADP	HADP
Vessel enhancement					
All arteries	+	+	+	+	+
Renal veins	−	−	+	+	+
Portal vein	−	−	−	+	+
Splenic vein	−	−	−	+	+
Superior mesenteric vein	−	−	−	−	+
Suprarenal IVC	−	−	±	+	+
Hepatic vein	−	−	−	−	−
Organ enhancement					
Renal cortex	No or slight	Mild or moderate	Moderate to intense	Moderate to intense	Moderate to intense
Spleen	No or slight	Mild or moderate	Moderate to intense	Moderate to intense	Moderate to intense
Pancreas	No or slight	Slight or mild	Mild or moderate	Moderate	Moderate
Liver	No or slight	Slight or mild	Slight or mild	Mild	Moderate

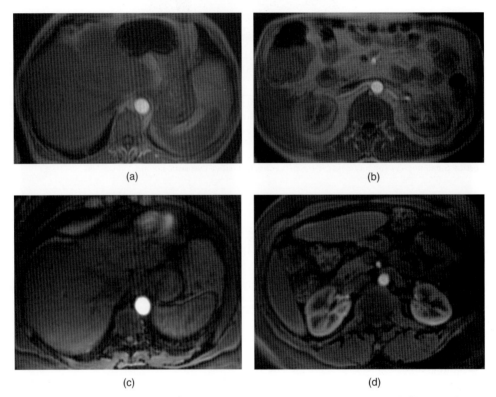

(a)

(b)

(c)

(d)

Figure 2.20 *EHAP and MHAP.* The early hepatic arterial phase (EHAP) was observed on transverse SGE images (a, b) acquired on 1.5 T. The mid hepatic arterial phase (MHAP) was observed on transverse 3D-GE images (c, d) acquired on 3.0 T. The contrast enhancement is seen in the aorta, renal arteries and superior mesenteric artery, but there is no contrast enhancement in the veins on both EHAP and MHAP. The renal cortex, spleen, pancreas and liver demonstrate slight enhancement on EHAP. The renal cortex, spleen and pancreas show mild enhancement and the liver shows slight enhancement on MHAP. The minimal enhancement of the normal pancreas reflects the too early acquisition of data in these sub-phases.

(d) SVHADP is characterized by the presence of contrast in the arteries including the hepatic arteries, and in the portal vein, splenic vein, renal veins, and suprarenal IVC; the absence of contrast in the superior mesenteric vein and hepatic veins; the presence of moderate to intense enhancement in the renal cortex and spleen; moderate enhancement in the pancreas; and mild enhancement in the liver (Figure 2.22).

(e) HADP is characterized by the presence of contrast in the hepatic arteries, portal vein, renal veins, splenic vein, superior mesenteric vein, and suprarenal IVC; the absence of contrast in the hepatic veins; the presence of moderate to intense enhancement in the renal cortex and spleen; and moderate enhancement in the pancreas and liver (Figure 2.22).

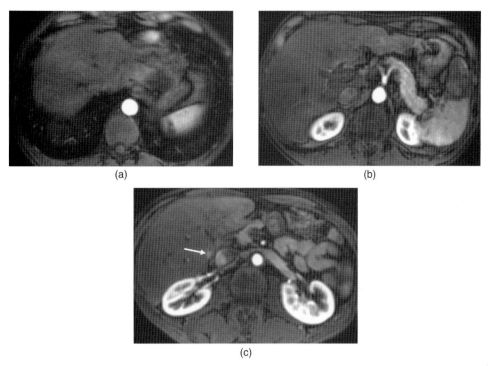

Figure 2.21 *LHAP.* The late hepatic arterial phase (LHAP) was observed on transverse 3D-GE images (a – c) acquired on 3.0 T. The contrast enhancement is seen in the aorta, celiac trunk, common hepatic artery and its branches, splenic, renal and superior mesenteric arteries; and renal veins. The renal cortex demonstrates intense enhancement, pancreas and spleen demonstrate moderate enhancement and the liver shows mild enhancement on LHAP. The moderate enhancement of the normal pancreas reflects the adequate timing of enhancement of LHAP. Contour irregularity of the liver, splenomegaly, patchy and nodular enhancement of the liver are also detected. Patchy enhancement of the liver is most pronounced in the left lobe (b, c) and consistent with acute-on-chronic hepatitis. Small nodular enhancement (arrow, c) is consistent with a dysplastic nodule.

The enhancement of parenchymal organs demonstrates variations in these subphases (13). It has been reported that the pancreas exhibits a capillary blush on the hepatic arterial dominant phase, which may act as surrogate for the determination of the timing of the examination, and for the enhancement of liver lesions (13). Therefore, it can be accepted that the phase of enhancement is optimal when the pancreas shows capillary brush (13). It has been reported that capillary blush is also observed in the LHAP and SVHADP sub-phases; and these phases are also the optimal phases of early enhancement (13). However, EHAP and MHAP are not optimal phases of early enhancement because the pancreas does not show capillary blush on these phases and these phases are too early for the evaluation of abdominal organs (13).

In our clinical experience, if the portal vein is not enhanced, it may be difficult to determine if the timing of liver enhancement is in the MHAP (too early) or the LHAP (adequate timing) (13). It has been reported that substantial enhancement of the pancreas is observed in combination with identification of the presence of contrast in renal veins in the LHAP (13). Therefore, the enhancement of renal vein may also be used as a landmark for the determination of optimal phase of enhancement in the presence of pancreatic pathology that reduces the enhancement of pancreatic tissue (13). We do however anticipate that this observation of renal vein enhancement may be influenced by cardiac output, vascular resistance of the lung parenchyma, and renal function (13).

The hepatic arterial dominant (capillary) phase is the single most important data set when using a nonspecific extracellular gadolinium chelate contrast agent (7,13). This technique is essential for imaging the liver as well as the spleen and pancreas, and also provides useful information on the kidneys, adrenals, vessels, bladder, and uterus. The timing for this phase of enhancement is the only timing for postcontrast sequences that is crucial. It is essential to capture the "first pass" or capillary bed enhancement of tissues during this phase. Demonstration of gadolinium in hepatic arteries and portal veins, and absence of gadolinium in hepatic veins are reliable landmarks. At this phase of enhancement, although contrast is present in portal veins, the majority of the gadolinium present in the liver has been delivered by hepatic arteries. The absolute volume of hepatic artery-delivered gadolinium is greater in this phase of enhancement than acquiring the data when gadolinium is only present in hepatic arteries; therefore more hepatic arterial enhancement information is available. This is important as most focal liver lesions, especially metastases and HCC, are fed primarily by hepatic arteries. Imaging slightly earlier than this, when only

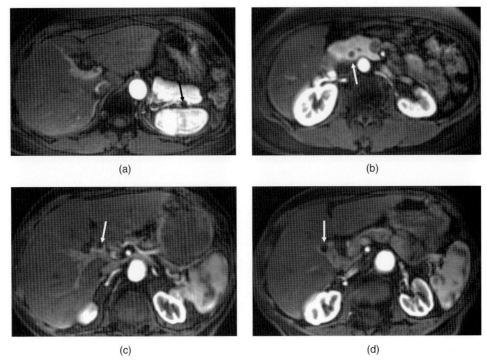

(a)   (b)

(c)   (d)

Figure 2.22 *SVHADP and HADP.* The splenic vein only hepatic arterial dominant phase (SVHADP) (a, b) and the hepatic arterial dominant phase (HADP) (c, d) were observed on transverse 3D-GE images acquired on 3.0 T. The contrast enhancement is seen in the aorta, renal arteries, splenic and superior mesenteric arteries; and renal, splenic and portal veins but not in the hepatic and superior mesenteric veins on SVHADP. The renal cortex and spleen demonstrate intense enhancement, the pancreas demonstrates moderate enhancement and the liver shows mild enhancement on SVHADP. Although there are two pseudocysts located in the pancreatic tail (arrow, a) and head (arrow, b); the moderate enhancement of the pancreas reflects the adequate timing of enhancement on SVHADP. In addition to the contrast enhanced vessels seen on SVHADP, the contrast enhancement is also observed in the superior mesenteric vein on HADP. The renal cortex demonstrates intense enhancement and the spleen, pancreas and liver demonstrate moderate enhancement. The moderate enhancement of the normal pancreas reflects the adequate timing of enhancement of HADP. Note that there are benign cystic lesions in the liver parenchyma (arrows, c, d).

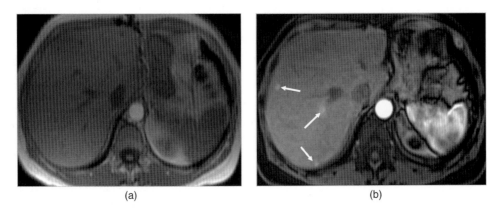

(a)   (b)

Figure 2.23 *Detection of hypervascular lesions on the LHAP.* Hypervascular colon carcinoma metastases (arrows, b) cannot be detected on the early hepatic arterial phase image but can be detected on the late hepatic arterial phase (b).

hepatic arteries are opacified (hepatic arteries-only phase) may approach the diagnostic utility of the hepatic arterial dominant phase if the data is acquired on the LHAP (Figure 2.23). It is very difficult to achieve these objectives on the hepatic arteries-only phases, particularly on EHAP and MHAP, and it is also difficult to judge if image acquisition is too early in this phase, when

the liver is essentially unenhanced (Figure 2.23). Appropriate timing, as judged by vessel enhancement, is also important for the evaluation of surrounding organs. Too little pancreatic enhancement is consistent with pancreatic fibrosis or chronic pancreatitis, and too little enhancement of renal cortex may imply ischemic nephropathy or acute cortical necrosis. This can be reliably judged on hepatic arterial dominant phase images by the fixed landmarks of contrast in portal veins and absence in hepatic veins. On hepatic arteries-only phases, particularly on EHAP and MHAP, minimal enhancement of pancreas or renal cortex may reflect too early image acquisition rather than disease process. As this immediate postgadolinium phase of enhancement is also used to diagnose adequate perfusion of these organs, it is oxymoronic to use enhancement of these organs as the determination of the appropriateness of the phase of image acquisition timing. Although enhancement of pancreas or renal cortex is used as ancillary information for assessment of timing, it is not the major determinant, as the extent of enhancement of these organs is also evaluated at this phase. In the liver, imaging too early on hepatic arteries-only phases, particularly on EHAP and MHAP, diminishes the ability to recognize the distinctive patterns of lesion enhancement for different lesion types, because the absolute volume of hepatic artery-delivered contrast may be too small and may cause lesions to be mischaracterized (7,13).

On hepatic arterial dominant phase T1-weighted SGE or 3D-GE images, various types of liver lesions have distinctive enhancement patterns: cysts show lack of enhancement, hemangiomas show peripheral nodules of enhancement in a discontinuous ring, nonhemorrhagic adenomas and focal nodular hyperplasia (FNH) show intense uniform enhancement, metastases show ring enhancement, and HCCs show diffuse heterogeneous enhancement (Figure 2.24). The ability to use this information to characterize lesions as small as 1 cm is unique to MRI. Appearances of less common liver lesions on immediate postgadolinium images have also been reported, many of which show overlap with the above described patterns of common liver lesions. To a somewhat lesser extent, appreciation of the capillary phase enhancement of lesions in the pancreas, spleen, and kidneys also provides information on lesion characterization. Clinical history is often important, despite the high diagnostic accuracy of current MRI imaging protocols. In addition, many different histologic types of liver lesions, when they measure less than 1 cm, demonstrate virtually identical uniform enhancement on the hepatic arterial dominant phase, for example, hemangiomas, adenomas, FNH, metastases, and HCC (Figure 2.25). However, these lesions may demonstrate different enhancement patterns on the early hepatic venous and interstitial phases such as maintaining the enhancement, fading, or washing out. Ancillary information to assist in characterization of lesions is crucial and includes T2-weighted images that demonstrate lesion fluid content (e.g., high for hemangioma and often high for hypervascular metastases, and relatively low for adenoma, FNH, and HCC) (Figure 2.19), T1-weighted images demonstrating fat, protein, and blood content (Figures 2.1–2.3, 2.7–2.10), appearance of other concomitant large lesions, and clinical history (e.g., history of known primary tumor that can result in hypervascular metastases, such as gastrointestinal leiomyosarcoma) (7).

Various enhancement patterns of liver and other organ parenchyma are also demonstrated on hepatic arterial dominant phase images. One of the most common perfusion abnormalities observed in the liver is transient increased segmental enhancement in liver segments with compromised portal venous flow due to compression or thrombosis (Figure 2.26). Other hepatic diseases that demonstrate perfusion abnormalities on immediate postgadolinium images include diffuse or focal parenchymal inflammation, inflammation around focal lesions, Budd–Chiari Syndrome with different enhancement patterns for acute, subacute, and chronic disease, severe acute hepatitis with hepatocellular injury, and ascending cholangitis (Figure 2.26) (7).

Imaging evaluation for liver metastases is a common indication for liver MR examination. Liver metastases have been classified as hypovascular (typical examples are colon cancer and transitional cell carcinoma) or hypervascular (typical examples are islet cell tumors, renal cell carcinoma, and breast cancer) (Figure 2.24). A third category of vascularity has not been described well in the past and that is near-isovascular with liver (Figure 2.27). *Near-isovascular* refers to lesion enhancement that is very comparable to that of liver on early and late postgadolinium images. Near isovascularity is most readily appreciated when lesions are poorly seen on postgadolinium images but well seen on precontrast images. Liver metastases from primaries of colon, thyroid, and endometrium may show this type of enhancement pattern. The most common setting is postchemotherapy, although this may also be observed in untreated patients. Fortunately, many of these tumors are moderately low signal intensity on T1-weighted images, rendering them readily apparent, and on occasion they may also be moderately high signal intensity on T2-weighted images. Rarely they may also be near isointense on T1-weighted and T2-weighted images, and therefore can escape detection. The rarity of this occurrence illustrates one of the great strengths of MRI over sonography and computed tomography. The greater the number of distinctly different data sets that are acquired, the less likely it is for disease to escape detection. MRI has more acquisitions of different types of data than ultrasound or CT (7).

Chemotherapy-treated liver metastases deserve special mention in that chemotherapy is routinely given to the majority of patients with liver metastases and chemotherapy alters the imaging features of metastases. Chemotherapy induces change in the signal intensity and imaging features of metastases such that they may resemble cysts, hemangiomas, or scar tissue (Figure 2.24). As mentioned above, they may also become near isovascular on postgadolinium images (7).

Early hepatic venous phase

This phase should be acquired following the hepatic arterial dominant phase and is customarily referred to as *portal venous phase*. However, it should be referred to as *early hepatic venous phase* more correctly, as contrast has just entered the hepatic veins at this time point. This phase is acquired at 45–60 s

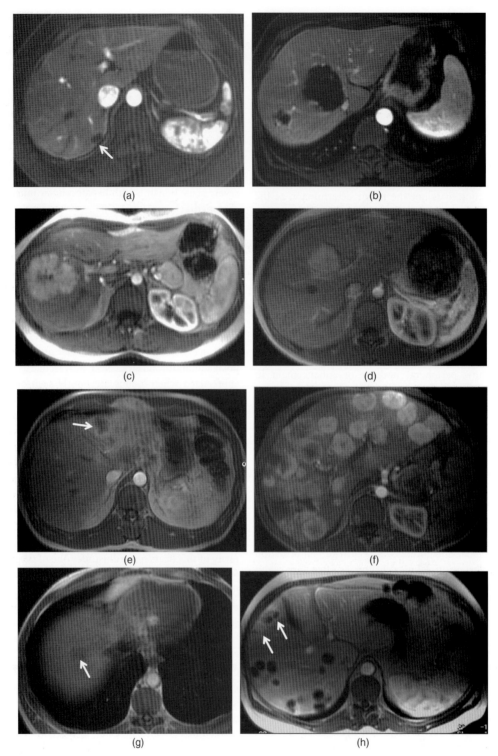

Figure 2.24 *Appearances of common lesions and their enhancement patterns on the hepatic arterial dominant phase.* simple cyst (arrow, a) does not show any enhancement. Hemangiomas (b) show peripheral nodular enhancement. FNHs (c) and adenomas (d) demonstrate homogeneous prominent enhancement. Hypovascular metastases (arrow, e) demonstrate peripheral enhancement. Hypervascular metastases (f) show intense peripheral enhancement or homogeneous enhancement. Chemotherapy treated liver metastases (arrow, g) demonstrate no enhancement or mild enhancement. Abscesses (arrow, h) show peripheral enhancement and associated peripheral parenchymal enhancement. Hepatocellular carcinoma (arrows, i) show heterogeneous prominent enhancement. Confluent fibrosis (arrow, j) and reticular fibrotic network (k) show mild enhancement. (Compare with Figure 2.19.)

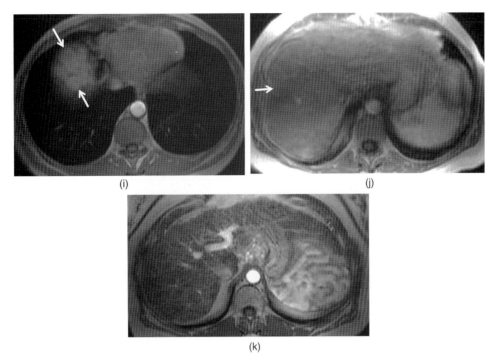

Figure 2.24 (*Continued*)

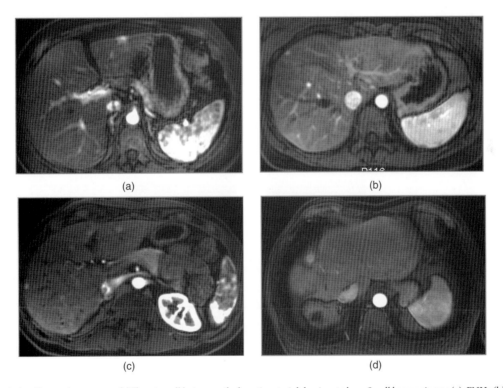

Figure 2.25 *Identical uniform enhancement of different small lesions on the hepatic arterial dominant phase.* Small hemangiomas (a), FNHs (b), hypervascular metastases (c) and HCCs (d) may show uniform homogeneous enhancement when they measure less than 1–1.5 cm.

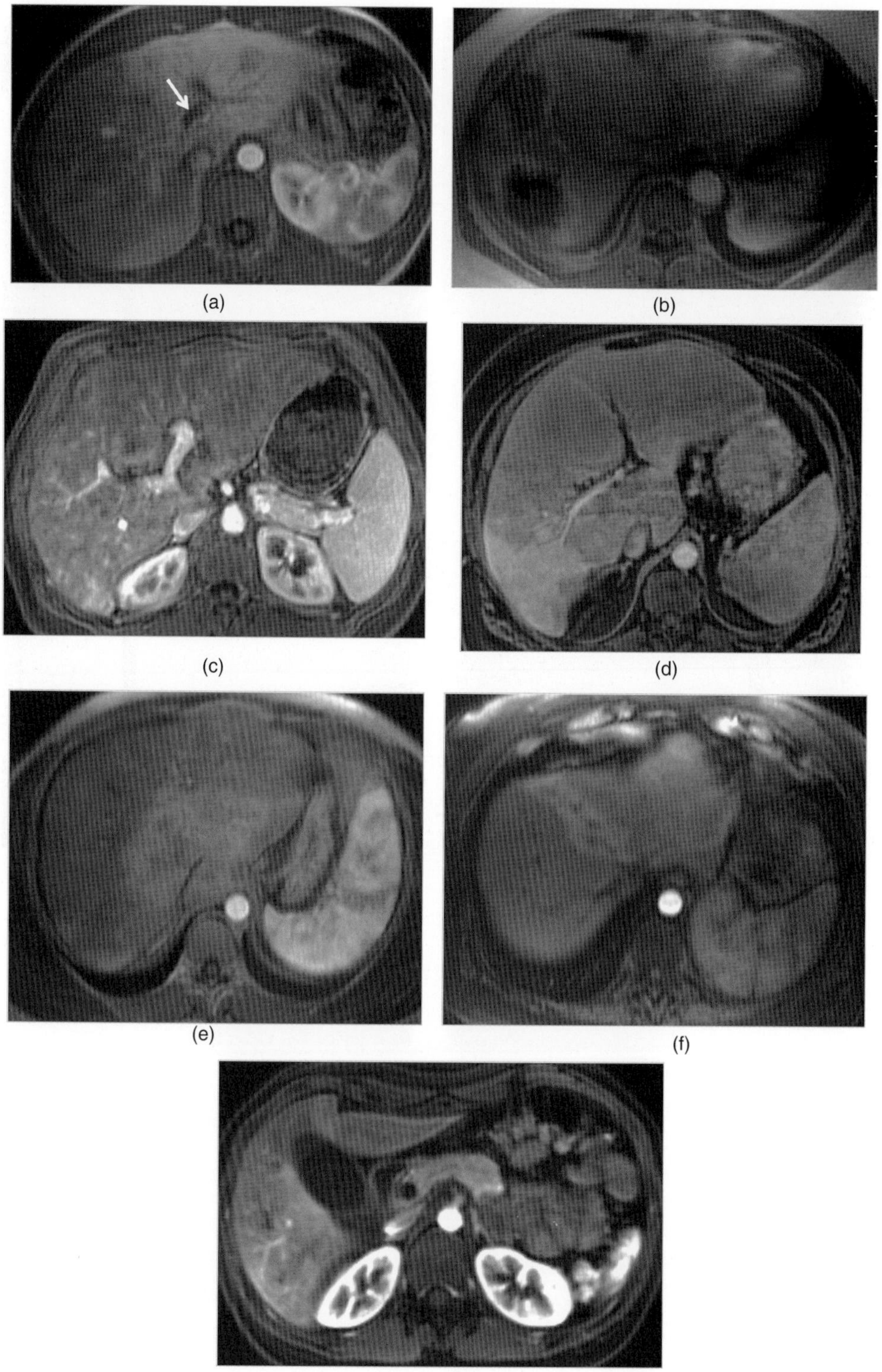

Figure 2.26 *Perfusion abnormalities on the hepatic arterial dominant phase.* Increased transient enhancement of the left lobe of the liver (a) develops due to the compensatory increase in the left hepatic arterial flow secondary to the hypointense bland thrombus (arrow, a) in the left portal vein. Increased transient enhancement around the hypointense abscesses containing air develops secondary to the parenchymal inflammation (b). Diffusely increased transient heterogeneous enhancement in the liver represents diffuse inflammation due to acute hepatitis (c). Focally increased transient heterogeneous enhancement in the right lobe of the liver develops due to acute on chronic hepatitis in a patient with chronic liver disease. Increased transient heterogeneous enhancement on the central portion of the liver may develop secondary to Budd–Chiari syndrome (e). Note that the IVC is compressed (e). Increased transient parenchymal enhancement may develop around dilated inflamed bile ducts in ascending cholangitis (f). Increased transient parenchymal enhancement may develop around inflamed gallbladder as in acute cholecystitis (g).

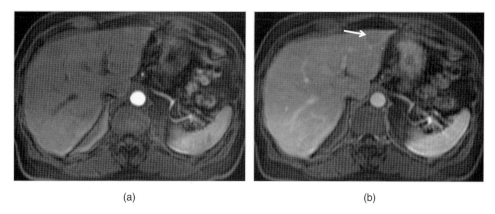

(a)   (b)

Figure 2.27 *Isovascular Metastases.* Both hypovascular and hypervascular type metastases may also present as isovascular metastases. Isovascular metastases demonstrate same amount of enhancement on the hepatic arterial dominant phase (a) as with the remaining liver parenchyma. Therefore, it may be difficult to differentiate these lesions on the hepatic arterial dominant phase. However, these lesions (arrow, b) usually enhance less than the remaining liver parenchyma on the hepatic venous or interstitial phases (b).

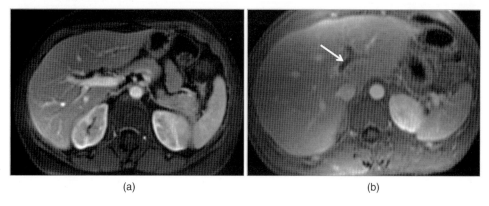

(a)   (b)

Figure 2.28 *Patent and thrombosed portal vein.* The right portal vein (a) is patent and the left portal vein (arrow, b) is thrombosed. The left portal vein thrombus is bland because of the absence of enhancement in the thrombus. Additionally, increased transient enhancement of the left lobe becomes isointense with the remaining liver parenchyma on the hepatic venous phase. (Compare with Figure 2.26a)

postinitiation of gadolinium injection. Patency or thrombosis of hepatic vessels are also best shown in this phase (Figure 2.28) (7). In this phase, hepatic parenchyma is maximally enhanced so hypovascular lesions (cysts, hypovascular metastases, and scar tissue) are best shown as regions of lesser enhancement similar to interstitial phase.

Interstitial phase

This phase should be acquired following the early hepatic venous phase and is customarily referred to as *equilibrium phase*. However, it should be referred to as *interstitial phase* more correctly, as there is no true equilibrium that occurs and the contrast is distributed into the interstitial space. Hepatic venous phase or interstitial phase is acquired 90 s–5 min following initiation of contrast injection. Late enhancement features of focal liver lesions on hepatic venous and interstitial phases aid in lesion characterization such as persistent lack of enhancement of cysts, coalescence and centripetal progression of enhancing nodules in

hemangiomas, homogeneous fading of enhancement of adenomas and FNH to near isointensity with liver, late enhancement of central scar in some FNHs, peripheral or heterogeneous washout of contrast in liver metastases, washout to hypointensity with liver in small liver metastases and HCC, heterogeneous washout of HCC, and delayed capsule enhancement in HCC (less commonly adenoma) (Figure 2.29). Fibrotic tissue enhances prominently in this phase. Inflammatory parenchymal tissue tends to be isointense with the remaining liver parenchyma on this phase (Figure 2.29). However, focal inflammatory lesions demonstrate prominent peripheral and wall enhancement such as abscess or wall of biliary ducts as in ascending cholangitis. Enhancement of peritoneal metastases, inflammatory disease, bone metastases and circumferential, superficial spreading cholangiocarcinoma are also well shown at this time frame. Enhancement patterns of small common lesions are also displayed on Figure 2.30. Concomitant use of fat suppression is essential for optimized demonstration of these findings. Additional documentation of vascular thrombosis is also provided on these images (7).

Hepatocyte phase

This phase can only be acquired following the administration of combined extracellular and hepatocyte specific agents, including gadobenate dimaglumine and gadoxetic acid. These agents are taken up by hepatocytes and excreted into the bile ducts. Hepatocyte phase can be acquired after 1 h following the administration of gadobenate dimeglumine and 20 min following the administration of gadoxetic acid (15). This phase is primarily used for the detection of metastases which do not contain hepatocytes and therefore metastases are seen as hypointense lesions. Additionally, these agents are used for the differentiation of FNH and hepatocellular adenoma.

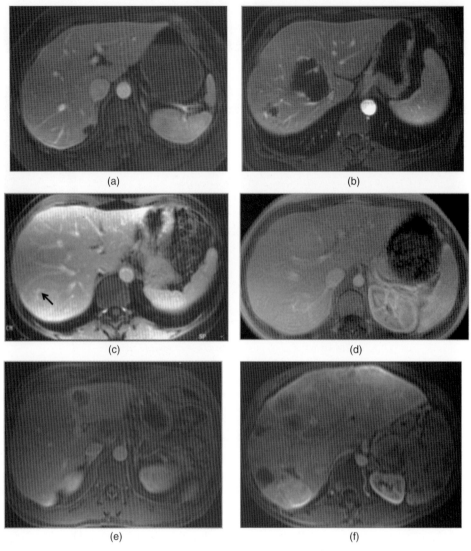

Figure 2.29 *Appearances of common lesions and their enhancement patterns on the interstitial phase.* Simple cysts (a) do not show any enhancement. Hemangiomas (b) show progressively increasing peripheral nodular and centripedal progressive enhancement. FNHs (c) and adenomas (d) generally demonstrate fading and become isointense or mildly hyperintense compared to the liver. Note that the central scar of FNHs enhance on this phase (arrow, c). Hypovascular metastases (e) show prominent peripheral enhancement and progressive enhancement toward the center. Hypervascular metastases (f) may show peripheral wash-out with central progressive enhancement or fading. Chemotherapy treated liver metastases (g) demonstrate progressive enhancement. Abscesses (h) show progressive prominent wall enhancement. Note that the peripheral parenchymal enhancement fades to isointensity with the remaining liver. Hepatocellular carcinoma (i) demonstrates wash-out with capsular enhancement. Confluent fibrosis (arrow, j) and diffuse fibrotic reticular network (k) show prominent progressive enhancement. Diffuse increased heterogeneous enhancement on the hepatic arterial dominant phase in a patient with acute hepatitis fades and becomes homogeneous on the interstitial phase (l). Focal increased heterogeneous enhancement on the hepatic arterial dominant phase in a patient with acute on chronic hepatitis becomes isointense with the remaining liver parenchyma on the interstitial phase (m). Progressive heterogeneous enhancement pattern is detected on the interstitial phase (n) in a patient with Budd–Chiari syndrome. Increased enhancement around dilated bile ducts in a patient with ascending cholangitis which tends to fade to isointensity with the remaining liver parenchyma on the interstitial phase (o). Increased transient enhancement around the gallbladder in a patient with acute cholecystitis becomes isointense with the remaining liver parenchyma on the interstitial phase (p). (Compare with Figures 2.19, 2.24 and 2.26.)

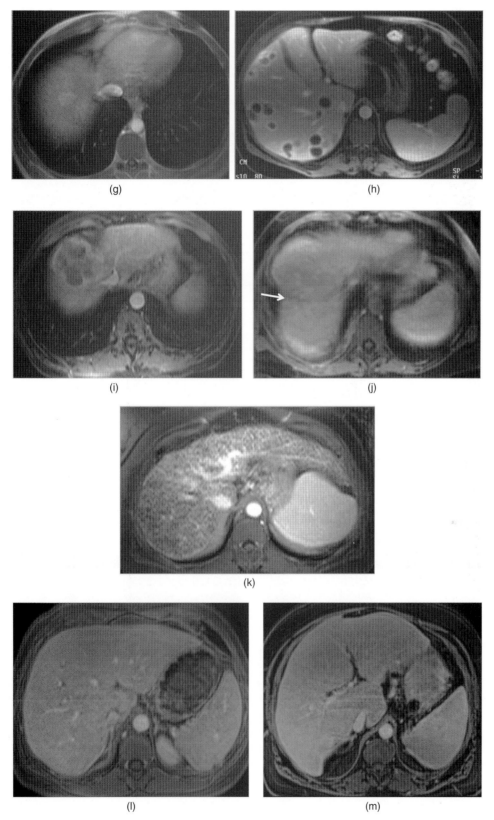

Figure 2.29 (*Continued*)

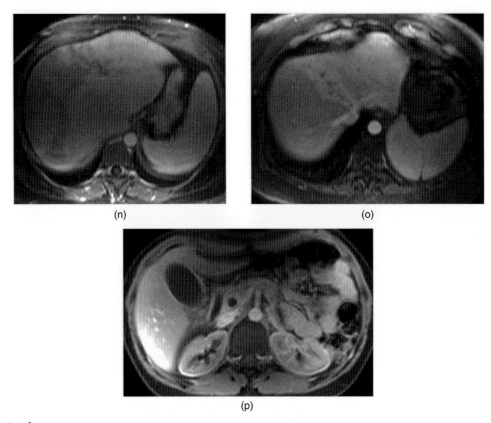

(n)

(o)

(p)

Figure 2.29 (*Continued*)

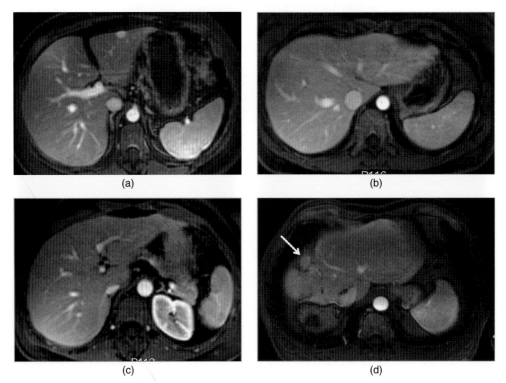

(a)

(b)

(c)

(d)

Figure 2.30 *Appearances of common small lesions and their enhancement patterns on the interstitial phase.* A small hemangioma maintains its prominent enhancement on the interstitial phase (a). FNH (b) and carcinoid metastases (c) fades to isointensity with the remaining liver parenchyma. Hepatocellular carcinoma shows wash out and peripheral capsular enhancement (arrow, d). (Compare with Figure 2.25)

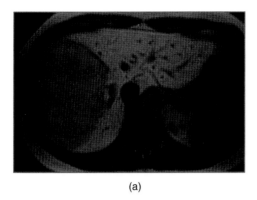
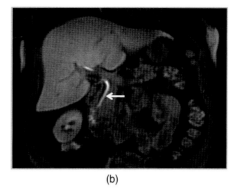

(a)   (b)

Figure 2.31 *Hepatocyte Phase.* T1-weighted transverse delayed phase SGE image acquired after the administration of gadobenate dimeglumine (Multihance) show a hepatocellular adenoma which do not enhance (a). T1-weighted coronal delayed phase 3D-GE image (b) acquired after the administration of gadoxetic acid (Eovist) demonstrate the common bile duct enhanced with biliary excretion of gadoxetic acid.

FNH enhances with hepatocyte specific agents but adenoma does not enhance (Figures 2.6 and 2.31).

MRI contrast agents

MR contrast agents are classified into three main types: (i) GBCAs, (ii) iron-based contrast agents, and (iii) manganese-based contrast agents.

GBCAs

GBCAs are overwhelmingly the most commonly used MR contrast agents. They are essential for the detection and characterization of tumors, detection of inflammation and fibrosis, assessment of organ perfusion, and delineation of vessels and related vascular pathologies. However, the phases of enhancement are critical for the detection and differentiation of these entities with the administration of GBCAs.

Classification of GBCAs

GBCAs are classified into three types according to their distribution in the body as follows: (i) extracellular agents, (ii) combined extracellular and intracellular agents, (iii) blood pool agents. GBCAs are classified into two types according to the backbone structure of their amine group, as linear or macrocyclic. Linear and macrocyclic GBCAs may be further subclassified according to their charges as ionic or non-ionic. Table 2.2 displays the categorization of GBCAs according to the distribution in the body, their chemical structure, elimination pathway, protein binding, thermodynamic stability, and dissociation rate (15–17).

Extracellular agents are distributed into the extracellular space, including vascular and interstitial spaces. They are the oldest and have been the most widely used GBCAs. Extracellular agents can be linear or macrocyclic and ionic or nonionic. All extracellular agents are eliminated by the kidneys and do not bind to proteins at all. They are generally used at their standard dose which is 0.1 mmol/kg. Gadobutrol has higher T1 relaxivity due to its structural difference. Marketed gadobutrol solutions

also have double the amount of gadolinium due to their 1 molar (M) concentrations compared to 0.5 M concentrations of the other GBCAs. Extracellular agents can be used for the acquisition of hepatic arterial dominant, early hepatic venous, and interstitial phases of standard gadolinium-enhanced MRI studies (15–17).

Combined extracellular and intracellular agents are distributed into the extracellular space, including vascular and interstitial spaces, and intracellular spaces of hepatocytes. Therefore, these agents can also be termed as *combined extracellular and hepatocyte-specific* agents. These agents are gadobenate dimaglumine and gadoxetic acid. These agents are taken up by hepatocytes and excreted into bile ducts. Therefore, they have dual elimination, including both renal and biliary eliminations. The phase that the liver shows the uptake of these agents is termed as *hepatocyte phase*. These agents, which are linear and ionic, have also higher T1 relaxivity due to their structural difference and protein binding. Less than 5% of gadobenate dimeglumine and 15% of gadoxetic acid bind serum albumin transiently and reversibly. Hepatocyte uptake and higher T1 relaxivity make these agents advantageous for liver imaging and MRAs. However, there is not sufficient data about the use of gadoxetic acid in MRAs. Hepatocyte phase is helpful for the detection of lesions which do not contain hepatocytes, including metastases, adenomas, or poorly differentiated HCCs. This phase is particularly helpful for the differentiation of FNH from adenoma. FNH contains hepatocytes and biliary canaliculi; therefore, hepatocyte-specific agents can be uptaken and excreted into the bile ducts in FNH. However, hepatic adenomas do not contain normal hepatocytes and biliary canaliculi; therefore, hepatocyte specific agents cannot be uptaken and excreted into the bile ducts. Thus, while FNH enhances in the hepatocyte phase, hepatic adenomas do not (Figures 2.6 and 2.31). This phase is also helpful for the evaluation of liver function and biliary system. Because of high T1 relaxivity, gadoxetic acid is used at ¼ dose (0.025 mmol/kg) of the standard dose of extracellular GBCAs. However, there is not sufficient data demonstrating the diagnostic efficacy of

Table 2.2 Categorization of GBCAs according to the distribution in the body, chemical structure, elimination pathway, protein binding.

Generic name	Chemical abbreviation	Product name	Distribution	Amine structure	Charge	Excretion	Protein binding	FDA approval	Standard dosage (mmol/kg)
Gadoversetamide	Gd-DTPA-BMEA	OptiMark (Mallinckrodt, St Louis, MO, USA)	Extracellular	Linear	Non-ionic	Renal	None	Yes	0.1
Gadodiamide	Gd-DTPA-BMA	Omniscan (GE Healthcare, Buckinghamshire, United Kingdom)	Extracellular	Linear	Non-ionic	Renal	None	Yes	0.1
Gadopentetate dimeglumine	Gd-DTPA	Magnevist (Bayer Schering Pharma AG, Germany)	Extracellular	Linear	Ionic	Renal	None	Yes	0.1
Gadobenate dimeglumine	Gd-BOPTA	MultiHance (Bracco Diagnostics, Milan, Italy)	Extracellular and intracellular (hepatocyte)	Linear	Ionic	Renal (%97), biliary (%3)	<5%	Yes	0.1*,†
Gadoxetic asit disodium	Gd-EOB-BOPTA	Eovist, (Bayer HealthCare Pharmaceuticals, Wayne, NJ, USA); Primovist (Bayer Schering Pharma AG, Germany)	Extracellular and intracellular (hepatocyte)	Linear	Ionic	Renal (%50), biliary (%50)	<15%	Yes	0.025*
Gadofosveset trisodium	Gd-DTPA	Vasovist (Epix Pharmaceuticals, Lexington, MA, USA)	Blood pool	Linear	Ionic	Renal (91%), biliary (9%)	>85%	Yes	0.025*
Gadobutrol	Gd-DO3A-butriol	Gadovist (Bayer Schering Pharma AG, Germany)	Extracellular	Macrocyclic	Non-ionic	Renal	None	Yes	0.1*,‡
Gadoteridol	Gd-HP-DO3A	ProHance (Bracco Diagnostics, Milan, Italy)	Extracellular	Macrocyclic	Non-ionic	Renal	None	Yes	0.1
Gadoterate meglumine	Gd-DOTA	Dotarem (Guerbet, Aulnay-sous-Bois, France)	Extracellular	Macrocyclic	Ionic	Renal	None	Yes	0.1

*Gadobenate dimeglumine, gadoxetic acid, gadofosveset, and gadobutrol have higher T1 relaxivity compared to the other agents.

†Gadobenate dimeglumine has been reported to be diagnostically effective at its half dose (0.05 mmol/kg).

‡Gadobutrol solution has double amount of gadolinium in its 1 M concentration compared to 0.5 M concentration of the other GBCAs' solutions.

this dose of gadoxetic acid compared to the standard doses of extracellular GBCAs. Gadobenate dimeglumine is used at 0.1 mmol/kg; however, it has been shown that gadobenate dimeglumine has comparable diagnostic efficacy at the half dose (0.05 mmol/kg) compared to the standard doses of extracellular GBCAs. Combined extracellular and hepatocyte specific agents can be used for hepatic arterial dominant, early hepatic venous, interstitial and hepatocyte phases of gadolinium-enhanced MRI studies (15–18).

An important difference between gadobenate dimeglumine and gadoxetic acid is the proportion that is eliminated through the biliary system in comparison to renal clearance. Approximately 5% of the administered dose of gadobenate dimeglumine is eliminated by the biliary system in patients with normal renal function, whereas approximately 50% of the dose of gadoxetic acid is eliminated by the biliary system. These proportions increase in the setting of renal failure, gadobenate dimeglumine to about 9%, and the fraction of gadoxetic acid not yet established. Image acquisition-wise this difference is manifest by the timing that hepatocyte phase occurs with these two agents, with gadobenate dimeglumine it is at about 1 h (lasting till at least 4 h) and with gadoxetic acid it is at about 20 min (lasting till about 4 h). Biliary elimination with visualization of high signal contrast in the biliary tree is also more pronounced with gadoxetic acid. The earlier hepatocyte phase that is achieved with gadoxetic acid permits ready acquisition of an entire postcontrast study, including hepatic arterial dominant, early hepatic venous, and interstitial phases, with hepatocyte-phase, in one imaging session. To avoid excessive dead-time between the interstitial phase and hepatocyte phase we recommend performing T2-weighted sequences following the interstitial phase and before the hepatocyte phase. Special note should be made that as the biliary elimination also results in T2-shortening, T2 sequence based MRCP should not be performed after contrast administration, but rather prior to it, as the T2 shortening can obscure the biliary tree. On the other hand, as the hepatocyte phase occurs at 1 h with gadobenate dimeglumine, it is unavoidable that two imaging sessions must be performed with a 1–2 h delay between the full MR study and the delayed hepatocyte phase (7,15–17).

In making a decision between the use of these agents for hepatocyte phase imaging, other considerations must be entertained: only gadoxetic acid is FDA-approved for liver imaging, gadobenate dimeglumine use is considered off-label, but on the other hand the cost of gadobenate dimeglumine is considerably less at the present time, and at the current recommended doses by the manufacturers. Gadobenate dimeglumine results in considerably greater signal increase on early postcontrast phases than gadoxetic acid (and our experience emphasizes the great importance of hepatic arterial dominant phase imaging), this is even the case if gadobenate dimeglumine is employed at half dose, as we routinely do for NSF considerations (7).

Blood pool agents mainly stay in the vascular space. Gadofosveset is a blood pool agent that has linear and ionic structure and more than 85% of gadofosveset binds serum albumin transiently and reversibly. A small amount of gadofosveset is also distributed into the extracellular space and hepatocytes. Binding to serum albumin provides higher T1 relaxivity and extended intravascular enhancement. Intravascular enhancement is higher and longer compared to the other protein binding GBCAs (gadobenate dimeglumine and gadoxetic acid) due to tighter and longer binding of gadofosveset. A small amount of gadofosveset is also taken up by hepatocytes and excreted into the bile ducts. Therefore, gadofosveset has dual elimination, including renal and biliary eliminations. Gadofosveset is administered with a dose of 0.025 mmol/kg. Blood pool agents may be advantageous for vascular imaging due to higher and longer intravascular enhancement and gadofosveset has recently been approved by FDA for body MRAs. However, the diagnostic role and safety profile of this agent need to be determined and we have no clinical experience with this agent.

Iron-based contrast agents

Iron-based contrast agents, which include superparamagnetic iron oxide particles and ultrasmall superparamagnetic iron oxide particles, are selectively taken up the Kupffer cells of the reticuloendothelial system (RES). RES cells are mainly present in the liver, spleen, and lymph nodes. These agents exert their effects both on T1 and T2 relaxation times, and therefore postcontrast imaging can be performed with T1- and T2-weighted sequences. They are generally used for problem solving in combination with GBCAs. Superparamagnetic iron oxide particles decrease the signal intensity of tissues containing RES cells on T1- and T2-weighted sequences, and therefore increase the conspicuity of lesions which do not contain RES cells such as metastases or primary tumors in the liver and spleen or hepatic fibrosis (Figure 2.32). Ultrasmall superparamagnetic iron oxide particles have been reported to be successful in the diagnosis of lymph node metastases. However, the roles of iron-based contrast agents in these assessments have not been well established yet (7).

Superparamagnetic iron oxide particles include ferumoxides (Feridex, Bayer Healthcare Pharmaceuticals, Wayne, NJ, USA) and ferucarbotran (Resovist, Bayer Schering Pharma Ag, Berlin, Germany). Both of these agents are FDA approved. Ultrasmall superparamagnetic iron oxide particles include ferumoxtran (Combidex), which has not been approved by FDA yet.

Ferumoxide particles are 50 to 180 nm in size, while ferucarbotran particles are about 60 nm in size (19). Ferumoxide particles are coated with dextran and ferucarbotran particles are coated with carboxydextran (19). The lower size of ferucarbotran particles increases the enhancement on T1-weighted sequences (19).

Resovist can be administered as a rapid bolus and imaging can be performed immediately following the administration (19). Both dynamic and delayed imaging can be performed. Accumulation of Resovist in RES cells begins at 10 min and is present upto 8 h following the administration. Vasodilatation and paraesthesia are the most common adverse events (19).

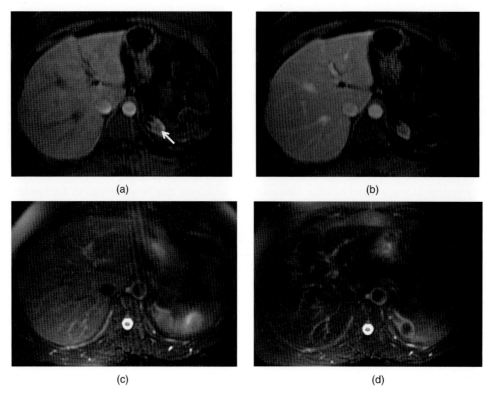

(a)

(b)

(c)

(d)

Figure 2.32 *Differentiation of Pancreatic Cancer from Intrapancreatic Splenule.* T1-weighted postgadolinium fat-suppressed hepatic arterial dominant phase (a) and hepatic venous phase (b) 3D-GE images and T2-weighted pre-superparamagnetic iron oxide (SPIO) (c) and post-SPIO (d) images demonstrate a lesion in the pancreatic tail in a patient with splenectomy. The pancreatic tail is located in the splenic fossa due to the operation. The lesion shows low signal on postgadolinium T1-weighted images. The differential diagnosis includes pancreatic cancer based on the findings of postgadolinium imaging. However, the lesion shows lower signal following SPIO administration. Therefore, the diagnosis is consistent with intrapancreatic splenule.

Feridex is diluted with 100 ml 5% dextrose solution administered as a slow infusion over 30 min. Postcontrast imaging can be performed immediately following the infusion upto 3.5 h. Leg and back pain are the most common adverse events (19).

Manganese-based contrast agents

Mangafodipir trisodium (Mn-DPDP, Teslascan) is a liver-specific contrast agent and postcontrast imaging is performed with T1-weighted sequences. However, it has not been reported that it is more accurate in the diagnosis of liver lesions compared to GBCAs. Additionally, mangafodipir chelate readily dissociates after injection to yield free manganese (Mn) ions (19). Free Mn is toxic, and therefore it has been considered that the instability of the chelate may lead to the toxicity (19). Chronic exposure to free Mn causes a Parkinsonism-like syndrome due to its accumulation in the brain (19). Furthermore, the neurological risk increases in patients with chronic liver failure as a result of decreased elimination of Mn by the liver (19). Free Mn ions dissociated from Mn-DPDP have also been reported to cause a depressive action on heart function (19). Mangafodipir trisodium (Mn-DPDP, Teslascan), which has FDA approval, was in the US market for a short period of time, but it is not marketed in the USA and many other parts of the world anymore.

General pitfalls

On MR images, it is common that multiple imaging properties are concurrently present. The contributions of these various properties must be separately determined in order that appropriate diagnosis is made. Table 2.3 displays the common imaging properties that should be recognized in precontrast sequences for different types of tissues. Table 2.4 displays the imaging properties of different stages of blood products on precontrast sequences. Table 2.5 displays the common imaging properties of different common pathologic processes on postgadolinium T1-weighted sequences.

Common potentially competing imaging characteristics include (i) fat suppression effects on precontrast T1- and T2-weighted images, (ii) magnetic susceptibility effects on T1- and T2-weighted images, (iii) out-of-phase effects on T1-weighted images, (iv) washout versus fat suppression effects on postgadolinium sequences, (v) enhancement of lesions containing subacute blood or high amounts of protein, and (vi) vessel enhancement problems.

Fat suppression effects can usually be separated by employing both non-suppressed and fat suppressed T1- and T2-weighted sequences. Low signal due to fat suppression effects can be correctly ascertained by the demonstration of higher signal intensity of the structure on non-fat-suppressed T1- and

Table 2.3 Common imaging properties of different types of tissues on precontrast sequences.

Precontrast sequences	Fluid	Fat	High protein content	Lesions or organs with abundant fat	Lesions or organs with lesser amount of fat	Lesions or organs with iron	Acute fibrosis	Chronic fibrosis
T1 in-phase	Markedly low	Markedly high	Variably high or intermediate	Markedly high	Variable	Variably low	Variably low	Variably low
T1 out-of-phase	Markedly low	Markedly high	Variably high or intermediate	Markedly high with peripheral chemical shift artifact	Lower compared to in-phase	Higher compared to in-phase	Variably low	Variably low
T1 fat suppressed	Markedly low	Markedly low	Variably high or intermediate	Markedly low	Variable	Variably low	Variably low	Variably low
T2	Markedly high	Markedly high	Variably low or intermediate	Moderate to markedly high	Variable	Variably low	Variably high	Variably low
T2 fat suppressed	Markedly high	Markedly low	Variably low or intermediate	Markedly low	Variable	Variably low	Variably high	Variably low

Table 2.4 Imaging properties of different stages of blood products on precontrast sequences.

Stage of blood products	Content of blood products	T1w sequences – including in-phase, out-of-phase, fat-suppressed sequences	T2w sequences – including fat-suppressed sequences
Hyperacute	Oxyhemoglobin/serum	Intermediate	High
Acute	Deoxyhemoglobin	Intermediate	Low
Early subacute	Intracellular methemoglobin	High	Low
Late subacute	Extracellular methemoglobin	High	High
Chronic	Hemosiderin	Low	Low

T2-weighted sequences, relative to the corresponding fat-suppressed sequences (Figures 2.2, 2.3, 2.10, and 2.16).

Signal loss due to magnetic susceptibility can be separated from signal loss from out-of-phase effects on T1-weighted in-phase and out-of-phase GE sequences by observing that susceptibility effects increase with increasing TE on GE sequences (Figures 2.9 and 2.11). Therefore, susceptibility effects which are seen as signal loss or decreased signal are prominent on T1-weighted in-phase GE sequence compared to T1-weighted out-of-phase GE sequence with shorter TE values. Additionally, susceptibility effects are also observed as low signal on T2-weighted ETSE sequences and these effects are less prominent on T2-weighted ETSE sequences compared to T1-weighted GE sequences (Figure 2.15). For example, susceptibility artifacts resulting from clips or prostheses are least prominent on T2-weighted ETSE sequences, and more prominent on in-phase T1-weighted compared to out-of-phase sequences. Additionally, iron deposition causes decreased signal on T2-weighted ETSE sequences, and also demonstrates loss of signal on T1-weighted in-phase image compared to out-of-phase image (Figures 2.9 and 2.15).

Out-of-phase effects cycle with in-phase and out-of-phase echo times on T1-weighted GE images. Lesions or tissues containing higher amounts of fat demonstrate signal loss on T1-weighted out-of-phase sequence compared to in-phase sequence (Figures 2.3, 2.9, and 2.10). Additionally, phase cancellation artifact forms around the lesions containing abundant amount of fat and these lesions do not demonstrate signal loss on out-of-phase T1-weighted sequences (Figure 2.10).

The distinction between washout and fat suppression effects on postgadolinium T1-weighted fat-suppressed GE sequences must also be established. This problem does not arise if precontrast T1-weighted GE images are acquired and postcontrast imaging is preformed with fat-suppression on all phases. However, if early postgadolinium imaging is performed with non-fat-suppressed sequences, the observation of low signal of a structure on later postgadolinium fat-suppressed sequences, that appeared as high signal on early postgadolinium non-suppressed sequences, may raise the question whether this reflects a fat suppression effect rather than a gadolinium washout effect. In the liver, this can usually be distinguished by the observation that a fatty lesion shows low signal on the interstitial phase postgadolinium fat-suppressed sequence, and isointense or hyperintense on both the hepatic arterial dominant or early hepatic venous phase non-suppressed GE sequences. Generally, if a liver lesion washes out on the interstitial phase, it has most often shown evidence of washout already by the early hepatic venous phase non-fat suppressed SGE images. Further supportive information of a fat effect is evidence that the lesion appears fatty on any of the other sequences employed in the imaging protocol (e.g.; out-of-phase or non contrast fat suppressed sequences).

Determination of enhancement on postgadolinium sequences may be difficult if the lesion contains a high amount of subacute blood or protein as the presence of high intensity blood or protein on T1-weighted images impairs the detection of gadolinium enhancement. The use of subtraction imaging is helpful for the detection of enhancement in these types of lesions.

Inhomogeneous signal intensity of vessels is a diagnostic problem not infrequently encountered on MR images. In general, we have found that image acquisition between 1 and 2 min postgadolinium on the interstitial phase using GE results in consistently high signal of patent arteries and veins. Unfortunately, data acquisition often falls beyond this range, particularly in the setting of acquiring images of the pelvis following images of the abdomen. If patency of vessels is a particular diagnostic concern then we employ sequences that consistently show high signal in patent vessels, often by combining intrinsic in-flow effects and gadolinium effects. Sequences we employ include: gadolinium-enhanced slice-selective MP-RAGE (particularly useful for non-cooperative patients), gadolinium-enhanced WE SGE, and GE sequences with GE refocusing (without gadolinium) (e.g., true FISP).

Non-cooperative patients

It is crucial to recognize that separate protocols are required for cooperative (Table 2.6) and non-cooperative patients (Table 2.7). In general, non-cooperative patients fall into two categories: (i) those who cannot suspend respiration, but breathe in a regular fashion, and (ii) those who cannot suspend respiration and cannot breathe in a regular fashion. The most common patient population that fits into the first group are sedated pediatric patients. Agitated patients are the most commonly encountered who fit

Table 2.5 Imaging properties of common pathologic processes on different phases on postgadolinium T1-weighted sequences.

Postgadolinium T1-weighted sequences	Inflammation	Fibrosis	Arterial compromise	Portal venous compromise	Hepatic venous compromise
Hepatic arterial dominant (capillary) phase	Increased homogeneous or heterogeneous hepatic parenchymal enhancement/Increased enhancement around inflammatory or infectious focal lesions	Decreased enhancement compared to normal liver parenchyma	Moderately decreased hepatic parenchymal enhancement in corresponding regions	Moderately or markedly increased hepatic parenchymal enhancement in corresponding regions	Increased or decreased heterogeneous peripheral hepatic enhancement with increased or decreased heterogeneous enhancement
Early hepatic venous phase	Increased hepatic parenchymal enhancement tends to become isointense with the remaining liver parenchyma	Variable enhancement	Mildly or moderately decreased hepatic parenchymal enhancement in corresponding regions	Mildly increased hepatic parenchymal enhancement in corresponding regions	Increased or decreased heterogeneous peripheral hepatic enhancement with increased or decreased heterogeneous enhancement
Interstitial phase	Increased hepatic parenchymal enhancement becomes isointense with the remaining liver parenchyma/increased enhancement in the walls of the bile ducts in case of ascending cholangitis	Increased enhancement or isointensity compared to normal liver parenchyma	Mildly decreased hepatic parenchymal enhancement in corresponding regions	Mildly increased hepatic parenchymal enhancement or isointensity in corresponding regions	Increased or decreased heterogeneous peripheral hepatic enhancement with increased or decreased heterogeneous enhancement

Table 2.6 Liver or general abdomen protocol for cooperative patients.

Sequence	Plane	TR	TE	Flip	Thickness/gap	FOV	Matrix
Cooperative patients at 1.5 T							
Localizer	3-plane						
SS-ETSE	Coronal	1500*	85	170	6–8 mm/20%	350–400	192 × 256
SS-ETSE	Axial	1500*	85	170	6–8 mm/20%	350–400	192 × 256
SS-ETSE fat suppressed	Axial	1500*	85	170	6–8 mm/20%	350–400	192 × 256
T1 SGE in/opposed phase	Axial	170	2.2/4.4	70	6–7 mm/20%	350–400	192 × 320
T1 3D SGE in/opposed phase	Axial	7.47	2.38/4.79	10	3 mm	380	320 × 200
SS-ETSE MRCP	Coronal	5000	700	180	50 mm	300	224 × 384
T1 3D SGE FS pre	Axial	3.8	1.7	10	3 mm	350–400	160 × 256
CONTRAST							
T1 3D SGE FS arterial	Axial	3.8	1.7	10	3 mm	350–400	160 × 256
T1 3D SGE FS venous	Axial	3.8	1.7	10	3 mm	350–400	160 × 256
T1 3D SGE FS interstitial	Axial	3.8	1.7	10	3 mm	350–400	160 × 256
Cooperative patients at 3.0 T							
Localizer	3-plane						
SS-ETSE	Coronal	1500*	70	170	6–8 mm/20%	350–400	192 × 256
SS-ETSE	Axial	1500*	70	170	6–8 mm/20%	350–400	192 × 256
SS-ETSE fat suppressed	Axial	1500*	70	170	6–8 mm/20%	350–400	192 × 256
T1 SGE in/opposed phase	Axial	170	2.2/4.4	70	6–7 mm/20%	350–400	192 × 320
T1 3D SGE in/opposed phase	Axial	7.47	2.38/4.79	10	3 mm	380	320 × 200
SS-ETSE MRCP	Coronal	5000	700	180	50 mm	300	224 × 384
T1 3D SGE FS pre	Axial	3.8	1.7	10	3 mm	350–400	180 × 288
CONTRAST							
T1 3D SGE FS arterial	Axial	3.8	1.7	10	3 mm	350–400	180 × 288
T1 3D SGE FS venous	Axial	3.8	1.7	10	3 mm	350–400	180 × 288
T1 3D SGE FS interstitial	Axial	3.8	1.7	10	3 mm	350–400	180 × 288

*TR between slice acquisitions.

Note: In-phase or opposed phase imaging can be performed in either SGE or 3D SGE techniques depending on the system features. Coronal T1-weighted SGE could be obtained for precontrast T1-weighted imaging. Postgadolinium coronal T1-weighted fat-suppressed imaging following the acquisition of axial images on the interstitial phase could be performed.

The delay time for the start of sequence acquisition for 3D SGE, following the contrast injection, can be calculated by the following formula: Contrast Arrival Time to the Liver/Portal Vein (35–40 s) − (Acquisition Time of 3D SGE Sequence/2).

into the second group. Optimal imaging strategies differ for each group.

In sedated patients, substitution of breath-hold images (e.g., SGE or 3D-GE sequences) can be made readily with breathing-averaged ETSE and SGE images, the image quality of which is improved by using fat suppression. Both SGE and ETSE have the ability to be gated to respiration. As SGE utilizes spoiling gradients within each TR interval, T1 information is preserved between respiratory periods, while T2 ETSE exploits the respiratory period into its inherent T2-weighting. With sedation, breathing is in a more regular pattern than that observed for all other patients. Additionally, breathing-independent T2-weighted SS-ETSE can be used, as is T1-weighted MP-RAGE or 3D-GE with radial sampling, if dynamic gadolinium-enhanced images are required (Figure 2.13) (10).

In patients who are agitated, only single-shot techniques should be used, including breathing-independent T2-weighted SS-ETSE, and pre- and postcontrast T1-weighted MP-RAGE or 3D-GE with radial sampling sequences (Figure 2.13) (10).

3D-GE with radial sampling has been used in routine clinical practice recently and has been replacing MP-RAGE sequences for fat-suppressed pre- and postgadolinium imaging due to its higher spatial resolution and image quality (Figure 2.13). Although the long acquisition time does not allow dynamic imaging, in the near future, dynamic imaging would also likely be available.

Emerging developments in MRI

There are several emerging developments in MR imaging that are important for body MR imaging. These include (i) recent technical developments in hardware and software, (ii) parallel MR imaging, and (iii) introduction of 3.0 T MR systems as whole body magnets.

Table 2.7 Liver or general abdomen protocol for non-cooperative patients.

Sequence	Motion	Plane	TR	TE	Flip	Thickness/gap	FOV	Matrix
Non-cooperative patients at 1.5 T								
Localizer		3-plane						
SS-ETSE	FB or RT	Coronal	1500*	85	170	6–8 mm/20%	350–400	192 × 256
SS-ETSE	FB or RT	Axial	1500*	85	170	6–8 mm/20%	350–400	192 × 256
SS-ETSE fat suppressed	FB or RT	Axial	1500*	85	170	6–8 mm/20%	350–400	192 × 256
T1 SGE in/opposed phase	RT	Axial	170	2.2/4.4	70	6–7 mm/20%	350–400	192 × 320
T1 2D MPRAGE in/opposed phase	FB	Axial	1540	2.33/4.07	15	6 mm/30%	380	256 × 156
SS-ETSE MRCP	FB	Coronal	5000	700	180	50 mm	300	224 × 384
T1 2D MP-RAGE fat suppressed	FB	Axial	3.5	1.2	15	6–8 mm/20%	350–400	150 × 256
T1 3D SGE FS with Radial Sampling	FB	Axial	3.83	1.6	10	3 mm	380	380 × 380
CONTRAST								
T1 3D SGE FS with Radial Sampling**	FB	Axial	3.83	1.6	10	3 mm	380	380 × 380
T1 2D MP-RAGE 15 s/1 min/5 min postinjection	FB	Axial	3.5	1.2	15	6–8 mm/20%	350–400	150 × 256
Non-cooperative patients at 3.0 T								
Localizer		3-plane						
SS-ETSE	FB or RT	Coronal	1500*	70	160	6–8 mm/20%	350–400	192 × 256
SS-ETSE	FB or RT	Axial	1500*	70	160	6–8 mm/20%	350–400	192 × 256
SS-ETSE fat suppressed	FB or RT	Axial	1500*	85	160	6–8 mm/20%	350–400	192 × 256
T1 SGE in/opposed phase	RT	Axial	170	2.2/4.4	70	6–7 mm/20%	350–400	192 × 320
T1 2D MPRAGE in/opposed phase	FB	Axial	1540	2.33/4.07	15	6 mm/30%	380	256 × 156
SS-ETSE MRCP	FB	Coronal	5000	700	180	50 mm	300	224 × 384
T1 2D MP-RAGE fat suppressed	FB	Axial	3.2	1.1	12	6–8 mm/20%	350–400	150 × 256
T1 3D SGE FS with Radial Sampling	FB	Axial	3.83	1.6	10	3 mm	380	380 × 380
CONTRAST								
T1 3D SGE FS with Radial Sampling**	FB	Axial	3.83	1.6	10	3 mm	380	380 × 380
T1 2D MP-RAGE 15 s/1 min/5 min postinjection	FB	Axial	3.2	1.1	12	6–8 mm/20%	350–400	150 × 256

*TR between slice acquisitions; FB, free breathe; RT, respiratory triggered; SSFP, steady state free precession.

**The acquisition time is around 80–85 s for fat-suppressed 3D SGE with radial sampling. Postcontrast acquisitions should be repeated two times. The contrast acquisition should be started after 45 s following the start of the sequence. The second acquisition on the axial plane should be done after the first acquisition.
Note: For precontrast and postcontrast imaging axial T1-weighted imaging either 2D MP-RAGE or 3D SGE with radial sampling technique should be preferred depending on the technical specifications of the system.
Coronal T1-weighted SGE could be obtained for precontrast T1-weighted imaging. Postgadolinium coronal T1-weighted fat-suppressed imaging following the acquisition of axial images on the interstitial phase could be performed with either 2D MP-RAGE or 3D SGE with radial sampling depending on the technical specifications of the system.

Recent technical developments

These developments have mainly occurred in the following areas:

(1) Increased main magnetic field strength (e.g., 3.0 T MRI systems).

(2) Improved radiofrequency coil design (from large single body or a single surface coil to arrays of multiple smaller (phased-array) coils containing 32 elements or higher).

(3) Improved bandwidth per receiver channel with faster readouts and faster reconstructions of k-space data sets.

(4) Increased gradient performance which can achieve lower TR and TE values and allow better spatial and temporal coverage.

(5) Newer and faster acquisition methods and sequences, like 3D-GE; 3D-GE with radial sampling; time resolved 3D-GE; MP-RAGE; bSSFP; SS-ETSE; EPI; and parallel imaging (7).

(6) Diffusion, perfusion, and spectroscopic imaging techniques have been developing although the role of perfusion and spectroscopy have not been established yet. Diffusion weighted imaging has the ability to detect more lesions or to show the lesions better due to its T2-weight compared to standard SS-ETSE T2-weighted sequences. The role of diffusion restriction in terms of sensitivity, specificity for the detection of lesions, characterization of lesions, and for the evaluation of treatment is still not clear.

Parallel MR imaging

Parallel MR imaging is comprised of a number of methods that can be used in combination with the majority of the MR imaging sequences in order to reduce scan time by acquiring less data than would otherwise be necessary to avoid aliasing. The current parallel imaging methods may evolve and very fast imaging eventually including the "massive" parallel MR imaging [in which the number of coil elements equals the number of k-space lines (20)], may become a reality.

In general, parallel imaging methods require the use of suitable phased-array coils. The key feature of parallel imaging methods is the simultaneous application and use of multiple independent receiver coils with distinct sensitivities across the object being imaged. In conventional MR imaging, the role of phased-array coils is merely to improve the SNR, whereas in parallel imaging the phased-array coils are also used to reduce the scan time. The application of parallel imaging allows (i) higher temporal resolution (faster imaging; e.g., MRI exams in non-cooperative patients, time-resolved MRA, and perfusion studies), (ii) higher spatial resolution (larger matrices, thinner slices; e.g., high-resolution MRA), (iii) reduced effective inter-echo spacing (less image blurring and image distortion in ETSE and echo planar imaging; e.g., high quality MRCP and single-shot EPI of the abdomen), and/or (iv) reduced SAR due to shorter echo-trains (important for optimization of body MRI sequences at 3 T) (7).

Body MR imaging at 3 T: general considerations compared to 1.5 T

3.0 T MR systems have been widely used in many institutions over the past few years. The main expected advantage of abdominal MRI at 3.0 T compared to 1.5 T is the gain in signal strength and SNR leading to higher spatial and temporal resolution (21–28). However, several potential disadvantages, such as an increase in imaging artifacts, prolonged T1 relaxation times, and SAR constraints have to be considered in abdominal MRI examinations at 3.0 T (21–28). Chemical shift artifacts of the first kind and susceptibility artifacts have been reported twice as large at 3.0 T compared to 1.5 T (21–28). Standing wave artifacts and conductivity effects that are usually not seen at 1.5 T may be seen at 3.0 T, particularly in patients with large body size, ascites or pregnancy (21–28). Prolonged T1 relaxation times cause a decrease in SNR and change the contrast resolution (21–28). The SAR, a measure for energy deposition within the human body, increases by a factor of 4 at 3.0 T compared to 1.5 T because the magnetic field strength is doubled (21–28).

3.0 T MRI enables the acquisition of very high quality post-gadolinium 3D-GE sequences, with thinner sections and higher spatial resolution compared to 1.5 T, allowing the detection and characterization of very small lesions (Figure 2.33). This high spatial resolution is comparable to the spatial resolution of current-generation multidetector CT, but with the advantage of higher intrinsic soft tissue contrast resolution (1). This capability gives potential advantages for the detection and characterization of small and ultra-small malignant and benign lesions (1).

Chemical shift artifacts of the first kind result from the difference between the resonance frequencies of fat and water protons and are directly proportional to the magnetic field (21–28). Chemical shift artifacts of the first kind are expected to be increased at 3.0 T imaging but generally not diagnostically compromising, although they are usually present on in-phase SGE images (Figure 2.34).

Differences in magnetic susceptibility within the body, which mostly occur at air–tissue interfaces or secondary to the presence of metallic objects, cause local inhomogeneities in the main magnetic field (B0) leading to shortened T2* relaxation times and resultant signal loss (21–24). At higher field strengths, the main magnetic field is more inhomogeneous and more sensitive to T2* dephasing; therefore, susceptibility artifacts are more pronounced at 3.0 T (Figure 2.34) (23). Susceptibility artifacts are usually more pronounced on T1-weighted in-phase sequences although they are not generally diagnostically compromising. Additionally, susceptibility artifacts may have diagnostic value in some cases, allowing better detection of blood products, intra-abdominal air or surgical clips (21–24).

Standing waves and conductivity effects are caused by B1 magnetic field inhomogeneity resulting from the use of higher frequency/decreased wavelength radiofrequency waves and shielding effects (21–24). These effects generate ill-defined areas with little or no signal, particularly in patients with a large body size or ascites (21–24). Standing wave/conductivity effects are most frequently observed on T2-weighted sequences (Figure 2.35). These artifacts generally represent a factor in image quality deterioration on all sequences except 3D-GE sequence (Figure 2.35). Dielectric pads may help to reduce this artifact.

Our results also show that 3D-GE sequences at 3.0 T were relatively robust to imaging artifacts, particularly standing wave/conductivity effects. It has previously been reported that this sequence generates higher SNR and more homogenous fat-suppression at 3.0 T and the effects of gadolinium are more pronounced, resulting in greater contrast and image quality compared to 1.5 T (3,24).

On T1-weighted SGE images, image quality, although still able to provide diagnostic information, is lower at 3.0 T compared to 1.5 T. A probable explanation for fair image quality is the change in contrast resolution at 3.0 T (21,24,29). This may reflect that the increase in T1 relaxation times differs from one tissue to another, which affects contrast resolution, and alters the appearance to that observed at 1.5 T MRI (Figure 2.36) (21,24,29). In our clinical experience, the detection of liver fibrosis on out-of-phase SGE sequence and the detection of fat content of the liver based on the comparison of in-phase and out-of-phase SGE sequences are more difficult at 3.0 T compared to 1.5 T (Figure 2.36). We believe that these problems may reflect the changes in contrast resolution at 3.0 T.

The image quality of T2-weighted sequences at 3.0 T is at least equal to that at 1.5 T if variable flip angle sequences such as hyperechoes or transition between pseudo steady states (TRAPS) are used. These new acquisition techniques have recently been developed to decrease SAR while maintaining acceptable SNR levels during the acquisition of T2-weighted sequences (6,22–24).

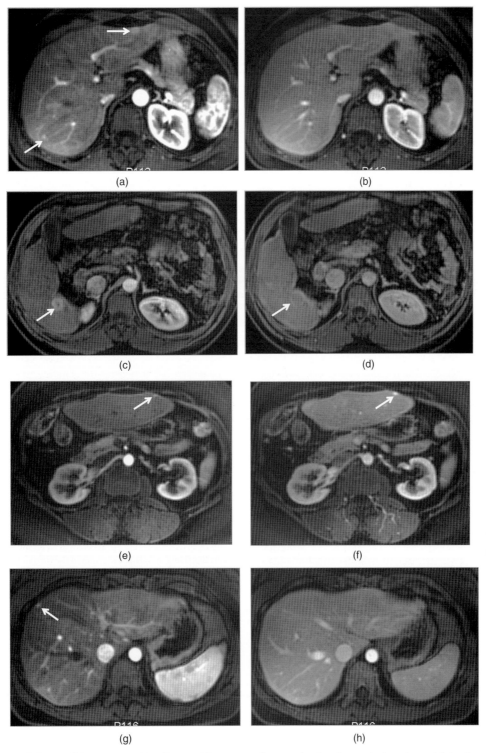

Figure 2.33 *Detection of ultra-small lesions at 3.0 T.* Small carcinoid metastases (arrows, a) enhancing on the hepatic arterial dominant phase (a) fade to isointensity with the remaining liver parenchyma on the interstitial phase (b). Small HCC (arrows; c, d) with central scar enhancing on the hepatic arterial dominant phase (c) shows washout with capsular enhancement on the interstitial phase (d). Small hemangioma (arrows; e, f) shows rapid filling on the hepatic arterial dominant phase (e) and maintains its enhancement on the interstitial phase (f). Small FNH (arrow, g) shows enhancement on the hepatic arterial dominant phase (g) and fades to isointensity with the remaining liver parenchyma on the interstitial phase (h).

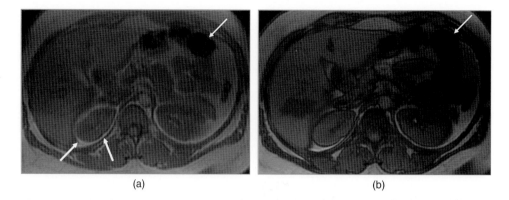

(a)   (b)

Figure 2.34 *Chemical shift artifacts of the first kind and susceptibility artifacts at 3.0 T.* Chemical shift artifacts of the first kind (thick arrows, a) are most commonly seen on in-phase (a) and out-of-phase (b) SGE images and most pronounced around the kidneys. Susceptibility artifacts (thin arrows; a, b) are most pronounced on SGE images.

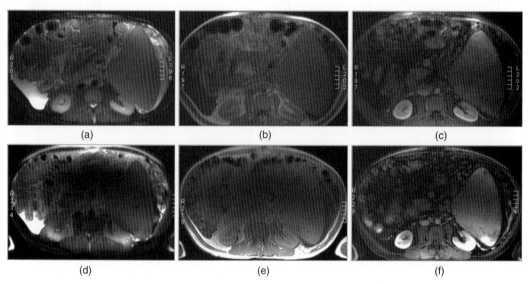

(a)   (b)   (c)

(d)   (e)   (f)

Figure 2.35 *Standing wave and conductivity artifacts at 3.0 T.* Standing wave and conductivity artifacts are not generally seen on single shot echo train spin echo (a), SGE (b) and 3D-GE (c) images at 1.5 T. However, these artifacts are seen as signal loss usually at the center of the image on single shot echo train spin echo (d) and SGE sequences (e) but not on 3D-GE images (f) at 3.0 T.

We believe that standing wave and conductivity artifacts and differences in contrast resolution, which constitute the major disadvantages of 3.0 T MR imaging, will be eliminated in the near future. The use of 3.0 T MR imaging will play a more essential role in the detection of very small lesions in the near future, especially on postgadolinium sequences.

CT imaging techniques

CT scanning of the liver is performed as a part of the upper or the whole abdomen study. CT is still being used for the imaging of liver, particularly in trauma patients, in some non-cooperative patients who are unable to hold their breath, in patients who require very fast imaging because of their unstable medical conditions, in patients with MR noncompliant medical equipment such as tubes, pacemakers or prostheses, and in some claustrophobic patients. CT scanning of the liver includes precontrast scanning followed by dual or triple phase contrast-enhanced scanning with non-ionic iodinated contrast media.

Precontrast imaging (Figure 2.37) may be performed as a baseline technique for the detection of blood, fat, calcification, or stones in the liver and biliary system, and for the better appreciation of enhancement on contrast-enhanced CT images. However, because of the radiation concern, precontrast imaging is not generally used anymore in major institutions. Postcontrast imaging (Figure 2.38) may be performed for different purposes, including the detection and differentiation of focal lesions, the

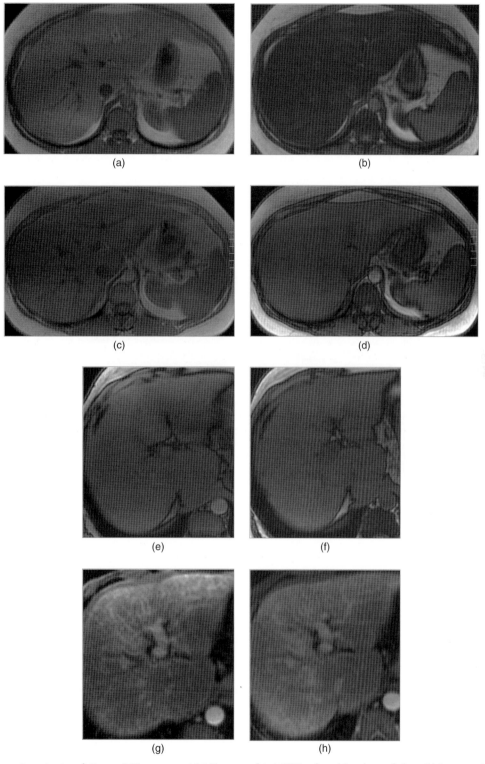

(a)

(b)

(c)

(d)

(e)

(f)

(g)

(h)

Figure 2.36 *Difference in contrast resolution on SGE sequences at 3.0 T compared to 1.5 T.* In-phase (a) and out-of-phase (b) images at 1.5 T demonstrate diffuse fatty liver. However, the signal drop on out-of-phase image (d) compared to in-phase image (c) at 3.0 T is not prominent compared to that of 1.5 T in the same patient due to the difference in contrast resolution at 3.0 T compared to 1.5 T. Fibrotic network of the liver on out-of-phase SGE image (e) at 3.0 T is not well appreciated compared to out-of-phase SGE image (f) at 1.5 T due to difference in contrast resolution. However, fibrotic network of the liver is better appreciated on post-gadolinium interstitial phase 3D-GE image (g) at 3.0 T compared to the corresponding image (h) at 1.5 T.

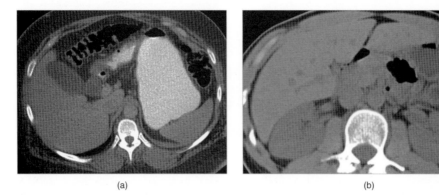

(a)   (b)

Figure 2.37 *Pre-contrast MDCT Images.*

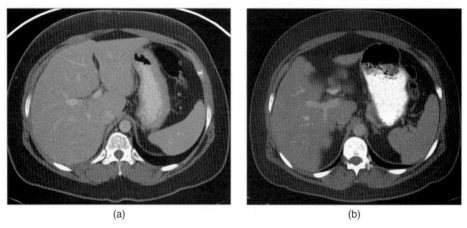

(a)   (b)

Figure 2.38 *Post-contrast MDCT Images.*

Table 2.8 Parameters of 64-slice multi-detector CT imaging of the liver.

Parameters	Precontrast	Hepatic arterial phase	Hepatic arterial dominant phase	Hepatic venous phase	Interstitial phase
KV/effective mAS/time per rotation (s)	120/250/0.33	120/250/0.33	120/250/0.33	120/250/0.33	120/1250/0.33
Detector collimation (mm)	0.6	0.6	0.6	0.6	0.6
Slice thickness (mm)	5	0.75–5	0.75–5	0.75–5	0.75–5
Data reconstruction interval (mm)	5	0.5–5	0.5–5	0.5–5	0.5–5
Pitch	0.75	0.75	0.75	0.75	0.75
Image order	Cranial-Caudal	Cranial-Caudal	Cranial-Caudal	Cranial-Caudal	Cranial-Caudal
IV Contrast volume (ml)	N/A	120	120	120	120
Injection rate (ml/s)	N/A	4	3	3	3
Scan delay (s)	N/A	25	35–40	50–60	90–120
3D technique	Volume rendering/MIP	Volume rendering/MIP	Volume rendering/MIP	Volume rendering/MIP	Volume rendering/MIP

evaluation of diffuse liver diseases, or the evaluation of vascular structures.

Dual phase study is performed on the hepatic arterial dominant and hepatic venous phases, whereas triple phase scanning is performed on the hepatic arterial dominant, hepatic venous, and interstitial phases as on MR studies. The hepatic arterial dominant phase is defined as the presence of contrast in the hepatic arteries and portal veins but not in the hepatic veins. The hepatic arterial dominant phase is acquired 25–30 s after the contrast media injection. The hepatic venous phase is the presence of contrast in the hepatic veins. The hepatic venous phase is acquired 50–60 s after the contrast media injection. The interstitial phase is the late phase and acquired 90–120 s after the contrast media injection. The important features of these phases are explained in the MR Imaging Techniques section. However, because of radiation concerns, only the hepatic venous imaging is generally performed in major institutions and MRI is usually used for further evaluation and characterization for equivocal lesions or cases, or for the detection of additional small lesions, or for the evaluation of the biliary system.

The parameters of CT imaging may vary depending on the purpose of imaging. However, it is prudent to use the techniques and parameters which will give the highest diagnostic accuracy and the lowest radiation dose in all patients. The detector collimation, slice thickness, data reconstruction interval and table speed should be decreased for the evaluation of vascular structures. The parameters of CT imaging technique are seen in Table 2.8.

Oral positive or negative contrast may also be used for the improved visualization of gastrointestinal tract.

References

1 Ramalho, M., Altun, E., Heredia, V. *et al.* (2007) Liver MR imaging: 1.5 T versus 3.0 T. Magn Reson Imaging Clin N Am, 15, 321–347.

2 Semelka, R.C., Balci, N.C., Op de Beeck, B., and Reinhold, C. (1999) Evaluation of a 10-minute comprehensive MR imaging examination of the upper abdomen. Radiology, 211, 189–195.

3 Lee, V.S., Hecht, E.M., Taouli, B. *et al.* (2007) Body and cardiovascular MR imaging at 3.0 T. Radiology, 244, 692–705.

4 Hussain, S.M., Wielopolski, P.A., and Martin, D.R. (2005) Abdominal magnetic resonance imaging at 3.0 T: problem or a promise for the future? Top Magn Reson Imaging, 16, 325–335.

5 Semelka, R.C., Martin, D.R., and Balci, N.C. (2006) Magnetic resonance imaging of the liver: How I do it. J Gastroenterol Hepatol, 21, 632–637.

6 Raman, S.S., Leary, C., Bluemke, D.A. *et al.* (2010) Improved characterization of focal liver lesions with liver-specific gadoxetic acid disodium-enhanced magnetic resonance imaging: a multicenter phase 3 clinical trial. J Comput Assist Tomogr, 34, 163–172.

7 Sharma, P., Martin, D.R., Semelka, R.C. *et al.* (2010) Diagnostic approach to protocoling and interpreting MR studies of the abdomen and pelvis, in Abdominal-pelvic MRI, 3rd edn (ed R.C. Semelka), Wiley-Blackwell, Hoboken, NJ, pp. 1–45.

8 Brown, M.A. and Semelka, R.C. (2010) Gradient echo sequences, in MRI: Basic principles and applications, 4th edn, Wiley-Blackwell, Hoboken, NJ, pp. 74–80.

9 Brown, M.A. and Semelka, R.C. (2010) Magnetization prepared sequences, in MRI: Basic principles and applications, 4th edn, Wiley-Blackwell, Hoboken, NJ, pp. 82–91.

10 Altun, E., Semelka, R.C., Dale, B.M., and Elias, J. Jr., (2008) Water excitation MPRAGE: an alternative sequence for postcontrast imaging of the abdomen in noncooperative patients at 1.5-T and 3.0-T MR. J Magn Reson Imaging, 27, 1146–1154.

11 Brown, M.A. and Semelka, R.C. (2010) Spin echo sequences, in MRI: Basic principles and applications, 4th edn, Wiley-Blackwell, Hoboken, NJ, pp. 71–74.

12 Brown, M.A. and Semelka, R.C. (2010) Signal suppression techniques, in MRI: Basic principles and applications, 4th edn, Wiley-Blackwell, Hoboken, NJ, pp. 101–110.

13 Goncalves Neto, J.A., Altun, E., Vaidean, G. *et al.* (2009) Early contrast enhancement of the liver: exact description of subphases using MRI. Magn Reson Imaging, 27, 792–800.

14 Sharma, P., De Becker, J., Beck, G.M. *et al.* (2006) Arterial-phase Bolus-track Liver Examination (ABLE): optimization of liver arterial phase gadolinium enhanced MRI using centric re-ordered 3D gradient echo and Bolus track real-time imaging. Proc Intl Soc Mag Reson Med, 14, 3318.

15 Altun, E., Martin, D.R., and Semelka, R.C. (2010) Contrast agents, in Abdominal-pelvic MRI, 3rd edn (ed R.C. Semelka), Wiley-Blackwell, Hooken, NJ, pp. 1767–1850.

16 Altun, E., Semelka, R.C., and Cakit, C. (2009) Nephrogenic systemic fibrosis and management of high risk patients. Acad Radiol, 16, 897–905.

17 Rofsky, N.M., Sherry, D.A., and Lenkinski, L.E. (2008) Nephrogenic systemic fibrosis: a chemical perspective. Radiology, 247, 608–612.

18 Grazioli, L., Morana, G., Kirchin, M.A., and Schneider, G. (2005) Accurate differentiation of focal nodular hyperplasia from hepatic adenoma at gadobenate dimeglumine-enhanced MR imaging: prospective study. Radiology, 236, 166–177.

19 Kirchin, M.A. and Runge, V.M. (2003) Contrast agents for magnetic resonance imaging: safety update. TMRI, 14, 426–35.

20 Hutchinson, M. and Raff, U. (1988) Fast MRI data acquisition using multiple detectors. Magn Reson Med, 6, 87–91.

21 Merkle, E.M. and Dale, B.M. (2006) Abdominal MRI at 3.0 T: the basics revisited. AJR Am J Roentgenol, 186, 1524–1532.

22 Soher, B.J., Dale, B.M., and Merkle, E.M. (2007) A review of MR physics: 3 T versus 1.5 T. Magn Reson Imaging Clin N Am, 15, 277–290.

23 Barth, M.M., Smith, M.P., Pedrosa, I. *et al.* (2007) Body MR imaging at 3.0 T: understanding the opportunities and challenges. Radiographics, 27, 1445–1464.

24 Akisik, F.M., Sandrasegaran, K., Aisen, A.M. *et al.* (2007) Abdominal MR imaging at 3.0 T. Radiographics, 27, 1433–1444.

25 Michaely, H.J., Kramer, H., Dietrich, O. *et al.* (2007) Intraindividual comparison of high-spatial-resolution abdominal MR angiography at 1.5 T and 3.0 T: initial experience. Radiology, 244, 907–913.

26 Zapparoli, M., Semelka, R.C., Altun, E. *et al.* (2008) 3.0 T MRI evaluation of patients with chronic liver diseases: initial observations. Magn Reson Imaging, 26, 650–660.

27 Tsurusaki, M., Semelka, R.C., Zapparoli, M. *et al.* (2008) Quantitative and qualitative comparison of 3.0 T and 1.5 T MR imaging of the

liver in patients with diffuse parenchymal liver disease. Eur J Radiol, 72, 314–320.

28 Ramalho, M., Heredia, V., Tsurusaki, M. *et al.* (2009) Qualitative and quantitative comparison of 3.0 T and 1.5 T MRI for the liver with chronic liver disease. J Magn Reson Imaging, 29, 869–879.

29 de Bazelaire, C.M., Duhamel, G.D., Rofsky, N.M., and Alsop, D.C. (2004) MR imaging relaxation times of abdominal and pelvic tissues measured in vivo at 3.0 T: preliminary results. Radiology, 230, 652–659.

CHAPTER 3
Safety of MRI and CT

Ersan Altun and Richard C. Semelka
The University of North Carolina at Chapel Hill, Department of Radiology, Chapel Hill, NC, USA

In recent years, diagnostic imaging safety has garnered considerable interest in medical literature because of concerns of health risks attributable to imaging investigation. Perhaps the greatest concern is the likelihood of cancer development, secondary to the use of increasing numbers and exposures of medical radiation, especially resulting from the increasing use of multislice CT scanners. Additional health concerns are the toxicity of iodine-based contrast agents (IBCAs) that are used in CT, and gadolinium-based contrast agents (GBCAs) that are used in MRI. The discovery in 2006, after 16 years of clinical use, of the association of the development of nephrogenic systemic fibrosis (NSF) in patients with renal impairment following the administration of GBCAs, stimulated unprecedented alarm in the imaging sphere among physicians and patients. This was especially vexing, as for many years GBCAS were considered the safe alternative to IBCAs.

Perhaps all of these concerns are sobering reminders that nothing is 100% safe, and we have to be constantly vigilant on the subject of patient safety. In this chapter we discuss many of these issues.

Toxicity of contrast agents

Iodine based contrast agents

IBCAs, which are the primary agents used in CT examinations, are the most commonly used contrast agents in routine daily practice. The risks of adverse reactions, contrast induced nephropathy (CIN), and possible drug interactions, have garnered attention, and may be especially important because of the large number of studies performed. Prevention or minimization of these complications is important.

Allergy-like acute adverse reactions

Allergy-like acute adverse reactions typically manifest themselves shortly after the administration of an IBCA, with signs ranging from urticaria to an anaphylactoid process characterized by life threatening bronchospasm, laryngeal edema, and hypotension (1,2). The majority of adverse side effects are mild to moderate, non-life-threatening events, occurring in about 30% of studies, and require only observation, reassurance, and support. Virtually all life-threatening reactions occur immediately, or within the first 20 min, after IBCA administration (3,4). Histories of allergies and previous reactions have served as predictors for the possible development of adverse reactions. Although a history of multiple severe allergies does increase the risk of a reaction following contrast agent injection, only a small percent of patients with severe adverse reactions to IBCAs have a strong history of allergies, and only a small percentage of patients with allergies will develop reactions to IBCA (1). Most reactions in these patients are also minor. A history of asthma is also considered to be a good predictor of increased risk of reactions to IBCAs (1–4). Fortunately, asthmatics are generally familiar with the use of β-agonist inhalers and usually have one with them. Nevertheless, such inhalers should be available where contrast media (CM) are administered (2). Patients who have experienced an allergy-like adverse event after IBCA injection are unlikely to experience a similar or more severe reaction if an IBAC is injected again (1). In fact, although a prior reaction remains the best predictor of a future adverse event, the likelihood of a recurrent reaction is in the range of 8–25%. If the previous reaction was caused by a true allergy, the risk would approach 100% (1,2). Therefore, if the patient has had a prior reaction to an IBCA, it is not necessary to avoid any further contrast agent injection in most cases, unless the reaction has been a major one. The use of a different IBCA is a reasonable approach, although it is often impossible to define either the specifics of a prior reaction or the specific contrast agent used. The use of non-ionic low osmolality contrast agents has been shown to reduce the risk of acute adverse reactions and CIN (5,6). The use of a pre-treatment regimen, including administration of corticosteroids with or without antihistamines or other medications, has been shown to be safe and effective in preventing minor adverse events (7,8). Prospective studies of pre-treatment have involved too few patient numbers, considering the rarity of life-threatening occurences, to determine whether pre-treatment with steroids prevents life-threatening reactions (7,9). There is evidence from a large prospective registry, however, that they do not (1). If pre-treatment is to be used, its use should begin about 12 h before contrast agent injection, to prevent minor adverse events (7), as shorter pretreatment regimen may not be effective. It is crucial that a trained health care worker be ready and able to treat an on-going life threatening reaction (3,4).

Contrast induced nephropathy (CIN)

CIN is defined as iatrogenic renal function impairment following exposure to CM, and the vast majority of cases have been related to IBCA use. Theoretically they also may occur with high dose GBCAs (10–12), but in the current era of NSF-concern, effectively no high dose GBCA studies are performed any more. CIN occurs much more commonly following the administration of IBCAs compared to GBCAs, but this likely reflects a dose-related phenomenon rather than intrinsic safety of the agent per se (13–15). CIN resulting from exposure to IBCAs is the third most common cause of acute renal failure in hospitalized patients, after impaired renal perfusion and the use of other nephrotoxic drugs (10–13,16).

The diagnosis of CIN includes three components: (i) an acute deterioration of renal function, (ii) a temporal relationship with the parenteral administration of CM, and (iii) the exclusion of alternative etiologic reasons which may result in the acute deterioration of renal function (10–12). The acute deterioration of renal function is described as a relative increase of 25% or more, or an absolute increase of 0.5 mg/dl or more from baseline in serum creatinine value (10–12). The acute deterioration of renal function in CIN develops within the first 24 h in 80% of patients, and may persist to 48–72 h in 20% of patients (10). Recently, caution has been suggested in the interpretation of an elevation of serum creatinine value, as fluctuations may occur in the normal state of the patient independent of CM use (17).

The pathophysiology of CIN remains uncertain (18,19). The proposed mechanisms include toxic injury to renal tubules, ischemic injury, or decreased renal medullary perfusion (18,19). It has also been reported that osmolality and viscosity of iodinated CM is also responsible in the pathophysiology, with higher viscosity having a greater likelihood of causing this condition (20). As the glomerular filtration rate (GFR) decreases, the risk of CIN increases; and the risk particularly increases when the GFR is below 60 ml/min/1.73 m^2 (10).

The incidence of CIN varies according to the type of IBCA used. Earlier literature emphasized a risk stratification based on IBCA osmolarity, with higher risk in high-osmolar compared to low- or iso-osmolar agents (13). The incidence of CIN is two times higher with the use of high-osmolality IBCA (HOCM) compared to that of low-osmolality IBCA (LOCM) (13).

HOCM has been largely replaced with LOCM because of their higher nephrotoxicity, lesser patient tolerance, and higher risk of adverse reactions (13).

The incidence of CIN following the intra-arterial or intravenous use of LOCM has been reported to vary between 0.6 - 2.3% in patients with normal renal function (10). In patients with decreased renal function, the incidence of CIN following the intra-arterial and intravenous use of LOCM has been reported to vary from 3% to 50% and 1% to 21%, respectively (13,21). The intra-arterial administration of LOCM has been reported to have a two times higher incidence of CIN compared to intravenous administration (10), which may in part reflect that administration rates and volumes are not as tightly controlled, and may be much higher than with intravenous administration.

The incidence of CIN following the use of iso-osmolality CM (IOCM) and LOCM is similar in patients with normal renal function (13,21). Although the incidence of CIN with IOCM has been reported to be lower in patients with decreased renal function compared to LOCM in a few studies, other studies have shown the opposite effect, apparently influenced in part by the sponsor of the study. There is no definite evidence that IOCM are safer in patients with decreased renal function compared to LOCM (21,22).

CIN is by definition an acute event, but the critical aspect of this condition is the long-term consequences and residual renal impairment. Few studies have been conducted to evaluate the long term outcome of CIN. Residual renal impairment may be seen in 30% of patients with CIN (16). CIN that requires dialysis may be observed in 3% of patients who have underlying renal impairment (16). Hospital mortality rate has been reported to be between 7 and 34% for in-patients secondary to CIN alone, 15% for patients with underlying renal impairment alone, and 36% for patients who require dialysis secondary to CIN (16,23). One-year mortality rate has been reported to be 38% for patients with renal impairment, and 45% for patients with renal impairment requiring dialysis (16). These numbers are comparable to the mortality rates of NSF.

The much lower incidence of CIN following exposure to GBCAs reflects primarily that in the doses that GBCAs are administered, these agents are less nephrotoxic than IBCAs at the dosages they are administered, which may be 10–20 times the volume of contrast compared to MRI (13–15).

Gadolinium-based contrast agents (GBCAs)

Toxicity can generally be categorized as acute, subacute, and chronic, where the time of occurrence of the complication determines this categorization. Acute toxicity generally occurs within 48 h (often within minutes) and these are generally manifest clinically as acute adverse events that are classified as mild, moderate, and severe. Subacute toxicity generally occurs from 1 week to several months. NSF is the major subacute toxicity. It is not known whether there is substantial chronic toxicity of GBCAs, and this may relate to bone deposition, and perhaps other organs like the liver.

Acute toxicity

The acute adverse reactions seen following GBCAs are allergy-like (urticaria), or unpleasant sensation-related, such as nausea, vomiting, headache, and altered taste sensation. Nausea, which is quite common with needle sticks in general, and vomiting, have served as a great source of concern with various GBCAs, and perhaps most of this is driven by sales individuals from the various manufacturers of these agents. Nausea and head-aches are also often referred to as *side-effects* and not adverse events, and these are relatively common. True acute adverse events are uncommon, and are usually mild to moderate in severity. Severe reactions, anaphylactoid types, are extremely rare (0.01–0.001%), which is a factor of 10 more safe than IBCAs (4). An increased frequency in adverse reactions has been observed in patients with a history of reactions to either GBCAs or IBCAs, and also a modest increased chance of adverse reactions is observed in patients with a history of allergies, as described with IBCAs. In patients with a history of previous GBCA reaction, a different MR contrast agent should be used, and 12–24 h of premedication with corticosteroids and antihistamines should be considered (4). This would be most prudent in patients with a prior moderate to severe reaction, because second reactions to GBCAs tend to be more severe than the first (4). Severe reactions should be treated very carefully and require the assistance of a resuscitation team.

GBCAs are generally considered to have no nephrotoxicity at approved dosages for MR imaging (4).

Subacute toxicity

Nephrogenic systemic fibrosis (NSF)

NSF is a systemic disease characterized by widespread tissue fibrosis (24–27). To date, it has been exclusively seen in patients with renal impairment (24–27). The progressive fibrosis results from the deposition of collagen in tissues, and initially and predominantly affects the skin (24–27). Systemic involvement, including the muscles and internal organs such as heart, lungs, and esophagus, generally follows after skin involvement (24–28). The incidence of NSF varies according to the type of GBCA administered (29). The incidence of NSF has been reported to be 2–7% in patients with renal impairment following the use of Omniscan, which has been the agent most often reported to be associated with the development of NSF (28,30).

Diminished renal function and GBCAs are the two crucial factors necessary for the development of NSF (31,32). Because NSF does not develop in all patients who have diminished renal function and prior GBCA exposure, it has been considered that additional cofactors might be involved in the pathophysiology (27), although most experts down-play the role of co-factors.

NSF is seen in patients with acute or chronic kidney disease (renal insufficiency), in whom the GFR is less than 30 ml/min/1.73 m^2 (29,33). Additionally, NSF is also seen in patients with acute renal insufficiency of any severity (29,33). More correctly though, the expression "of any severity" reflects that the actual dysfunction of kidneys in the acute setting is difficult to impossible to ascertain as it may be a rapidly changing/evolving process, hence acute renal sufficiency may represent 'extreme' renal failure, despite what lab values may suggest. Patients with GFR above 60 ml/min/1.73 m^2 have not been reported to develop NSF (29,33). More than 95% of NSF patients have stage 4 and 5 chronic kidney disease, with the great majority of these having stage 5 chronic renal disease and/or on renal dialysis (Table 3.1) (27,33).

Diminished renal function has the effect of decreasing renal excretion of gadolinium, which results in an increased half-life in the body (30,34). The level of renal dysfunction is correlated with the risk of developing NSF, and the severity of NSF; that is, the worse the renal function, the higher the risk and severity of NSF (29,33,36).

Extreme caution is also recommended in pregnancy and in children < 1 year of age. Because GBCAs can cross the placenta, enter fetal circulation, and stay in the amniotic fluid for a long time in pregnant patients, the half-life of gadolinium is longer in pregnant patients and in embryos or fetuses (29,35). The half-life of gadolinium is likely longer in children under age of 1 as well due to their immature renal function (29).

The dissociation of gadolinium ions from gadolinium-chelate complexes varies for different types of GBCAs and can be defined by the thermodynamic stability constant and dissociation constant (38). Thermodynamic stability constant determines the concentration at which gadolinium ions will dissociate from gadolinium-chelate complexes (38). The rate of this dissociation reaction is dependent on the dissociation constant. Taken together, these two constants define the affinity of ligands for gadolinium ions at the physiological pH (38). Each GBCA has a different thermodynamic stability constant and dissociation rate (Table 3.2) (38). Because the specific type of GBCAs with lower thermodynamic stability and higher dissociation constants are more commonly associated with the development of NSF, the dissociation of gadolinium ion from gadolinium-chelate complexes has been considered the trigger

Table 3.1 Stages of chronic kidney disease.

Stage	Description	GFR, ml/min/1.73 m^2
1	Slight kidney damage with normal or increased filtration	More than 90
2	Mild decrease in kidney function	60–89
3	Moderate decrease in kidney function	30–59
4	Severe decrease in kidney function	15–29
5	Kidney failure requiring dialysis or transplantation	Less than 15

Table 3.2 Categorization of GBCAs according to the distribution in the body, chemical structure, elimination pathway, thermodynamic stability, and dissociation rate

Generic name	Chemical abbreviation	Product name	Distribution	Amine structure	Charge	Excretion	Standard dosage, mmol/kg	Thermodynamic stability constant	Dissociation rate
Gadoversetamide	Gd-DTPA-BMEA	OptiMark (Mallinckrodt, St Louis, MO, USA)	Extracellular	Linear	Non-ionic	Renal	0.1	16.8	$>2.2 \times 10^{-2}$
Gadodiamide	Gd-DTPA-BMA	Omniscan (GE Healthcare, Buckinghamshire, United Kingdom)	Extracellular	Linear	Non-ionic	Renal	0.1	16.8	$>2 \times 10^{-2}$
Gadopentetate dimeglumine	Gd-DTPA	Magnevist (Bayer Schering Pharma AG, Germany)	Extracellular	Linear	Ionic	Renal	0.1	22.2	1.2×10^{-3}
Gadobenate dimeglumine	Gd-BOPTA	MultiHance (Bracco Diagnostics, Milan, Italy)	Extracellular and intracellular (Hepatocyte)	Linear	Ionic	Renal (%97), biliary (%3)	0.1*, †	22.6	–**
Gadoxetic asit disodium	Gd-EOB-BOPTA	Eovist, (Bayer HealthCare Pharmaceuticals, Wayne, NJ, USA); Primovist (Bayer Schering Pharma AG, Germany)	Extracellular and intracellular (Hepatocyte)	Linear	Ionic	Renal (%50), biliary (%50)	0.025*	23.4	–**
Gadofosveset trisodium	Gd-DTPA	Vasovist (Epix Pharmaceuticals, Lexington, MA, USA)	Blood pool	Linear	Ionic	Renal (91%), biliary (9%)	0.025*	–**	–**
Gadobutrol	Gd-DO3A-butirol	Gadovist (Bayer Schering Pharma AG, Germany)	Extracellular	Macrocyclic	Non-ionic	Renal	0.1*, ‡	21.0	2.8×10^{-6}
Gadoteridol	Gd-HP-DO3A	ProHance (Bracco Diagnostics, Milan, Italy)	Extracellular	Macrocyclic	Non-ionic	Renal	0.1	23.8	6.4×10^{-5}
Gadoterate meglumine	Gd-DOTA	Dotarem (Guerbet, Aulnay-sous-Bois, France)	Extracellular	Macrocyclic	Ionic	Renal	0.1	25.6	8.4×10^{-7}

*Gadobenate dimeglumine, gadoxetic acid, gadofosveset, and gadobutrol have higher T1 relaxivity compared to the other agents.

†Gadobenate dimeglumine has been reported to be diagnostically effective at its half dose (0.05 mmol/kg).

‡Gadobutrol solution has double the amount of gadolinium in its 1 molar (M) concentration compared to 0.5 M concentration of the other GBCAs' solutions.

**Not available.

in NSF development (27,39). GBCAs with higher thermodynamic stability constant and lower dissociation rate have an extremely low or nonexistent likelihood of NSF development. Another factor associated with the risk of NSF development and the severity of the disease is the increased total volume of GBCA administered either as a single or cumulative dose (30,40).

GBCAs are classified into two types according to the backbone structure of their amine group, linear or macrocyclic (41). Linear and macrocyclic GBCAs may be further subclassified according to their charges as ionic or non-ionic (41). In contrast to the linear GBCAs, macrocyclic GBCAs create tighter bonds with gadolinium, as the structure resembles a cage, and therefore have higher thermodynamic stability constants and lower dissociation rates (41). This supports the observation that macrocyclic agents have a much lesser or near nonexistent association with the development of NSF, compared to linear GBCAs, in particular nonionic linear agents (30,41). It has also been postulated that electrostatic charges present in ionic GBCAs render tighter bonding than nonionic GBCAs, and therefore ionic GBCAs are more stable than non-ionic GBCAs (42). This may also be reflected by the lower incidence of NSF with ionic linear GBCAs (Magnevist, Multihance, Eovist) than nonionic linear GBCAs (Omniscan, Optimark [gadoversetamide, (Mallinckrodt, St Louis, MO, USA)]) (29,31). Our opinion is that agents that also exhibit hepatocyte elimination (Multihance, Eovist) have an additional protective feature of a route of elimination when renal function is poor, which may be of paramount importance.

NSF is diagnosed by clinical findings, deep skin biopsy, and histopathology (29,31). There is no known effective treatment method for NSF (27). The correction of renal impairment with treatment or renal transplantation may either stop the progression of the disease, or reverse the signs and symptoms (27). Dialysis has not been shown to be useful in the treatment of NSF (27). Currently, there is no medication with a proven efficacy for the treatment of NSF. Fulminant progression of disease is seen in approximately 5% of patients, and may result in death in a short time period. The mortality of NSF has been reported as 30%, although only limited data is available (43). The most common causes of NSF-related mortality include complications that develop secondary to restricted joint movement, and respiratory insufficiency developing secondary to the involvement of respiratory muscles.

Recommended guidelines to minimize the risk of NSF

1 Pros and cons of the use of GBCAs should be assessed very carefully for high-risk patients prior to GBCA administration (33). Noncontrast techniques including US, CT, or MRI should be used for the examination whenever the patient's medical problem can be evaluated safely and diagnostically with these techniques (33). It should be remembered that even noncontrast CT carries with it the risk of radiation-induced malignancy; therefore, noncontrast ultrasound and MRI are generally the safest alternatives.

2 Omniscan, Magnevist, and Optimark should not be administered to patients with acute renal diseases or chronic renal diseases of all stages (29,33). Because of the risk of bone deposition, it may be prudent to avoid these agents in young children in general.

3 When GBCA administration is considered diagnostically important for the evaluation of high-risk patients, GBCAs that do not have proven associations with NSF development should be used (29). Macrocyclic GBCAs due to their relatively stable structure, or linear GBCAs with biliary elimination (Multihance and Eovist) may be preferred for these high risk patients (29,32).

4 The minimum dose of GBCA which generates a diagnostic MR examination should be administered to patients at high risk (29). Multihance and Eovist can be administered at lower doses than the standard doses of other GBCAs due to their high T1 relaxivity, and are therefore advantageous. Multihance and Eovist may be administered at 0.05 mmol / kg (half dose of standard dose of Multihance) and at 0.025 mmol / kg (standard dose of Eovist) to high-risk patients, respectively. There is insufficient data about the use of Eovist in subjects under age 18. Their additional property of biliary elimination is advantageous as well (30).

5 GBCAs should not be administered in the first and second trimesters of pregnancy unless maternal survival may depend upon it (35). The use of GBCAs is controversial in the third trimester of pregnancy and should be employed sparingly (35). The pros and cons of GBCA administration to these patients should also be assessed very carefully; the most stable GBCAs should be administered at the lowest possible doses, and should be used primarily if maternal survival depends upon it (29,35).

6 For traditional high dose gadolinium procedures, such as MRA, GBCAs with high T1 relaxivity (e.g., Multihance) should be used at doses as low as reasonable (29).

7 Determination of renal function may be necessary in certain groups, generally by obtaining serum creatinine levels, and calculating estimated GFR (eGFR) (30). Kidney function diminishes with increasing age. GFR below 60 ml/min/1.73 m^2 is observed in 11% of the population older than 60 years of age, and this circumstance may not be recognized in many patients. Patients should be questioned about their medical history, especially for renal diseases including solitary kidney, renal transplantation, renal tumors, and renal surgery; hypertension; and diabetes prior to MR examination (44). Serum creatinine or eGFR values should be determined in these patients and perhaps also in patients over 60 years of age (44). In general for these patients, GBCAs with high T1 relaxivity should be administered at low doses.

8 There is no evidence documenting when a repeat GBCA-enhanced study should be performed in at-risk patients. It

may be prudent to wait at least 48 h between consecutive GBCA-enhanced examinations for patients who are not at risk to low risk, and at least 1 week, or perhaps longer, for patients who are at risk (29,45).

9　Hemodialysis is effective at lowering the serum concentrations of GBCAs; however, hemodialysis is unlikely to be effective at eliminating GBCAs or deposited gadolinium in tissue (45–47). Because there is a strong dose–response relationship between GBCAs and NSF development, GBCAs should be eliminated from the body as much as, and as soon as, possible, before substantial transmetallation and deposition of gadolinium in tissues occur (45–47). Since there is no consistent effective treatment for NSF, immediate hemodialysis after the administration of GBCAs, as a potential preventive approach, should be recommended for patients who are already on hemodialysis and receive GBCAs (45–47). No patient who is not already on hemodialysis should receive hemodialysis , if the indication for dialysis is the MR study alone, because the mortality and morbidity of hemodialysis is higher than the risk of developing NSF following the exposure to stable GBCAs (29,45–47). Ongoing research suggests two sessions of hemodialysis spaced closely together (e.g., within 24 h) may be important, as the first session may remove free chelate, that could also rebind with free gadolinium.

10　GBCAs should not be used in high dose as a substitute for iodinated CM on CT, on angiography, or on other X-ray procedures (29).

11　GBCAs should not be administered to patients who already have NSF (27).

NSF versus CIN

NSF is a disease process with high morbidity and probably mortality (27,33). The risk of developing NSF is high in patients with stage 4 and 5 chronic renal disease and in patients with acute renal insufficiency, although most studies show that the great majority of patients have stage 5 disease and / or are on hemodialysis (33,48). The risk of developing NSF is nearly nonexistent in patients with stage 3 chronic renal disease. NSF has not been reported in patients with GFR above 60 ml/min/1.73 m^2 (64). More importantly, NSF develops following the exposure to specific types of GBCAs, including Omniscan, Optimark, and Magnevist (29,33). Other GBCAs, in solitary use settings, have very minimal to nonexistent association with the development of NSF (29).

CIN also has high morbidity and mortality (16). The incidence of CIN is much higher than NSF (10,13,28,30). CIN also is seen in patients of all renal functional levels, including patients with normal renal function, following the exposure to IBCAs (10,13,50). Importantly, the risk of developing CIN is also substantial in patients with stage 2 and 3 chronic renal diseases, and in patients with acute renal insufficiency (10,28,44). The risk of CIN increases as the GFR decreases (10,28). CIN develops following all types of IBCAs (16,51). Furthermore,

it is recognized that further deterioration of renal function, even in patients on hemodialysis for CIN, worsens the patient's prognosis (16,52).

In patients with acute renal failure, IBCAs should not be used in order to preserve recoverable renal function (44). The risk of NSF is also high in this patient group (44). Therefore, if CM administration is necessary, the lowest doses of macrocyclic GBCAs, or linear GBCAs with high T1 relaxivity, should be used in this patient group (44).

The risk of CIN following the administration of IBCAs is vastly higher in patients with stage 2 and 3 chronic kidney disease, compared to the risk of NSF following the administration of macrocyclic GBCAs, or linear GBCAs with high T1 relaxivity, the latter likely being nonexistent (32,44,53). The risk of CIN is higher in patients with stage 4 and 5 chronic kidney disease, who have residual renal function and are not regularly on dialysis, compared to the risk of NSF following the administration of macrocyclic GBCAs, or linear GBCAs with high T1 relaxivity (44).

Both GBCAs and iodinated CM should be used cautiously in all patients, particularly in patients with renal impairment. Risk benefit analysis should be performed prior to the administration of all CM, and the best combination of safety and diagnostic accuracy should be sought. Concern of NSF or CIN should not prevent the use of contrast agents in MRI or CT when they are deemed essential. The risk of NSF may be minimized or avoided with the use of GBCAs which are not associated with the development of NSF. The risk of CIN may also be reduced with the use of appropriate management techniques.

Chronic toxicity

It is not known whether there is chronic toxicity of GBCAs or not. There is no identified disease process as yet related to chronic toxicity of GBCAs. Processes such as bone deposition or liver deposition of GBCA may fit into this category. At present the importance of this is unknown. It may be prudent to avoid the use of nonionic linear GBCAs in the young pediatric patient.

Breast feeding and IBCAs / GBCAs

The literature on the excretion of GBCAs and IBCAs into breast milk, and the gastrointestinal absorption of these agents from breast milk is very limited. A review of the literature, however, reveals important facts: (i) less than 1% of the administered maternal dose of contrast agent is excreted into breast milk; and (ii) less than 1% of the contrast medium in breast milk ingested by an infant is absorbed from the gastro-intestinal tract. Therefore, the expected dose of contrast medium absorbed by an infant from ingested breast milk is extremely low (4). At the present time, the use of a pump to remove breast milk after contrast agent administration, and discarding breast milk for 24 h before resuming normal breast-feeding, is no longer recommended. This should be considered optional according to the mother's wishes. Since the biologic half-life of contrast agents is less than 120 min, the amount remaining in the mother (assuming her renal function is normal) after 24 h is essentially undetectable (54).

Medical radiation and cancer

Ionizing radiation arising from medical imaging studies has been recognized to have the potential to result in cancer (55–58). The utilization of CT studies has dramatically increased in recent years, especially following the use of multi-slice CT scanners. Increased use of CT studies in combination with the other medical imaging studies utilizing ionizing radiation has contributed to the increasing burden of ionizing radiation world-wide (59–67).

Based on data from the biological effects of ionizing radiation (BEIR) VII report of the National Academy of Sciences, 1 in 1000 patients may develop cancer following an exposure to 10 mSv of radiation, which is the amount of radiation delivered in a single phase upper abdominal CT study (55,57). Many recent studies (59–67) and the American College of Radiology (68) raised concerns about the use of the increasing amount of radiation. Large population-based data from nation-wide studies in Australia and UK have shown an increased incidence of malignancies in patients undergoing high dose radiation imaging studies such as CT (69,70)

The critical aspects of these concerns are as follows: (i) the greater sensitivity of children and young adults, particularly young women (due to breast and reproductive organ exposure especially in pulmonary embolism CT studies and cardiac CT studies), to develop radiation-induced malignancies, (ii) the burgeoning problem of overuse of CT, (iii) the importance of attention to and control of radiation dose in individual studies, and (iv) seeking alternative imaging strategies that do not involve ionizing radiation, specifically MRI and ultrasound.

CT is a very useful diagnostic tool that has been an extremely important part of modern health care. Its great strengths are in acute major trauma, diagnosis of diffuse parenchymal diseases of the lung including interstitial lung diseases, renal stones, and determination of the localization of tubes and catheters, particularly in intensive care patients. However, the use of CT must be carefully evaluated in individuals in whom the likelihood of an important medical diagnosis is low, and the risk of developing cancer from radiation is especially high. Average radiation doses associated with common imaging studies are given in Table 3.3.

The recommendations to lower the risk of development of cancer associated with medical radiation, especially radiation from CT, might be as follows:

a. Carefully consider the appropriate use of CT in each patient recommended to be imaged by a diagnostic study.

b. Carefully evaluate patients who have received multiple body CT equivalents in 1 year, and assess them for alternative imaging studies in the future.

Table 3.3 Average radiation doses associated with common imaging studies.

Diagnostic examination	Effective dose, mSv
X-rays	
Chest (PA film)	0.02
Head	0.07
Cervical spine	0.3
Thoracic spine	1.4
Lumbar spine	1.8
Abdomen	0.53
Pelvis/hip	0.83
Limbs/joints	0.06
Upper GI	3.6
Lower GI	6.4
Screening mammogram	0.13
CT	
Head	2.0
Abdomen	10.0
Chest	20–40
Pulmonary angiography	20–40
PET–CT	25

c. Specific crisis intervention should be entertained in patients who have received multiple body CT equivalents, and a protocol developed for surveying for cancer in the future.

d. Be very circumspect in all cases of body CT studies and repeat CT studies in children, unless it is the initial investigation of major trauma.

e. Be very circumspect in all cases of chest CTs in women aged 15–40 years.

f. Be very circumspect in ordering/performing renal CTs and pulmonary embolism CTs, as these are the most over-ordered of all CT examinations with relatively low yield.

g. CT of the liver should generally be avoided as the dose is especially high, and MRI is a diagnostically superior study for this organ.

h. It must also be remembered that Positron Emission Tomography and Nuclear medicine studies are also high radiation producing diagnostic tests, and similar scrutiny, as with CT, must be employed in their use (66,67).

References

1 Bettmann, M.A., Heeren, T., Greenfield, A., and Goudey, C. (1997) Adverse events with radiographic Contrast agents: results of the SCVIR Contrast Agent Registry. Radiology, 203, 611–620.

2 Bettmann, M.A. (2004) Frequently asked questions: iodinated contrast agents. RadioGraphics, 24, S3–S1.

3 American College of Radiology (1998) American College of Radiology Manual on Contrast Media, 4th edn, American College of Radiology, Reston, VA.

4 American College of Radiology Committee on Drugs and Contrast Media (2013) Manual on contrast media, 9th edn, American College of Radiology, Reston, VA.

5 Katayama, H., Yamaguchi, K., Kozuka, T. *et al.* (1990) Adverse reactions to ionic and nonionic contrast media: a report from the Japanese Committee on the Safety of Contrast Media. Radiology, 175, 621–628.

6 Rudnick, M.R., Goldfarb, S., Wexler, L. *et al.* (1995) Nephrotoxicity of ionic and nonionic contrast media in 1196 patients: a randomized trial. Kidney Int, 47, 254–261.

7 Lasser, E.C., Berry, C.C., Talner, L.B. *et al.* (1987) Pre-treatment with corticosteroids to alleviate reactions to intravenous contrast material. N Engl J Med, 317, 845–849.

8 Greenberger, P.A. and Patterson, R. (1991) The prevention of immediate generalized reactions to radiocontrast media in high risk patients. J Allergy Clin Immunol, 87, 867–872.

9 Lasser, E.C., Berry, C.C., Mishkin, M.M. *et al.* (1994) Pretreatment with corticosteroids to prevent adverse reactions to nonionic contrast media. AJR Am J Roentgenol, 162, 523–526.

10 Mehran, R. and Nikolsky, E. (2006) Contrast-induced nephropathy: definition, epidemiology, and patients at risk. Kidney Int, 69, S11–S15.

11 Gleeson, T.G. and Bulugahapatiya, S. (2004) Contrast-induced nephropathy. AJR, 183, 1673–1689.

12 Murphy, S.W., Barrett, B.J., and Parfrey, P.S. (2000) Contrast nephropathy. J Am Soc Nephrol, 11, 177–182.

13 Solomon, R., Biguori, C., and Bettmann, M. (2006) Selection of contrast media. Kidney Int, 69, S39–S45.

14 Tombach, B., Bremer, C., Reimer, P. *et al.* (2002) Using highly concentrated gadobutrol as an MR contrast agent in patients also requiring hemodialysis: safety and dialysability. AJR Am J Roentgenol, 178, 105–109.

15 Ergun, I., Keven, K., Uruc, I. *et al.* (2006) The safety of gadolinium in patients with stage 3 and 4 renal failure. Nephrol Dial Transplant, 21, 697–700.

16 McCullough, P., Adam, A., Becker, C.R. *et al.* (2006) Epidemiology and prognostic implications of contrast-induced nephropathy. Am J Cardiol, 98, 5K–13K.

17 Bruce, R.J., Djamali, A., Shinki, K. *et al.* (2009) Background fluctuation of kidney function versus contrast-induced nephrotoxicity. Am J Roentgenol AJR, 192, 711–718.

18 Perrson, P.B. and Tepel, M. (2006) Contrast medium-induced nephropathy: the pathophysiology. Kidney Int, 69, S8–S10.

19 Persson, P.B., Hansell, P., and Liss, P. (2005) Pathophysiology of contrast medium-induced nephropathy. Kidney Int, 68, 14–22.

20 Katzberg, R.W. and Haller, C. (2006) Contrast-induced nephrotoxicity: Clinical landscape. Kidney Int, 69, S3–S7.

21 Katzberg, R.W. and Barrett, B.J. (2007) Risk of iodinated contrast material-induced nephropathy with intravenous administration. Radiology, 243, 622–628.

22 Thomsen, H.S., Morcos, S.K., Erley, C. *et al.* (2008) The ACTIVE trial: comparison of the effects on renal function of iomeprol-400 and iodixanol-320 in patients with chronic kidney disease undergoing abdominal computed tomography. Invest Radiol, 43, 170–178.

23 Levy, E.M., Viscoli, C.M., and Horwitz, R.I. (1996) The effect of acute renal failure on mortality. A cohort analysis. JAMA, 275, 1489–1494.

24 Cowper, S.E., Robin, H.S., Steinberg, S.M. *et al.* (2000) Scleromyxoedema-like cutaneous diseases in renal-dialysis patients. Lancet, 356, 1000–1001.

25 Cowper, S.E., Su, L.D., Bhawan, J. *et al.* (2001) Nephrogenic fibrosing dermopathy. Am J Dermatopathol, 23, 383–393.

26 Daram, S.R., Cortese, C.M., and Bastani, B. (2005) Nephrogenic fibrosing dermopathy / nephrogenic systemic fibrosis: report of a new case with literature review. Am J Kidney Dis, 46, 754–759.

27 Kuo, P.H., Kanal, E., Abu-Alfa, A.K., and Cowper, S.E. (2007) Gadolinium-based MR contrast agents and nephrogenic systemic fibrosis. Radiology, 242, 647–649.

28 Thomsen, H.S. (2007) Enhanced computed tomography or magnetic resonance imaging: a choice between contrast medium-induced nephropathy and nephrogenic systemic fibrosis. Acta Radiologica, 48, 593–596.

29 Thomsen, H.S. (2007) ESUR Guideline: gadolinium-based contrast media and nephrogenic systemic fibrosis. Eur Radiol, 17, 2692–2696.

30 Lauenstein, T.C., Salman, K., Morreira, R. *et al.* (2007) Nephrogenic systemic fibrosis: center case review. J Magn Reson Imaging, 26, 1190–1197.

31 Wertman, R., Altun, E., Martin, D.R. *et al.* (2008) Risk of nephrogenic systemic fibrosis: evaluation of gadolinium chelate contrast agents by four American universities. Radiology, 248, 799–806.

32 Altun, E., Martin, D.R., Wertman, R. *et al.* (2009) Nephrogenic systemic fibrosis: change in the incidence following a switch in gadolinium agents and adoption of a gadolinium policy – a report from two American universities. Radiology, 253, 689–696.

33 U.S. Food and Drug Administration. Public health advisory: gadolinium-containing contrast agents for magnetic resonance imaging (MRI): Omniscan, OptiMARK, Magnevist, ProHance, and MultiHance. U.S. Food and Drug Administration. www.fda.gov/cder/drug/advisory/gadolinium_agents.htm. Published June 8, 2006. Updated May 23, 2007. Accessed July 12, 2008.

34 Joffe, P., Thomsen, H.S., and Meusel, M. (1998) Pharmacokinetics of gadodiamide injection in patients with severe renal insufficiency and patients undergoing hemodialysis or continuous ambulatory peritoneal dialysis. Acad Radiol, 5, 491–502.

35 Kanal, E., Barkovich, J.A., Bell, C. *et al.* (2007) ACR Guidance document for safe MR practices: 2007. AJR Am J Roentgenol, 188, 1–27.

36 Marckmann, P. (2008) Nephrogenic systemic fibrosis: epidemiology update. Curr Opin Nephrol Hypertens, 17, 315–319.

37 Prince, M.R., Zhang, H., Morris, M. *et al.* (2008) Incidence of nephrogenic systemic fibrosis at two large medical centers. Radiology, 248, 807–816.

38 Lin, S.-P. and Brown, J.J. (2007) MR contrast agents: physical and pharmacologic basics. J Magn Reson Imaging, 25, 884–899.

39 Grobner, T. (2006) Gadolinium – a specific trigger for the development of nephrogenic fibrosing dermopathy and nephrogenic systemic fibrosis. Nephrol Dial Transplant, 21, 1104–1108.

40 Marckmann, P., Skov, L., Rossen, K. *et al.* (2007) Case–control study of gadodiamide-related nephrogenic systemic fibrosis. Nephrol Dial Transplant, 22, 3174–3178.

41 Thomsen, H.S. (2008) Nephrogenic systemic fibrosis. Imaging Decisions MRI, 11, 13–18.

42 Morcos, S.K. (2008) Extracellular gadolinium contrast agents: differences in stability. Eur J Radiol, 66, 175–179.

43 Sadowski, E.A., Bennett, L.K., Chan, R.M. *et al.* (2007) Nephrogenic systemic fibrosis: risk factors and incidence estimation. Radiology, 243, 148–157.

44 American College of Radiology (2008) Manual on contrast media version 6 2008. Nephrogenic systemic Fibrosis, American College of Radiology, Reston, VA, pp. 53–57.

45 Shellock, F.G. and Spinazzi, A. (2008) MRI safety update 2008: Part 1, MRI contrast agents and nephrogenic systemic fibrosis. AJR, 191, 1–11.

46 Saab, G. and Abu-Alfa, A. (2007) Will dialysis prevent the development of nephrogenic systemic fibrosis after gadolinium-based contrast administration? AJR, 189, W169.

47 Broome, D.R., Cottrell, A.C., and Kanal, E. (2007) Response to "Will dialysis prevent the development of nephrogenic systemic fibrosis after gadolinium-based contrast administration?". AJR, 189, W234–235.

48 Rydahl, C., Thomsen, H.S., and Marckmann, P. (2008) High prevalence of nephrogenic systemic fibrosis in chronic renal failure patients exposed to gadodiamide, a gadolinium-containing magnetic resonance contrast agent. Invest Radiol, 43, 141–144.

49 Thomsen, H.S., Morcos, S.K., Erley, C. et al. (2008) The ACTIVE trial: comparison of the effects on renal function of iomeprol-400 and iodixanol-320 in patients with chronic kidney disease undergoing abdominal computed tomography. Invest Radiol, 43, 170–178.

50 Cheruvu, B., Henning, K., Mulligan, J. et al. (2007) Iodixanol: risk of subsequent contrast nephropathy in cancer patients with underlying renal insufficiency undergoing diagnostic computed tomography examinations. J Comput Assist Tomogr, 31, 493–498.

51 Coresh, J., Astor, B.C., Greene, T. et al. (2003) Prevalence of chronic kidney disease and decreased kidney function in the adult US population: Third National Health and Nutrition Examination Survey. Am J Kidney Dis, 41, 1–12.

52 Levy, E.M., Viscoli, C.M., and Horwitz, R.I. (1996) The effect of acute renal failure on mortality. A cohort analysis. JAMA, 275, 1489–1494.

53 Halvorsen, R.A. (2008) Which study when? Iodinated contrast-enhanced CT versus gadolinium-enhanced MR imaging. Radiology, 249, 9–15.

54 Bettmann, M.A.M.D. (2004) Frequently asked questions: iodinated contrast agents. RadioGraphics, 24, S3–S1.

55 U.S. Food and Drug Administration. What are the radiation risks from CT? U.S. Food and Drug Administration, Center for Devices and Radiological Health Web site. http://www.fda.gov/cdrh/ct/risks.html. Updated May 4, 2005. Accessed July 29, 2008.

56 Valentin, J. (2000) Effects of in utero irradiation. Ann ICRP, 30, 9–12.

57 Nuclear and Radiation Studies Board (2006) Committee on the Biological Effects of Ionizing Radiation Board on Radiation Effects Research Division on Earth and Life Studies National Research Council of the National Academies. Estimating cancer risk. Health effects of exposure to low levels of ionizing radiation: BEIR VII Phase 2, National Academy Press, Washington, DC, pp. 267–312.

58 UNSCEAR. United Nations Scientific Committee on the Effects of Atomic Radiation UNSCEAR 2000 Report to the General Assembly, 2000, pp. 1–17.

59 Semelka, R.C., Armao, D.M., Elias, J. Jr., and Huda, W. (2007) Imaging strategies to reduce the risk of radiation in CT studies, including selective substitution with MRI. J Magn Reson Imaging, 25, 900–909.

60 Martin, D.R. and Semelka, R.C. (2006) Health effects of ionizing radiation from diagnostic CT. Lancet, 367, 1712–1714.

61 Martin, D.R. and Semelka, R.C. (2007) Health effects of ionizing radiation from diagnostic CT imaging: consideration of alternative imaging strategies. Applied Radiology, 36, 20–29.

62 Brenner, D.J. and Hall, E.J. (2007) Computed tomography – an increasing source of radiation exposure. N Engl J Med, 357, 2277–2284.

63 Hurwitz, L.M., Reiman, R.E., Yoshizumi, T.T. et al. (2007) Radiation dose from contemporary cardiothoracic multidetector CT protocols with an anthropomorphic female phantom: implications for cancer induction. Radiology, 245, 742–750.

64 Hurwitz, L.M., Yoshizumi, T.T., Reiman, R.E. et al. (2006) Radiation dose to the female breast from 16-MDCT body protocols. AJR Am J Roentgenol, 186, 1718–1722.

65 Einstein, A.J., Henzlova, M.J., and Rajagopalan, S. (2007) Estimating risk of cancer associated with radiation exposure from 64-slice computed tomography coronary angiography. JAMA, 298, 317–323.

66 Picano, E. (2004) Sustainability of medical imaging. BMJ, 328, 578–580.

67 Picano, E. (2004) Informed consent and communication of risk from radiological and nuclear medicine examinations: how to escape from a communication inferno. BMJ, 329, 849–851.

68 Amis, E.S. Jr., Butler, P.F., Applegate, K.E. et al. (2007) American College of Radiology white paper on radiation dose in medicine. J Am Coll Radiol, 4, 272–284.

69 Mathews, J.D., Forsythe, A.V., Brady, Z. et al. (2013) Cancer risk in 680.000 people exposed to computed tomography scans in childhood or adolescence: data linkage study of 11 million Australians. BMJ, 21, 346–360.

70 Pearce, M.S., Salotti, J.A., Little, M.P. et al. (2012) Radiation exposure from CT scans in childhood and subsequent risk of leukemia and brain tumors: a retrospective cohort study. Lancet, 380, 499–505.

CHAPTER 4
Cystic diseases of the liver

Ersan Altun[1], Mohamed El-Azzazi[1,2,3,4], Richard C. Semelka[1], and Miguel Ramalho[1,5]

[1]The University of North Carolina at Chapel Hill, Department of Radiology, Chapel Hill, NC, USA
[2]University of Dammam, Department of Radiology, Dammam, Saudi Arabia
[3]King Fahd Hospital of the University, Department of Radiology, Khobar, Saudi Arabia
[4]University of Al Azhar, Department of Radiology, Cairo, Egypt
[5]Hospital Garcia de Orta, Department of Radiology, Almada, Portugal

Cystic focal liver lesions can be classified as

- Developmental
- Neoplastic
- Inflammatory or
- Miscellaneous.

The identification and recognition of different types of cystic focal liver lesions are extremely important in order to determine the clinical implications, treatment, and management strategies (1–5).

Cystic focal liver lesions may be benign or malignant. Morphologically, they may be classified as

- Simple or complex.
- Solitary or multiple.
- Sporadic or hereditary.

Developmental cystic lesions

Benign developmental hepatic cysts

- Benign developmental hepatic cysts are the most common benign masses of the liver.
- Liver cysts are generally unilocular (95%). However, they may occasionally be multilocular.
- They may be solitary or multiple, with the latter being the more frequent situation.
- They are generally asymptomatic and incidentally discovered at the fifth to seventh decades of life.
- They are generally simple; however, they may occasionally be complicated with internal hemorrhage and infection, and may be symptomatic due to the presence of pain and fever.
- Large cysts may be symptomatic due to stretching of the liver capsule.
- Asymptomatic cysts require no further workup or treatment (1–5).

- **Causes:** They are benign congenital and developmental cysts deriving from biliary endothelium that does not communicate with the biliary tree. The current theory is that true hepatic cysts originate from the hamartomatous tissue (4,5).
- **Pathology:** The lining of a true hepatic cyst shows a single layer of cuboidal to columnar epithelial cells that rest on an underlying fibrous stroma. A true hepatic cyst contains serous fluid (4,5).
- **Imaging:**
- *Simple Cysts*
- **On CT:**
  - ° Ovoid or round homogeneous lesions of near-water attenuation value (−10 to 20 HU) with sharply defined margins and smooth thin walls (Figure 4.1). They may occasionally contain a few thin septations.
  - ° Usually do not contain multiple or thick septations, mural nodularity, calcifications, or fluid-debris level.
  - ° Show no enhancement or negligible subtle enhancement after IV contrast in the hepatic arterial dominant, hepatic venous, or interstitial phases of enhancement.
  - ° Small lesions may have a density higher than 20 HU due to partial volume averaging with adjacent hepatic parenchyma, especially on contrast enhanced scans. However, this is generally not a problem for the diagnosis of small cysts on MRI because of the higher soft tissue contrast resolution compared to CT (4,5).
- **On MRI:**
  - ° Ovoid and round homogeneous well-defined lesions with smooth thin wall, possessing sharp margin with liver.
  - ° Demonstrate moderate to prominent low signal on T1-WIs due to high fluid content.
  - ° Demonstrate prominent high signal on T2-WIs due to high fluid content.

Liver Imaging: MRI with CT Correlation, First Edition. Edited by Ersan Altun, Mohamed El-Azzazi and Richard C. Semelka.
© 2015 John Wiley & Sons, Inc. Published 2015 by John Wiley & Sons, Inc.

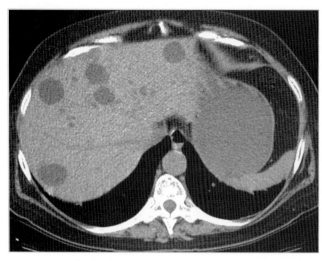

Figure 4.1 *Simple cysts.* Transverse non-contrast CT scan shows multiple rounded hypodense lesions scattered in both right and left lobes.

° Show no enhancement or negligible subtle wall enhancement in the early and late phases of enhancement on post-gadolinium sequences; show no change in shape, margination, and appearance from early to late postcontrast images (Figures 4.2–4.4). This observation ensures that lesions are simple cysts and not poorly vascularized metastases that show gradual enhancement (1–5).

- *Complex Cysts*
  ° Complex cysts contain hemorrhage or high protein levels, and fluid-debris level; thickened and irregular walls may be seen with complicated cysts.
- **On CT:**
  ° Complicated cysts with internal protein or hemorrhage show high attenuation on pre-contrast CT images and show no enhancement or subtle negligible enhancement on post-contrast images including all phases (Figure 4.5).
- **On MRI:**
  ° Hemorrhagic cysts and cysts containing high protein levels demonstrate similar imaging features.
  ° Hemorrhagic cysts may show variable signal intensities on pre-contrast T1-WI and T2-WI according to the age of hemorrhage.
  ° Hemorrhagic cysts and cysts with high internal protein levels commonly display high signal on T1-WI and may also show very low signal on T2-WI.
  ° They show no enhancement or negligible wall enhancement (Figures 4.5 and 4.6) (1–5). Comparison of appearance between early and late postcontrast images is essential.

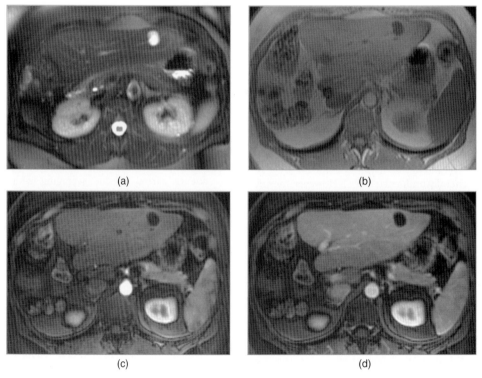

(a)   (b)

(c)   (d)

Figure 4.2 *Solitary simple cyst.* Transverse T2-weighted fat-suppressed single shot ETSE (a), T1-weighted 2D-GE (b), T1-weighted post-gadolinium fat-suppressed hepatic arterial dominant phase (c) and hepatic venous phase (d) 3D-GE images acquired at 3.0 T demonstrate a small solitary simple cyst. The cyst which illustrates markedly high signal on T2-weighted image (a) and low signal on pre-contrast T1-weighted image (b) shows no enhancement on post-gadolinium images (c, d).

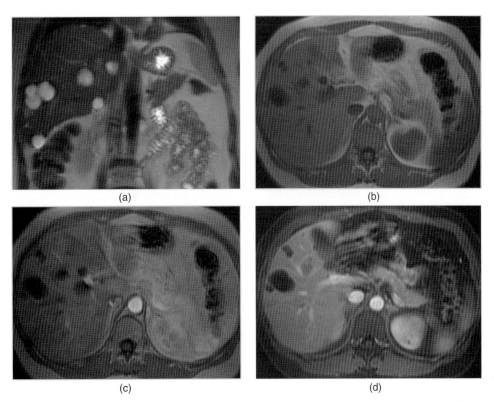

Figure 4.3 *Multiple simple cysts.* Coronal T2-weighted single shot ETSE (a), T1-weighted 2D-GE (b), T1-weighted post-gadolinium hepatic arterial dominant phase (c) and fat-suppressed hepatic venous phase 2D-GE (d) images acquired at 1.5 T show multiple intermediate size cysts. The cysts which illustrate markedly high signal on T2-weighted image (a) and low signal on pre-contrast T1-weighted image (b) show subtle cyst wall enhancement on post-gadolinium images (c, d).

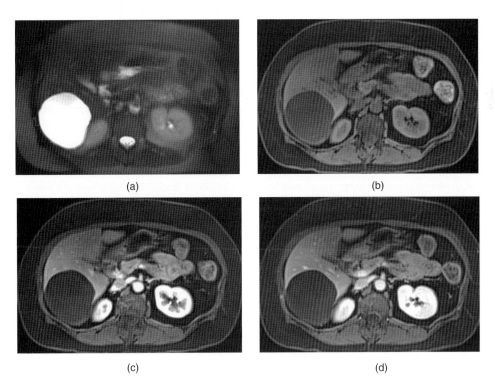

Figure 4.4 *Solitary large simple cyst.* Transverse T2-weighted fat-suppressed SS-ETSE (a), T1-weighted fat-suppressed 3D-GE (b), T1-weighted fat-suppressed post-gadolinium hepatic venous phase (c) and interstitial phase 3D-GE (d) images acquired at 1.5 T show a large liver cyst. The large cyst which demonstrates markedly high signal on T2-weighted image (a) and low signal on pre-contrast T1-weighted image (b) shows no wall enhancement on post-gadolinium images (c, d).

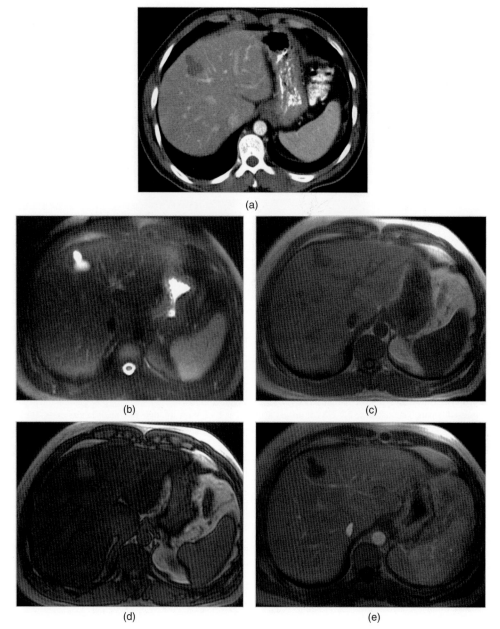

(a)

(b)

(c)

(d)

(e)

Figure 4.5 *Solitary small complex cyst.* Transverse hepatic venous phase contrast-enhanced CT scan (a) shows a lobulated cyst with no enhancement. Transverse T2-weighted fat-suppressed single shot ETSE (b), T1-weighted in-phase (c) and out-of-phase (d) 2D-GE, T1-weighted post-gadolinium hepatic venous phase 2D-GE (e) images acquired at 1.5 T demonstrate a lobulated complex cyst with high protein content. Due to its high protein content, the cyst displays high signal on in-phase and out-of-phase SGE images (c, d) without any signal loss on out-of-phase image (d). The cyst does not show any enhancement on post-gadolinium sequences (e). Note the diffuse signal drop on out-of-phase SGE image (d) compared to in-phase image (c) due to diffuse fatty infiltration of the liver.

- **Differential Diagnosis and Pearls:**
  - ○ The presence of heterogeneous content, mural nodules, enhancing thick and irregular septations, calcifications, and significantly enhancing cyst wall should raise the suspicion that the cystic lesion may be inflammatory and neoplastic. The differential diagnosis of inflammatory cystic lesions includes abscesses and hydatid cysts. The differential diagnosis of neoplastic cystic lesions includes biliary cystadenoma / biliary cystadenocarcinoma and cystic metastases (such as ovarian cancer, pseudomyxoma peritonei) (1–5).

Ciliated hepatic foregut cyst

- Ciliated hepatic foregut cysts are developmental solitary unilocular cysts. They are uncommon benign cysts.

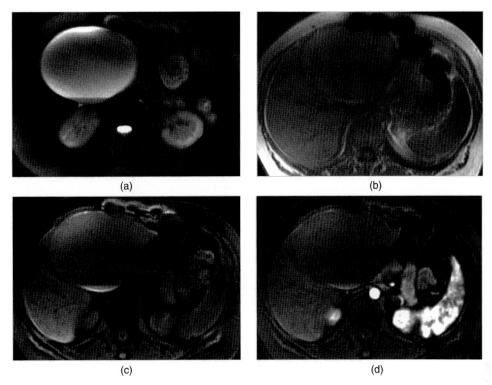

(a)   (b)

(c)   (d)

Figure 4.6 *Solitary large complex cyst.* Transverse fat-suppressed single shot ETSE (a), T1-weighted in-phase 2D-GE (b), T1-weighted fat-suppressed 3D-GE (c), T1-weighted post-gadolinium hepatic arterial dominant phase 3D-GE (d) images acquired at 3.0 T show a large cyst with high protein content. The cyst shows high signal intensity on T1-weighted SGE image (b), and fluid-fluid level with dependant low signal on T2-weighted (a) and high signal on T1-weighted images (b–d); which are consistent with high protein content. Note that the cyst wall does not show any enhancement.

- They arise from the embryonic foregut and differentiate towards bronchial tissue in the liver.
- **Pathology:**
- The cyst wall consists of four layers, including the innermost layer with pseudostratified ciliated columnar epithelium containing mucous cells, subepithelial connective tissue, abundant smooth muscle, and outermost fibrous capsule.
- They are most commonly located at the anterosuperior margin of the liver or at intersegmental locations and usually bulge (extend beyond) the liver contour (1–5).
- **Imaging**
- **On CT:**
  ° Ciliated hepatic foregut cysts are also well circumscribed oval lesions which show near-water attenuation on pre-contrast CT images with no enhancement or subtle wall enhancement on contrast enhanced CT images (Figure 4.7) (4,5).
- **On MRI:**
  ° Ciliated hepatic foregut cysts demonstrate markedly high signal on T2-weighted image and variable signal intensity on T1-weighted image, including intermediate and high signal, depending on the internal protein content (Figures 4.7 and 4.8). They may show prominent uniform thickness wall enhancement (Figures 4.7 and 4.8) (1–5).

- **Differential diagnosis and Pearls:**
  ° Typical location of these cysts is generally suggestive of the diagnosis (Figures 4.7 and 4.8). They may also rarely demonstrate high density or wall calcifications (Figure 4.8g–i). The differential diagnoses of benign developmental hepatic cysts are also true for ciliated hepatic foregut cysts (1–5).

Polycystic liver disease

- Isolated polycystic liver disease is a rare distinct autosomal dominant genetic disease in which multiple cysts are present in the liver without any or substantial involvement of the kidneys.
- Most often, polycystic liver disease is associated with autosomal dominant polycystic kidney disease (ADPKD).
- Hepatic cysts are found in 40% of patients with ADPKD.
- Liver dysfunction occurs only rarely even despite extensive involvement. Advanced disease may result in hepatomegaly and compression of vascular structures, and, occasionally, in liver failure.
- Cysts tend to be multiple and smaller than the renal cysts.
- Cysts may undergo hemorrhage and may contain variable amounts of protein; however, this is much less common in the liver than in the kidney.

- Cysts exhibit similar CT and MR features to simple cysts and foregut cysts (Figures 4.9 and 4.10). However, complicated cysts which may contain hemorrhage or variable amounts of protein demonstrate variable signal intensities on T2-WI and T1-WI (Figure 4.10) (6,7).

Biliary hamartomas

- Biliary hamartomas (also known as von Meyenburg complexes) are common benign malformations of the biliary tract

and they are considered to arise from bile ducts that fail to involute.
- Present in approximately 5–10% of patients.
- Biliary hamartomas are generally asymptomatic and detected incidentally.
- Biliary hamartomas are often multiple, in most cases a few in number, but may be extensively scattered throughout the liver (Figure 4.11).
- Biliary hamartomas are round or oval lesions usually sizing less than 1.5 cm in diameter and have a thin appreciable wall,

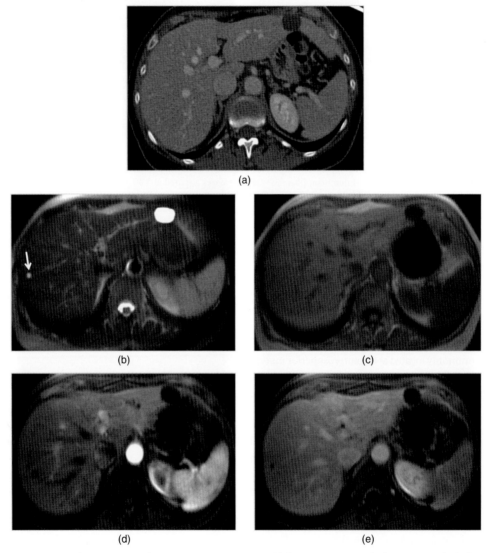

Figure 4.7 *Foregut cyst.* Transverse hepatic venous phase post-contrast CT image (a) demonstrates a simple foregut cyst, which does not show any wall enhancement, located at the anterior margin of the left lateral segment. Transverse T2-weighted single shot ETSE (b), T1-weighted 2D-GE (c), T1-weighted post-gadolinium hepatic arterial dominant phase (d) and interstitial phase (e) 3D-GE images acquired at 3.0 T demonstrate the foregut cyst located in the left lateral segment. The cyst shows markedly high homogeneous signal on T2-weighted image (b) and low signal on T1-weighted images without any wall enhancement (c–e). Note the presence of a small cyst (arrow, b) in the right liver lobe. Coronal T2-weighted single shot ETSE (f), T1-weighted 2D-GE (g), T1-weighted post-gadolinium hepatic arterial dominant phase (h) and hepatic venous phase (i) fat-suppressed 3D-GE images acquired at 3.0 T show a simple foregut cyst situated at the intersegmental location between segments 7 and 8, in another patient.

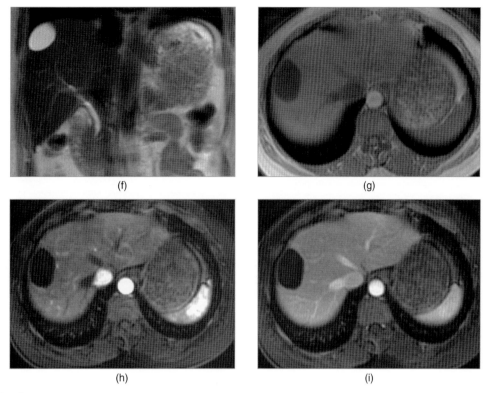

(f)   (g)

(h)   (i)

Figure 4.7 (*Continued*)

representing a thin layer of compressed liver tissue. Often, biliary hamartomas are smaller, more uniform, and numerous compared to simple cysts.

- They are usually predominantly cystic although they may be occasionally predominantly solid (4,5).
- Biliary hamartomas may be large in size (Figure 4.11j–l), where they would be termed giant cystic biliary hamartomas, and may be complicated with hemorrhage (8).
- Pathology:
  ° Biliary hamartomas consist of a collection of small, sometimes dilated, irregular, and branching bile ducts embedded in a fibrous stroma.
  ° Biliary hamartomas may contain inspissated bile, with no or few vascular channels (4,5).
- **Imaging**
- **On CT:**
  ° Multiple hypoattenuating lesions (<1.5 cm) are detected.
  ° Biliary hamartomas usually do not enhance and are seen as hypoattenuating lesions on postcontrast CT examinations.
  ° Biliary hamartomas may show peripheral rim enhancement (Figure 4.11) (4,5).
- **On MR images:**
  ° Markedly high signal on T2-WIs.
  ° Low signal on T1-WIs.
  ° Biliary hamartomas usually show no central enhancement and a subtle thin rim of enhancement, that persists unchanged on the hepatic arterial dominant,

hepatic venous, and interstitial phases of enhancement (Figure 4.11). They may sometimes show homogeneous enhancement on postgadolinium images and may become isointense with the remaining liver parenchyma.

  ° MR imaging is superior to CT, demonstrating the high fluid content of these lesions (1–6).
  ° Large or giant biliary hamartomas may show high signal on T1-WI if they become complicated with hemorrhage (8).
- **Differential Diagnosis and Pearls:**
  ° Multiple small cystic lesions in the liver without any renal involvement favor the diagnosis of biliary hamartomas.
  ° Biliary cystadenoma or cystadenocarcinoma are in the differential diagnosis of large biliary hamartomas. Small biliary hamartomas may always be present in the setting of large biliary hamartomas, which aids the diagnosis and distinction from other entities.

Peribiliary cysts

- Peribiliary cysts are cystic dilatation of glands in the bile duct walls and are uncommon but most often associated with cirrhosis, especially in patients with portal hypertension.
- They are commonly seen around central portal tracts and within the portal hilum.
- These cysts are generally asymptomatic, although larger cysts may occasionally cause focal biliary obstruction (9).

- **On CT:**
  ◦ Hypoattenuating lesions on pre- and post-contrast CT examinations.
  ◦ No enhancement on post-contrast CT examinations (9).
- **On MRI:**
  ◦ Prominently hypointense lesions on T1-WI.
  ◦ Markedly hyperintense lesions on T2-WI.
  ◦ No enhancement or subtle wall enhancement on post-gadolinium T1-WI (Figure 4.12) (9).

- **Differential Diagnosis and Pearls:**
  ◦ Their location is typical.

Caroli disease

- A rare condition, 0.8 in 100,000 individuals.
- An autosomal recessive disorder characterized by multifocal saccular dilation of the non-obstructed intrahepatic bile ducts.
- The disease may be segmental or diffuse.

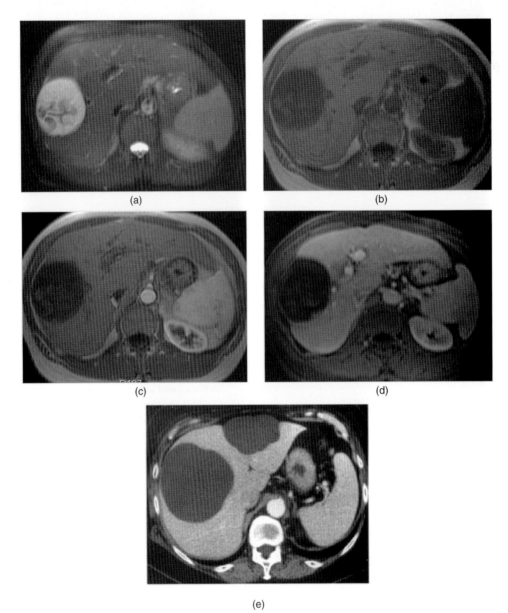

(a)

(b)

(c)

(d)

(e)

Figure 4.8 *Complex foregut cyst.* Transverse T2-weighted fat-suppressed single shot ETSE (a), T1-weighted 2D-GE (b), T1-weighted post-gadolinium fat-suppressed hepatic arterial dominant phase 2D-GE (c) and hepatic venous phase 3D-GE (d) images demonstrate a foregut cyst situated at the intersegmental location, in another patient. The cyst shows non-enhancing heterogeneous internal content with low signal on T2-weighted image (a) and relatively high signal on T1-weighted image (b). Large foregut cysts. Transverse contrast enhanced hepatic venous phase CT examination (e) shows two large foregut cysts which are located at the anterior margin of the liver and bulge the liver. Foregut cyst with rim calcification. Transverse non-contrast CT examination (f) and transverse US images (g) show a foregut cyst with rim calcification which shows high attenuation on CT (f) and high echogenicity on US (g). MR image (h) confirms the typical intersegmental location.

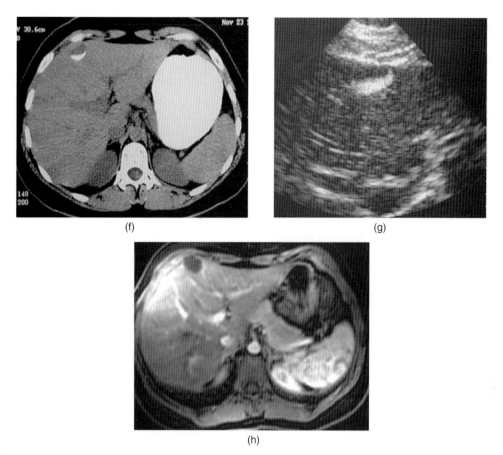

(f)   (g)

(h)

Figure 4.8 (*Continued*)

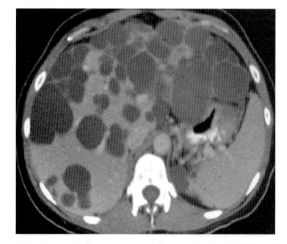

Figure 4.9 *Liver cysts due to autosomal dominant polycystic kidney disease.* Transverse hepatic venous phase contrast-enhanced CT examination shows multiple liver cysts due to autosomal dominant polycystic kidney disease.

- The left lobe of liver is more commonly involved.
- Caroli disease may be associated with cystic renal disease, especially medullary sponge kidney.
- The incidence of cholangiocarcinoma is increased in patients with Caroli disease and cholangiocarcinoma may be seen in up to 7% of patients.
- Two forms of Caroli disease have been defined.

- **Types:**
  - **Type 1:**
    - The less common form, also known as the pure or simple form.
    - Associated with intrahepatic stone formation, cholangitis, and abscess formation.
    - Patients usually present with recurrent attacks of cholangitis with right upper quadrant pain, fever, and sometimes, jaundice.
  - **Type 2:**
    - More common form, also known as the complex form or Caroli Syndrome.
    - Associated with periportal fibrosis and may progress to portal hypertension and cirrhosis.
    - Patients usually present with symptoms of hepatic fibrosis and portal hypertension.
- **Imaging:**
- **On CT:**
  - Multiple hypoattenuating fluid-filled cystic structures of various sizes that communicate with the biliary system tree on pre-contrast and post-contrast CT examinations.
  - A characteristic finding that is suggestive of Caroli disease is "central dot sign". The central dot sign is described as the presence of tiny foci of contrast enhancement,

corresponding to intraluminal portal vein radicals, within dilated intrahepatic bile ducts (4,5).

- **On MRI:**
  ° Multiple fluid-filled cystic structures of various sizes that communicate with biliary system on MRCP images (Figure 4.13).
  ° Markedly high signal on T2-WI and markedly low signal on T1-WI.
  ° Bridging internal septations (which are insufficiently resorbed and malformed ductal plate surrounding the portal vein radicals) may be seen crossing dilated intrahepatic ducts.

° The central dot sign may be seen on post-gadolinium images (4,5).

- **Differential Diagnosis and Pearls:**
  ° The demonstration of multiple cystic saccular structures communicating with the biliary tree on T2-WI and MRCP images is critical.

Neoplastic cystic lesions

- Neoplastic cystic lesions may be primary or secondary. The most common primary neoplastic cystic lesions are biliary

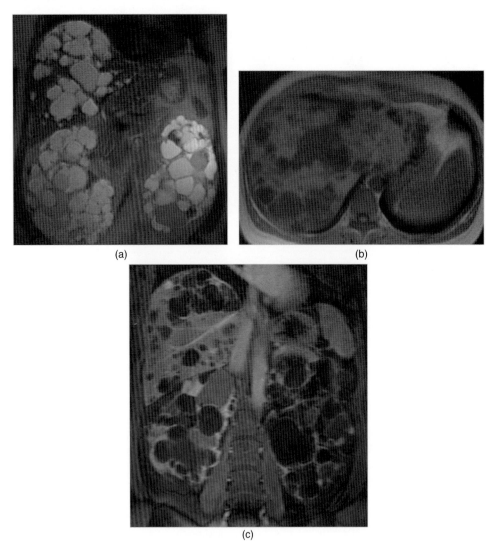

(a)   (b)

(c)

Figure 4.10 *Liver cysts due to autosomal dominant polycystic kidney disease.* Coronal T2-weighted single shot echo train spin echo (a), transverse T1-weighted 2D-GE (b), coronal T1-weighted fat-suppressed hepatic venous phase 3D-GE (c) images acquired at 3.0 T demonstrate multiple cysts in the kidneys and liver. The enlarged kidneys are replaced with innumerable cysts. Multiple cysts replacing a significant portion of normal liver are present in the liver. Due to their variable protein content, the cysts in the kidneys and liver show variable signal intensity ranging from markedly hypointense to markedly hyperintense signal on T2-weighted image (a) while the liver cysts show intermediate to markedly low signal intensity on T1-weighted image (b). The cysts show no enhancement or subtle wall enhancement on post-gadolinium hepatic venous phase 3D-GE (c). Coronal (d) and transverse (e) T2-weighted single shot ETSE, transverse T1-weighted water excitation MPRAGE (f) and T1-weighted postgadolinium water excitation MPRAGE (g) images demonstrate multiple liver and renal cysts with variable protein content in another noncooperative patient.

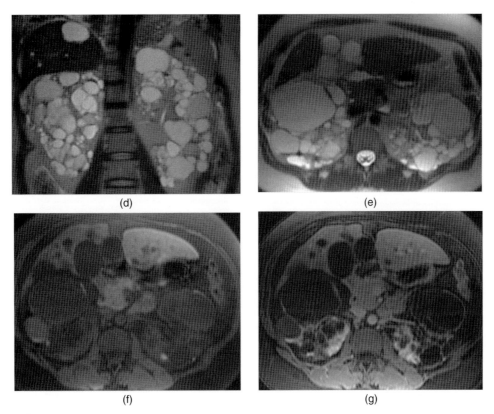

(d)   (e)

(f)   (g)

Figure 4.10 (*Continued*)

cystadenoma and cystadenocarcinoma. Undifferentiated embryonal sarcoma (UES) of the liver, which is a rare type of mesencyhmal malignant neoplasm, may contain cystic spaces. Additionally, cystic subtypes of primary liver neoplasms including hepatocellular carcinoma and giant cavernous hemangioma may sometimes be seen.

- UES of the liver, cystic subtypes of hepatocellular carcinoma, and hemangioma with central cystic spaces are explained in corresponding chapters and sections. Cystic metastases, which are secondary neoplastic cystic lesions, are explained in the corresponding chapter and sections.

Biliary cystadenoma and cystadenocarcinoma

- Biliary cystadenoma is a benign and at times premalignant biliary ductal neoplasm.
- Biliary cystadenocarcinoma is a malignant biliary ductal neoplasm.
- Both represent less than 5% of intrahepatic cystic masses of biliary origin.
- Rare, usually slow-growing, multilocular complex cystic neoplasms.
- Frequently found in the right lobe (55%) but also found in the left lobe (29%) or in both lobes (16%).
- Biliary cystadenomas are predominantly seen in middle-aged white women.

- Their presentation is related to the mass effect of the lesion and its biliary obstruction and they may present with abdominal pain, nausea, vomiting, and obstructive jaundice (3–5).
- **Pathology:**
  ° Cystic and stromal components are present in variable degrees.
  ° A fibrous capsule is present.
  ° A single layer of mucin-secreting cells line the cyst wall.
  ° Malignant lesions exhibit pronounced cytologic atypia with evidence of stromal invasion.
  ° These tumors are typically multilocular and typically contain internal septations and mural nodules (Figure 4.14).
  ° The fluid within the tumor can be proteinaceous, mucinous, and occasionally gelatinous, purulent, or hemorrhagic (3–5).
- **On CT:**
  ° The characteristic CT appearance of biliary cystadenoma is a cystic lesion with lobulated contours and septa.
  ° The characteristic CT appearance of biliary cystadenocarcionoma is a solitary complex cystic mass with a well-defined thick fibrous capsule, mural nodules, internal septa, and, sometimes capsular calcification (Figure 4.15).
  ° Although mural nodules or polypoid, pedunculated excrescences are more common in biliary cystadenocarcinoma compared to biliary cystadenoma, mural nodules may also be present in biliary cystadenoma.

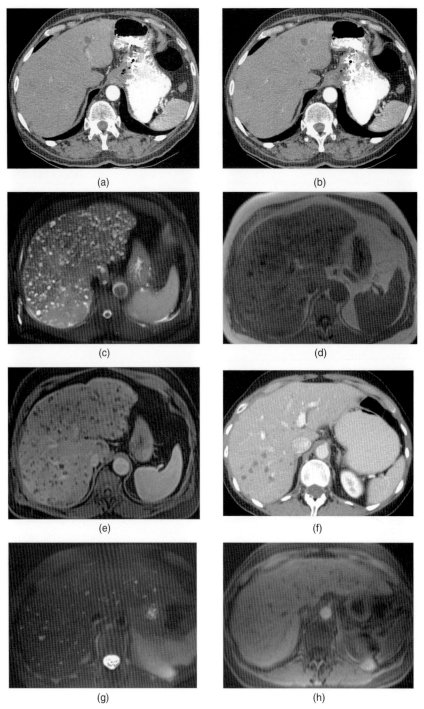

(a)   (b)

(c)   (d)

(e)   (f)

(g)   (h)

Figure 4.11 *Biliary hamartomas.* Transverse hepatic arterial dominant phase contrast enhanced CT examinations display the presence of multiple small-sized hypodense lesions (a, b) with low attenuation levels, showing no enhancement. The lesions are consistent with biliary hamartomas. Transverse T2-weighted fat-suppressed single shot ETSE (c), T1-weighted in-phase 2D-GE (d) and post-gadolinium fat-suppressed hepatic venous phase 3D-GE (e) images acquired at 3.0 T show multiple small biliary hamartomas in another patient. Transverse contrast enhanced hepatic venous phase CT image (f), T2-weighted fat-suppressed single shot ETSE (g), T1-weighted fat-suppressed hepatic arterial phase (h) and hepatic venous phase 3D-GE (i) images acquired at 1.5 T show multiple small biliary hamartomas in another patient. Transverse T2-weighted fat-suppressed single shot ETSE (j), T1-weighted in-phase 2D-GE (k) and T1-weighted post-gadolinium fat-suppressed hepatic venous phase 3D-GE (l) images acquired at 3.0 T show multiple small and large biliary hamartomas in another patient. Large biliary hamartomas show similar imaging features. Transverse T2-weighted fat-suppressed single shot ETSE (m), T1-weighted 2D-GE (n), T1-weighted post-gadolinium fat-suppressed hepatic arterial dominant phase (o) and hepatic venous phase (p) 3D-GE images acquired at 3.0 T demonstrate a large lobulated biliary hamartoma and multiple small biliary hamartomas in another patient. Note the presence of a small amount of pleural effusion at the left side.

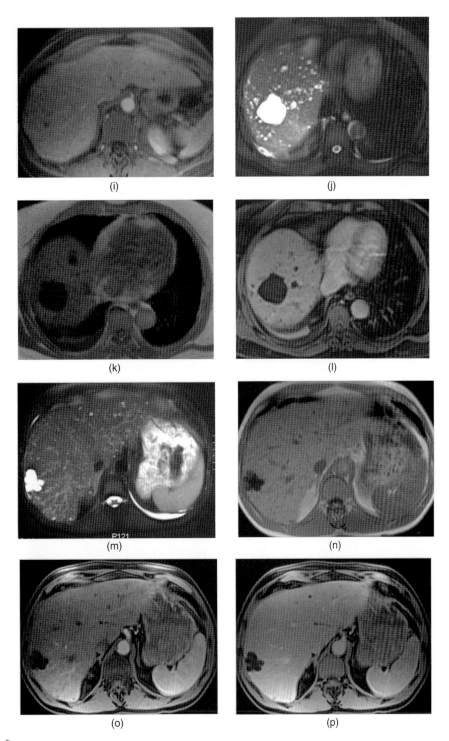

(i)

(j)

(k)

(l)

(m)

(n)

(o)

(p)

Figure 4.11 (*Continued*)

○ These tumors may show higher attenuation due to the mucinous or proteinaceous fluid on pre-contrast CT examinations.

○ The fibrous capsule, internal septations, or mural nodules demonstrate contrast enhancement on post-contrast CT examinations (3–5).

- **On MRI:**

  ○ Biliary cystadenoma appears as a lobulated cystic lesion with thin septa (Figure 4.14).

  ○ Biliary cystadenoncarcinoma appears as a solitary multilocular complex mass with solid components (Figure 4.15).

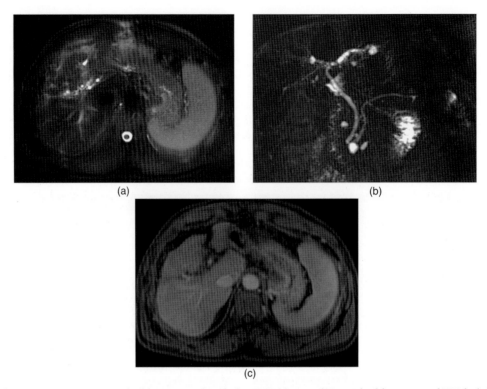

Figure 4.12 *Peribiliary cysts.* Transverse T2-weighted fat-suppressed single shot ETSE (a), coronal T2-weighted fat-suppressed TSE thick slab MRCP (b) and transverse T1-weighted fat-suppressed hepatic venous phase 3D-GE (c) images acquired at 3.0 T demonstrate peribiliary cysts located along the biliary ducts within the portal hilum in a patient with chronic liver disease and portal hypertension. Note that the cysts do not show any enhancement on post-gadolinium image (c). There are also pancreatic cysts located adjacent to the common bile duct and pancreatic duct.

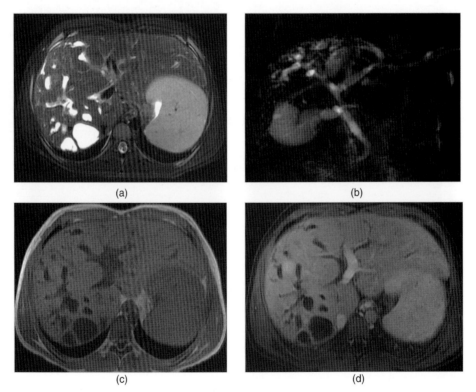

Figure 4.13 *Caroli disease.* Transverse T2-weighted single shot ETSE (a), coronal 3D MIP reconstructed MRCP (b), transverse T1-weighted in-phase 2D-GE (c), transverse T1-weighted post-gadolinium 3D-GE (d) images acquired at 1.5 T demonstrate cystic saccular dilatations of intrahepatic bile ducts. The communication of cystic structures with the biliary tree is seen on MRCP image (b).

° Biliary cystadenomas and cystadenocarcinomas usually appear low signal on T1-WI and high signal on T2-WI (Figures 4.14 and 4.15).

° These lesions may demonstrate variable signal intensities depending on their protein and hemorrhage content, and solid components on T1-WI and T2-WI. Therefore, they may show high signal on T1-WI and low signal on T2-WI on pre-contrast sequences.

° The solid components of the tumor, including the fibrous capsule, internal septations, and mural nodules, demonstrate heterogeneous progressive enhancement in all phases of enhancement on post-gadolinium sequences (Figure 4.15) (3–5).

- **Differential Diagnosis and Pearls:**
° Imaging findings and characteristics of biliary cystadenoma show less irregular stroma and mural nodules than cystadenocarcinoma; however, there is considerable overlap.

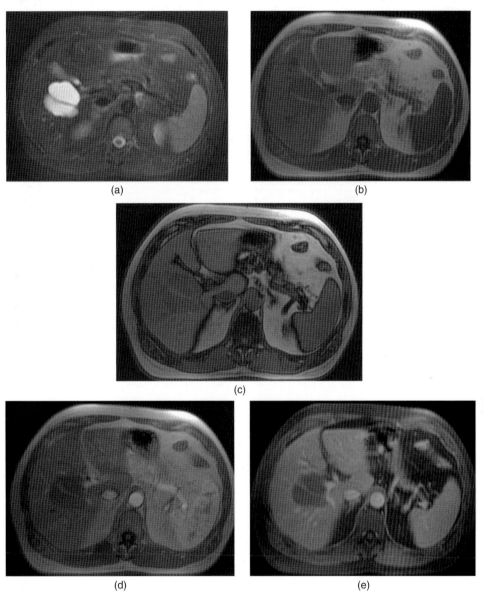

Figure 4.14 *Biliary cystadenoma.* Transverse T2-weighted single shot ETSE (a), T1-weighted in-phase 2D-GE (b), T1-weighted out-of-phase 2D-GE (c), T1-weighted hepatic arterial dominant phase 2D-GE (d) and hepatic venous phase 3D-GE (e) images acquired at 1.5 T demonstrate an intermediate size biliary cystadenoma. The cystic lesion contains a thick internal septum (a-e) and shows mild capsular enhancement on postgadolinium images (d, e). Transverse T2-weighted single shot ETSE (a), T1-weighted in-phase 2D-GE (b), T1-weighted out-of-phase 2D-GE (c), T1-weighted postgadolinium hepatic arterial dominant phase 2D-GE (d) and hepatic venous phase 3D-GE (e) images acquired at 1.5 T demonstrate an intermediate size biliary cystadenoma. The cystic lesion contains a thick internal septum (a–e) and shows mild capsular enhancement on postgadolinium images (d, e). Ultrasound image (f), transverse T2-weighted single shot ETSE (g), transverse T1-weighted 2D-GE (h) and transverse T1-weighted postgadolinium hepatic venous phase 3D-GE (i) images acquired at 3.0 T demonstrate biliary cystadenoma in another patient. Note that the lobulated cystic lesion contains internal septations and the capsule enhances on postgadolinium image (i).

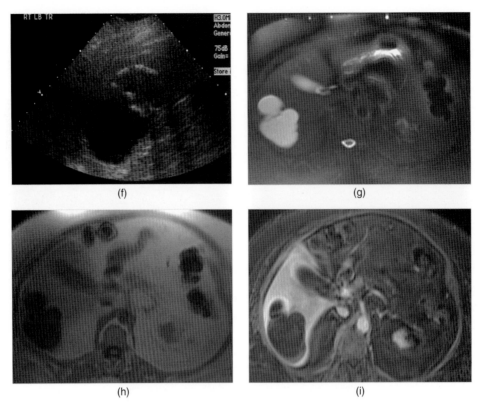

Figure 4.14 (*Continued*)

○ The presence of contrast enhancement of multiple internal septations and mural nodules in biliary cystadenoma and cystadenoncarcinomas may help to distinguish them from hemorrhagic or infected cysts, in which septations and mural nodules are usually not present.

○ UES is a rare malignant neoplasm of the liver predominantly seen in children, and age represents a major distinction. Although cystadenoma/carcinoma is rare, UES is extremely rare.

Inflammatory cystic lesions

Hydatid cyst

- Hepatic echinococcosis is an endemic disease in the Mediterranean region and other sheep-raising countries. Hydatid disease is caused by the larval form of the tapeworm *Echinococcus granulosis* or *Echinococcus multilocularis*. *E. granulosis* is much more common compared to *E. multilocularis*, especially in North America. *E. multilocularis* is the more aggressive form.

- After the ingestion of eggs of *E. granulosis* or *E. multilocularis* with contaminated food, the larvae invade the intestinal wall, migrate to the liver via the portal vein, and form hepatic hydatid cysts. Each hydatid cyst consists of three layers, including an outer pericyst, middle laminated membrane or ectocyst, and inner germinal layer. The middle laminated membrane and inner germinal layer are together also referred to as the endocyst. Daughter cysts develop on the periphery as a result of germinal layer invagination in the mother cyst.

- The patients are usually asymptomatic, although the cysts may cause pain or jaundice (3–5).

- **On CT:**

○ Hydatid cysts are seen as intermediate or large sized unilocular or multilocular hypoattenuating liver cysts. Hydatid cysts may appear as a unilocular cyst with a thick or thin wall. They may also appear as multilocular–multivesicular cysts with multiple daughter cysts or septations. Daughter cysts may be seen as round peripheral structures that may have lower attenuation compared to the fluid within the mother cyst. A cyst with a detached membrane, known as the water lily sign, is a specific finding for hydatid cysts. Coarse calcifications may be present in the wall of the cysts and within the cysts. Hydatid cysts do not show contrast enhancement on post-contrast examinations (3–5).

- **On MRI:**

○ Pericyst appears as a hypointense rim on both T1-WI and T2-WI. The signal intensity of internal fluid content of the pericyst, including the hydatid sand or matrix, is variable on T2-WI and T1-WI. Therefore, the mother cysts may be seen as hyperintense or hypointense on both T1-WI and

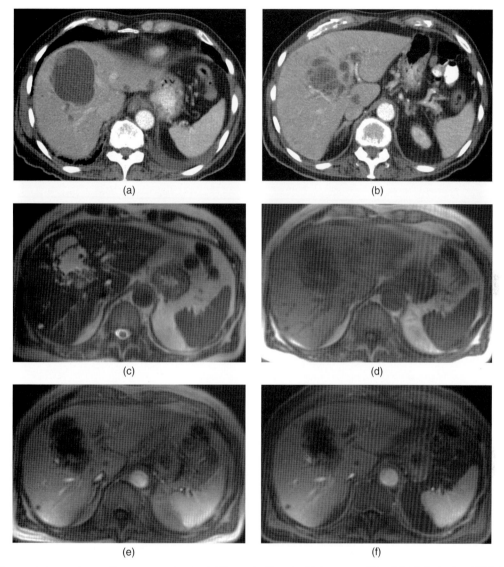

Figure 4.15 *Biliary cystadenocarcinoma.* Transverse postcontrast CT examinations (a, b), transverse T2-weighted single shot ETSE (c), T1-weighted MPRAGE (d), T1-weighted postgadolinium non-fat-suppressed (e) and fat-suppressed (f) MPRAGE images acquired at 3.0 T demonstrate a heterogeneous lobulated cystic structure with enhancing thick septations and enhancing heterogeneous mural nodules. Note the presence of a few small cystic structures in the liver. Transverse T1-weighted out-of-phase MPRAGE (g), transverse T1-weighted postgadolinium fat-suppressed (h, i) and coronal non-fat-suppressed (j) MPRAGE images acquired at 3.0 T demonstrate the presence of left adrenal gland metastasis (thick arrow; g, h), peritoneal metastases (thin arrow, h) and pleural metastases (arrow, i), and metastatic lung nodules (arrow; i, j) in the same patient with biliary cystadenocarcinoma. Coronal T2-weighted single shot ETSE (k), transverse T2-weighted fat-suppressed single shot ETSE (l), coronal 3D MIP MRCP (m), transverse T1-weighted fat-suppressed 3D-GE (n), transverse T1-weighted postgadolinium hepatic arterial dominant (o) and hepatic venous (p) phase 3D-GE images acquired at 3.0 T demonstrate a heterogeneous lobulated cystic structure with thick internal septations (k–p), mural nodules and solid components (k–p), and fluid-fluid level (l). The lesion compresses the biliary tree at the portal hilus and causes intrahepatic biliary ductal dilatation (m). The fibrous capsule, mural solid components, and internal septations show contrast enhancement on postgadolinium images (o, p).

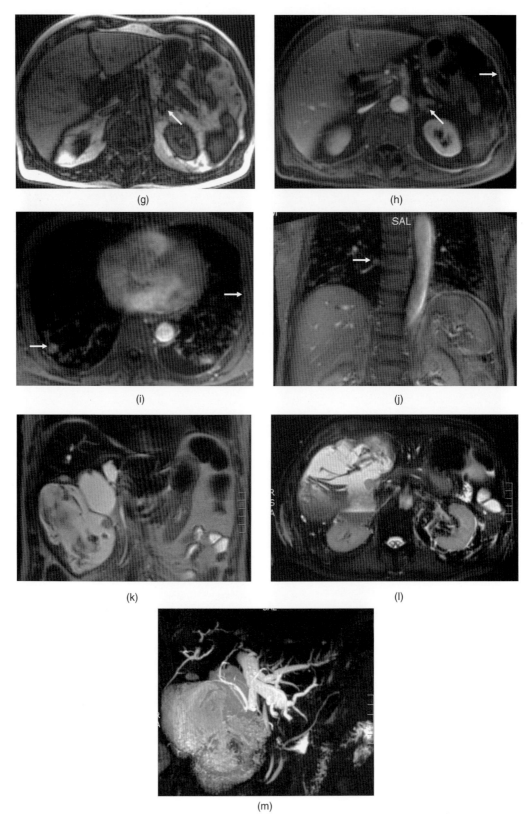

Figure 4.15 (*Continued*)

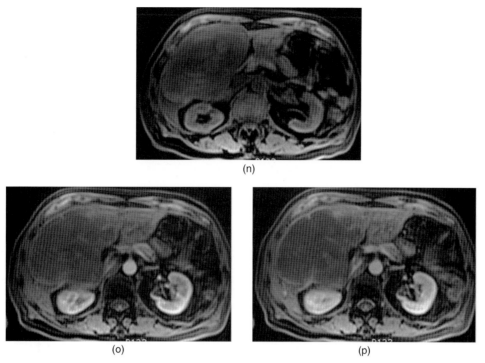

(n)

(o)   (p)

Figure 4.15 (*Continued*)

T2-WI depending on the protein content. Daughter cysts usually show individually high or low signal on T2-WI and T1-WI, respectively, and they often show lower signal compared to the internal matrix of mother cysts on T2-WI and T1-WI. Daughter cysts are often arranged peripherally within the mother cyst. Detached germinal membrane may also show high signal on T2-WI and low signal on T1-WI (Figure 4.16). Hydatid cysts do not show substantial contrast enhancement on post-gadolinium images except the pericyst, which may show subtle enhancement (Figure 4.16) (3–5). The demonstration of internal cystic characteristics, including daughter cysts, are most clearly defined on single shot T2-weighted images, and are considerably better shown than on CT.

- **Differential Diagnosis and Pearls:**
  - Unilocular cysts with thin or thick walls may be confused with simple cysts, cystic metastases, or pyogenic abscesses. Cystic metastases usually demonstrate considerably more mural enhancement than hydatid cysts on post-contrast examinations. Pyogenic abscesses usually demonstrate progressively intense mural enhancement on post-contrast examinations and are usually associated with the presence of early perilesional hepatic parenchymal enhancement on the hepatic arterial dominant phase.
  - Clinical and serologic data help to differentiate these entities.

Abscess

- Hepatic abscesses may be classified as amebic, pyogenic, or fungal.
- They may occur as single or multiple lesions.
- Infectious agents reach the liver through the hepatic artery, portal vein, biliary tract, and by direct extension from contiguous organs.
- **General Imaging Features**
- **On CT:**
  - Round or irregularly shaped hypoattenuating mass with a peripheral capsule that exhibits contrast enhancement.
  - Double-target appearance: consists of a hypodense central area surrounded by a hyperdense ring, which is surrounded by a hypodense zone (localized edema).
  - Cluster of grapes sign: small abscesses coalescing into and forming a multiloculated larger abscess cavity.
- **MRI findings:**
  - Usually high signal intensity on T2-WI, but often some are low signal, reflecting increased protein content (Figures 4.17 and 4.18).
  - Low signal intensity on T1-WI (Figure 4.17).
  - Moderate perilesional enhancement with indistinct outer margins on the hepatic arterial dominant phase post-gadolinium images that rapidly fade to isointensity with the remaining liver parenchyma and nearly resolve by 1-min

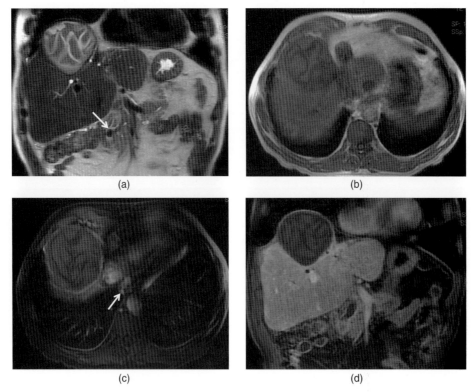

(a)　　　(b)

(c)　　　(d)

Figure 4.16 *Hydatid Cyst.* Coronal T2-weighted single shot ETSE (a), transverse T1-weighted 2D-GE (b), transverse (c) and coronal (d) T1-weighted fat-suppressed hepatic venous phase post-gadolinium 3D-GE images acquired at 1.5 T demonstrate a cystic lesion with water lily sign. The cystic lesion is located in the dome of the liver and abuts the diaphragm. The cystic lesion shows low signal on T2-weighted (a) and intermediate signal on T1-weighted (b) images. The detached germinal membrane shows high signal on T2-weighted image (a). The pericyst shows subtle enhancement on postgadolinium images (c, d) although no enhancement is detected inside the hydatid cyst. Note the presence of common bile duct stones (arrow, a) and esophageal varices (arrow, c).

post injection (Figure 4.17). This reflects a hyperemic inflammatory response in adjacent liver parenchyma, and is almost invariably present in bacterial abscesses, but is more variable in fungal, depending in part on the host's ability to mount an immune response.

° Progressively increasing enhancement of the wall and internal septations in all phases of postgadolinium sequences, forming a continuous ring. No new stroma is enhanced over time.

° Double target or cluster of grapes signs may be present (Figure 4.17).

° With or without layering of gas (signal void on both T2- and T1-WIs) and debris (variable signal on T1-WI or T2-WI, mostly low signal on T2- and high signal on T1-WI due to high protein) within the abscess cavity (Figure 4.17o–q).

• The differentiation of amebic abscesses from pyogenic abscesses is based on the clinical, radiologic, and serologic data. Amebic abscesses have a propensity to be situated superiorly in the liver and invade the diaphragm, causing a pleural reaction.

• Pyogenic, amebic, and fungal abscesses are explained in depth in the chapter on infectious diseases of the liver.

• **Differential Diagnosis and Pearls:**

° Clinical history and laboratory findings are critical.

° Metastases may mimic abscesses as both may show perilesional enhancement and peripheral rim type enhancement. Metastases can be distinguished from abscesses by the observation that metastases show progressive centripetal enhancement of internal stroma, not initially enhanced, in late phases of contrast enhancement. Abscesses show progressively more intense enhancement of tissue that was already enhanced on initial images, with no enhancement of previously unenhanced central tissue on late images. The enhancement of internal septations of abscesses should not be confused with the centripetal enhancement of solid metastatic tissue.

° Metastases with large necrotic components or cystic metastases may mimic the appearance of hepatic abscesses more closely. Absence of clinical features of infection and history of a known tumor that results in cystic metastases (e.g., ovarian cancer) aid in the distinction.

° Metastases may also mimic abscesses clinically if they become secondarily infected. Infected metastases often have a history of a primary tumor (typically colon cancer) and the wall of an infected metastasis is thicker and more shaggy than an abscess.

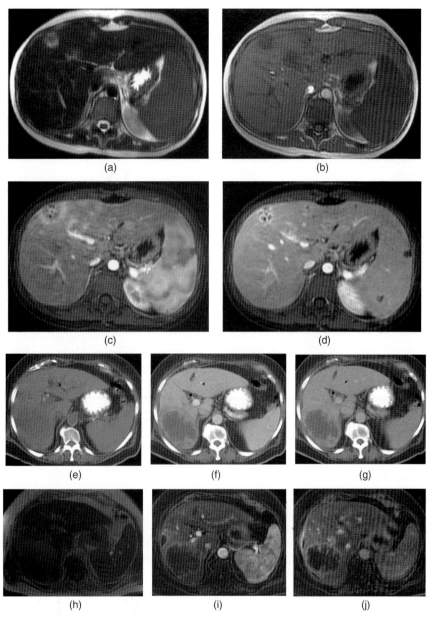

Figure 4.17 *Abscess.* Transverse T2-weighted single shot ETSE (a), transverse T1-weighted 2D-GE (b), transverse T1-weighted hepatic arterial dominant phase (c) and hepatic venous phase (d) 3D-GE images acquired at 1.5 T demonstrate a pyogenic abscess in an immunocompromised patient. The lesions shows high signal on T2-weighted images (a), peripheral parenchymal transient enhancement on the hepatic arterial dominant phase images (c) and progressive enhancement on postgadolinium images (c, d). The lesions display the "cluster of grapes" sign. Progressive rim enhancement and enhancement of internal septations are seen on post-gadolinium images (c, d). The lesions are composed of small abscesses coalescing into and forming a multiloculated larger abscess cavity. Note the presence of small infarcts in the spleen (d). Transverse precontrast (e), postcontrast hepatic venous (f) and interstitial (g) phase CT images show a large abscess with surrounding hypodense edema and thick peripheral wall enhancement. Transverse T1-weighted (h), postgadolinium hepatic arterial dominant phase (i) and hepatic venous phase (j) fat-suppressed 3D-GE images show the large abscess with high T1 signal due to its high protein content. The lesion shows moderately high T2 signal (not shown). Peripheral parenchymal mild transient enhancement is seen on the hepatic arterial dominant phase. The lesion shows thick wall enhancement. Note the presence of peripheral cystic lesion which shows peripheral enhancement, which is secondary to biopsy / drainage attempt. Transverse T2-weighted fat-suppressed single shot ETSE (k), transverse T1-weighted 2D-GE (l), transverse T1-weighted fat-suppressed postgadolinium hepatic arterial phase (m) and hepatic venous phase (n) 3D-GE images acquired at 3.0 T demonstrate a number of cystic lesions located in the right lobe of the liver. The larger cystic lesion contains an air bubble. Peripheral transient parenchymal enhancement is seen on the hepatic arterial phase image (m). Abscess cavities show progressive rim type of enhancement on postgadolinium images (m, n). Note the development of bland thrombus in the right hepatic vein due to adjacent inflammation. Transverse T2-weighted fat-suppressed single shot ETSE (o), transverse T1-weighted 2D-GE (p), transverse fat-suppressed postgadolinium hepatic venous phase 2D-GE (q) images acquired at 1.5 T demonstrate an abscess containing an air-fluid level in a patient with recent liver transplantation. The wall of abscess cavity shows mild contrast enhancement (q).

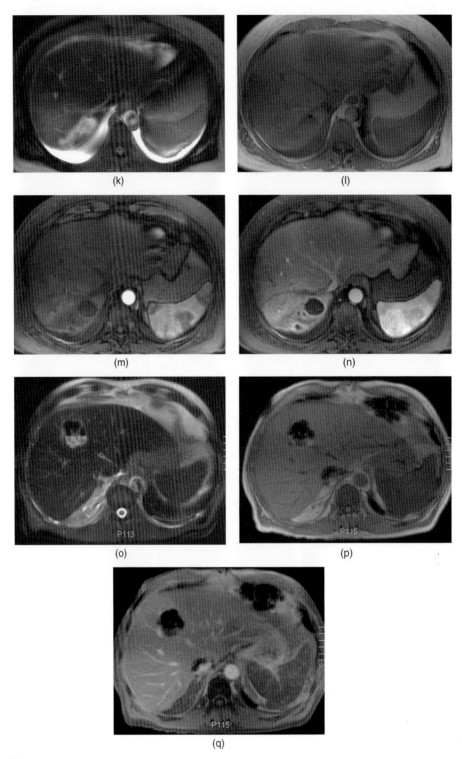

(k)

(l)

(m)

(n)

(o)

(p)

(q)

Figure 4.17 *(Continued)*

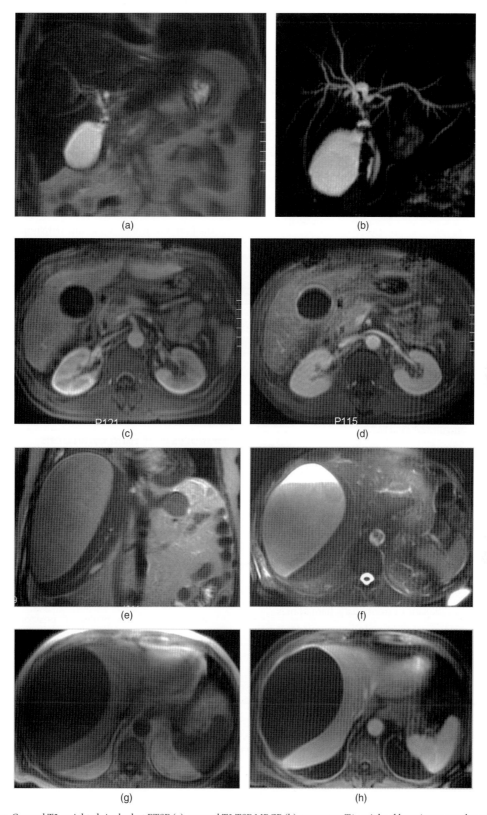

Figure 4.18 *Biloma*. Coronal T2-weighted single shot ETSE (a), coronal T2 TSE MRCP (b), transverse T1-weighted hepatic venous phase (c) and interstitial phase (d) fat-suppressed 3D-GE images acquired at 1.5 T show a fluid collection located following cholecystectomy operation. The fluid collection contains bile and shows high signal on T2-weighted images (a, b) and pseudocapsular enhancement on postgadolinium images (c, d). Note that the biliary tree is mildly dilated. Coronal T2-weighted single shot ETSE (e), transverse fat-suppressed T2-weighted single shot ETSE (f), T1-weighted 2D-GE (g) and fat-suppressed hepatic venous phase 2D-GE (h) images acquired at 1.5 T demonstrate a large subcapsular bile containing fluid collection with fluid-fluid level in another patient.

Miscellaneous cystic lesions

Biloma

- Bilomas are encapsulated collections of bile outside the biliary tree.
- May be spontaneous, traumatic, or iatrogenic secondary to surgical or interventional procedures.
- May be intrahepatic or perihepatic.
- Leakage of bile from the biliary tree provokes an intense inflammatory reaction resulting in the formation of a well-defined pseudocapsule (3–5).
- Imaging
  - **On CT and MRI**, a biloma appears as a well-defined or slightly irregular cystic lesion without septations and calcifications.
  - **On CT**, a biloma is seen as a non-enhancing hypoattenuating cystic lesion with mild to moderate wall enhancement on postcontrast examinations.
  - **On MRI**, a biloma is seen as a non-enhancing cystic lesion with high T2 signal, with mild to moderate wall enhancement on postgadolinium examinations (Figure 4.18) (3–5).
- **Differential Diagnosis and Pearls:**
  - Clinical history and location of the lesion in combination with the imaging findings are critical for the diagnosis.

Hematoma

- Hematomas can be intrahepatic or perihepatic.
- Hematomas are usually secondary to trauma, surgery, interventional procedures, or neoplasms.
- Neoplasms including hepatocellular adenomas and carcinomas may lead to intrahepatic or perihepatic hematomas.
- Clinical presentation consists of right upper quadrant pain and tenderness, signs and symptoms of blood loss and peritoneal irritation, and elevated liver enzymes (3–5).
- Imaging
  - The appearance of an intra or perihepatic hemorrhage depends on the age of blood products within the fluid collection. Therefore, imaging findings depend on the lag time between the formation of hematoma and imaging procedure.
  - On CT, acute or subacute hematoma or hemorrhage has higher attenuation compared to pure fluid, due to the presence of aggregated fibrin. Chronic hematoma has identical attenuation to that of pure fluid. Chronic hematoma may contain septations and debris.

- **On MRI**, a hyperacute hematoma has signal intensity of fluid, low signal on T1-WI, and high signal on T2-WI, and the appearance of oxyhemoglobin. Acute hematoma at day 1–2, contains deoxyhemoglobin and possesses the distinctive feature of very low signal on T2-WI, with intracellular methemoglobin at day 3, showing high T1-WI in conjunction with very low T2 signal. Subacute hematomas, day 4–7, show high signal on T1-WI and T2-WI, reflecting extracellular methemoglobin. Chronic hematoma often shows similar signal intensity to fluid centrally but often possesses a thick, very low signal, hemosiderin-laden rind (Figure 4.19). On both CT and MRI, hematomas do not show enhancement on postcontrast examinations, although the pseudocapsules of chronic hematomas may show slight enhancement, especially on hepatic venous and interstitial phases. Chronic hematoma may contain septations and debris on CT and MRI (3–5).
- **Differential Diagnosis and Pearls:**
  - Hepatic lacerations, rib fractures, and perihepatic fluid may coexist in posttraumatic patients. Hematoma following surgery or interventional procedure is seen along the surgical plane.
  - Perihepatic or intrahepatic hematomas may be associated with hemorrhagic neoplasms, including hepatocellular carcinomas and adenomas (Figure 4.19i–l).

Pseudocysts or fluid collections

- Hepatic extrapancreatic pseudocysts or fluid collections occur frequently in or around the left lobe of the liver and are secondary to an extension of fluid from the lesser sac into the gastrohepatic ligament.
- Clinical signs and symptoms of acute pancreatitis should be present.
- Imaging
  - **On CT:** acute fluid collections, subacute or chronic pseudocysts are seen as hypoattenuating fluid collections with enhancing pseudocapsules on postcontrast examinations (Figure 4.20). Higher attenuation due to high protein content or hemorrhage may be seen in acute fluid collections or subacute pseudocysts.
  - **On MRI:** acute fluid collections, subacute or chronic pseudocysts usually show high signal on T2-WI, low signal on T1-WI, and enhancing pseudocapsule on postgadolinium images (Figure 4.20). Pseudocapsules typically exhibit progressive intensification of enhancement from early to late postcontrast images. High signal on T1-WI due to high protein content or hemorrhage may be seen in acute fluid collections or subacute pseudocysts (3–5).
- **Differential Diagnosis and Pearls:**
  - Associated imaging findings of acute pancreatitis.
  - Peripheral inflammatory stranding may be associated with acute fluid collections or subacute pseudocysts.

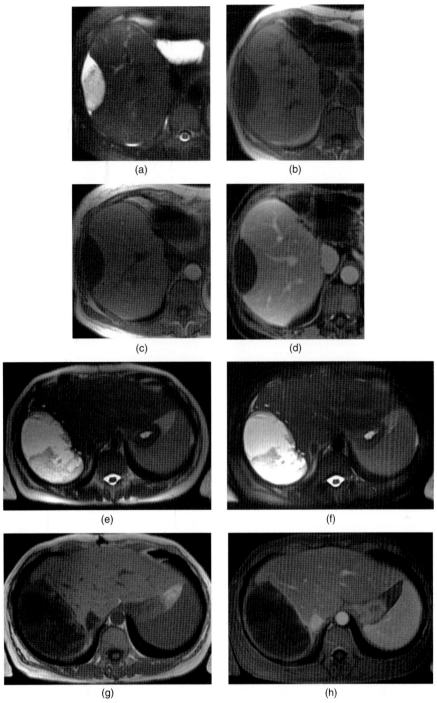

Figure 4.19 *Hematoma.* Transverse T2-weighted single shot ETSE (a), transverse T1-weighted 2D-GE (b), transverse T1-weighted hepatic arterial dominant phase (c) and hepatic venous phase (d) 3D-GE images demonstrate a chronic subcapsular hematoma following liver biopsy in a patient with liver transplantation. The subcapsular fluid collection shows layering of high fluid signal above coagulated blood products with relatively lower signal on T2-WI (a). The fluid collection shows prominently low signal on T1-WI (b) and no enhancement except mild capsular enhancement on postgadolinium images (c, d). Transverse T2-weighted single shot non-fat-suppressed (e) and fat-suppressed (f) ETSE, transverse T1-weighted 2D-GE (g), transverse T1-weighted fat-suppressed hepatic venous phase 3D-GE (h) images demonstrate a chronic hematoma-biloma complex in a patient with hepatic segmentectomy. The fluid collection is along the surgical plane. The fluid collection shows high signal on T2-WI (e, f) and heterogeneous signal due to coagulated blood products on both T2- (e, f) and T1-WI (g). Note that the internal content of fluid collection does not show enhancement while its pseudocapsule enhances (h). Transverse T2-weighted single shot ETSE (i), transverse T1-weighted 2D-GE (j), transverse T1-weighted non-fat-suppressed hepatic arterial dominant phase (k) and fat-suppressed hepatic venous phase (l) 2D-GE images demonstrate a subacute to chronic large hematoma occurring due to a hemorrhagic hepatocellular carcinoma. The hematoma shows relatively high but heterogeneous signal on T2-WI (i) and relatively high and intermediate signal on T1-WI (j). The hematoma displays capsular enhancement on postgadolinium images (k, l). Note that there is a heterogeneously enhancing hemorrhagic tumor (arrows, k, l) leading to the formation of hematoma. Source: Semelka 2010. Reproduced with permission of Wiley.

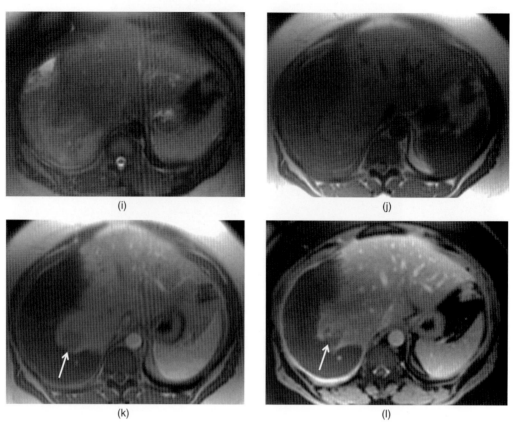

(i)

(j)

(k)

(l)

Figure 4.19 (*Continued*)

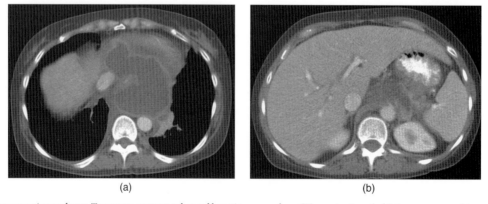

(a)

(b)

Figure 4.20 *Extrapancreatic pseudocyst.* Transverse contrast enhanced hepatic venous phase CT examinations (a, b), transverse non-fat-suppressed and coronal fat-suppressed T2-weighted single shot ETSE (c, d), transverse and coronal T1-weighted MPRAGE postgadolinium hepatic venous phase (e, f) images demonstrate a fluid collection in a patient with acute pancreatitis. The fluid collection is located adjacent to the left lobe of the liver, diaphragm, stomach, esophagus, and heart, and extends into the posterior mediastinum. The fluid collection shows prominent pseudocapsular enhancement on postcontrast CT examinations (a, b) and postgadolinium images (e, f). The fluid collection shows heterogeneous high signal on T2-WI (c, d) due to respiration artifacts and the presence of debris.

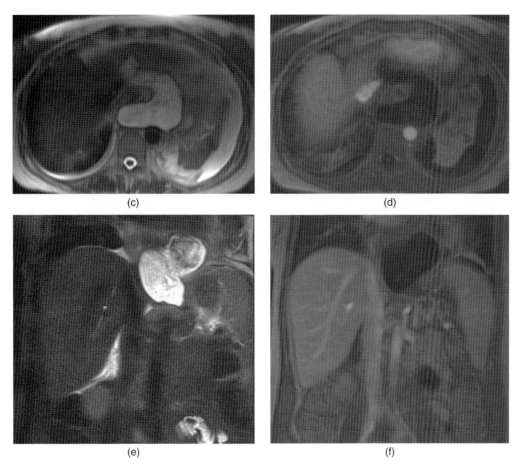

(c)

(d)

(e)

(f)

Figure 4.20 (*Continued*)

References

1 Semelka, R.C., Martin, D.R., and Balci, N.C. (2006) Magnetic resonance imaging of the liver: How I do it. J Gastroenterol Hepatol, 21, 632–637.

2 Ramalho, M., Altun, E., Heredia, V. *et al.* (2007) Liver MR Imaging: 1.5 T versus 3 T. Magn Reson Imaging Clin N Am, 15, 321–347.

3 Braga, L., Armao, D., El Azzazi, M., and Semelka, R.C. (2010) Liver, in Body MRI, 3rd edn (ed. R.C. Semelka), Wiley-Blackwell, Hoboken, NJ, pp. 45–455.

4 Mortele, K.J. and Ros, P.R. (2001) Cystic focal liver lesions in the adult: differential CT and MR imaging features. Radiographics, 21, 895–910.

5 Vacha, B., Sun, M.R., Siewert, B., and Eisenberg, R.L. (2011) Cystic lesions of the liver. Am J Roentgenol, 196, W668–W677.

6 Brancatelli, G., Federle, M.P., Vilgrain, V. *et al.* (2005) Fibropolycystic liver disease: CT and MR Imaging Findings. Radiographics, 25, 659–670.

7 Morgan, D.E., Lockhart, M.E., Canon, C.L. *et al.* (2006) Polycystic liver disease: Multimodality imaging for complications and transplant evaluation. Radiographics, 26, 1655–1668.

8 Martin, D.R., Kalb, B., Sarmiento, J.M. *et al.* (2010) Giant and complicated variants of cystic bile duct hamartomas of the liver: MRI findings and pathological correlations. J Magn Reson Imaging, 31, 903–11.

9 Anderson, S.W., Kruskal, J.B., and Kane, R.A. (2009) Benign hepatic tumors and iatrogenic pseudotumors. Radiographics, 29, 211–229.

10 Crider, M.H., Hoggard, E., and Manivel, J.C. (2009) Undifferentiated (embryonal) sarcoma of the liver. Radiographics, 29, 1665–1668.

CHAPTER 5
Benign solid liver lesions

Ersan Altun[1], Mohamed El-Azzazi[1,2,3,4], Richard C. Semelka[1], and Mamdoh AlObaidy[1,5]
[1]The University of North Carolina at Chapel Hill, Department of Radiology, Chapel Hill, NC, USA
[2]University of Dammam, Department of Radiology, Dammam, Saudi Arabia
[3]King Fahd Hospital of the University, Department of Radiology, Khobar, Saudi Arabia
[4]University of Al Azhar, Department of Radiology, Cairo, Egypt
[5]King Faisal Specialist Hospital & Research Center, Department of Radiology, Riyadh, Saudi Arabia

Hemangiomas

- Hemangiomas are:
  ° Most common benign hepatic neoplasm, with an incidence between 2% and 10% (Figure 5.1).
  ° More frequent in females (F : M; 2–5 : 1).
  ° Usually multiple, rarely produce symptoms, usually detected incidentally, and remain stable in size in adults over time.
  ° Are fed by hepatic artery branches.
  ° Are generally cavernous.
- Pathologically: They are well circumscribed, sponge-like blood-filled mesenchymal tumors.
- Microscopically: They reveal numerous large vascular channels lined by a single layer of flat endothelial cells, separated by slender fibrous septa. Foci of thrombosis, extensive fibrosis/scarring, and calcification may be present.
- **Imaging of Appearance of Hemangiomas:**
  ° **On US:**
    - **Typical features:**
      (a) Well defined, homogeneous, and hyperechoic lesions with posterior acoustic enhancement (80%) (Figure 5.1).
    - **Atypical features:**
      (a) Thin or thick echogenic border with hypoechoic center.
      (b) Heterogeneously or homogeneously hypoechoic.
      (c) May be seen as hypoechoic lesions with hepatic steatosis.
  ° **On CT:**
    - **Unenhanced CT findings:**
    - Hemangiomas are sharply defined oval/round masses that are usually hypoattenuating on noncontrast images.
    - They may be iso- or hyperattenuating on noncontrast images in patients with hepatic steatosis.
    - Hemorrhage may complicate giant hemangiomas and hemorrhagic areas may then be seen as hyperattenuating areas in giant hemangiomas. Calcifications may also be detected.
    - The vascular components of hemangiomas have similar attenuation value as blood vessels. The postcontrast enhancement level may approach the enhancement of venous structures.
    - Thrombosed, fibrotic, or degenerated areas that are frequently present within large hemangiomas are initially lower and remain lower in attenuation on delayed images compared to the vascular components.
  ° **On MRI:**
    - **Unenhanced MRI findings:**
    - Hemangiomas are sharply defined round/oval masses which have long T2 and T1 values, so they show moderately high signal on T2-weighted images and low signal on T1-weighted images (Figure 5.1). Note that if lesions are not bright on T2-weighted images, they are very unlikely to be hemangiomas.
    - Hemorrhage/cystic changes/fibrosis may complicate giant hemangiomas and hemorrhage may be seen as hyperintense areas on T1-weighted images, although the signal intensity may change according to the age of hemorrhage on T1- and T2-weighted images.

Liver Imaging: MRI with CT Correlation, First Edition. Edited by Ersan Altun, Mohamed El-Azzazi and Richard C. Semelka.
© 2015 John Wiley & Sons, Inc. Published 2015 by John Wiley & Sons, Inc.

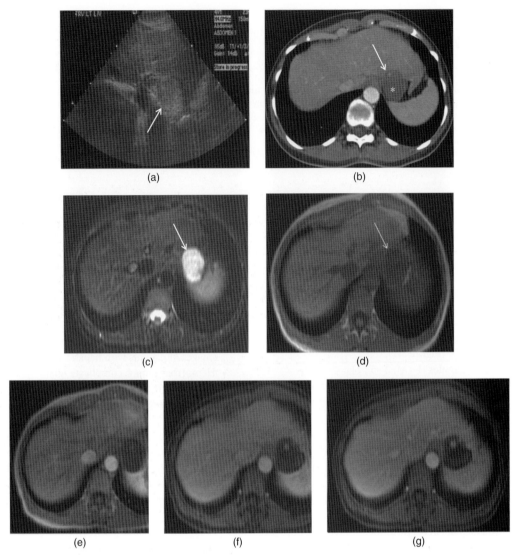

Figure 5.1 *Transverse image from the liver (a) shows a hyperechoic well-defined exophytic mass (arrow, a) arising from the left lobe of the liver, which is seen as a rounded well-defined hypoattenuating lesion (asterisk, b) on transverse postcontrast hepatic venous phase CT image (b).* The lesion shows peripheral nodular enhancement (arrow, b). Transverse T2-weighted STIR (c), T1-weighted 2D-GE (d), postgadolinium T1-weighted 2D-GE hepatic arterial dominant phase (e), fat-suppressed 3D-GE progressive hepatic venous phase (f, g) images show characteristic features of a liver hemangioma. The hemangioma shows markedly high signal due to its high water content and peripheral discontinuous nodular enhancement (e, f) with progressive coalescence of nodules (g).

Enhancement features on CT and MRI

There are three patterns of enhancement of hemangiomas on CT and MRI.

1 **Pattern I.** Uniform enhancement immediately after contrast administration on the hepatic arterial dominant phase (Figures 5.2–5.5).
   ° Observed only in small tumors which are less than 1 cm.
   ° May be difficult to distinguish from hypervascular liver metastases.
   ° Usually maintain their enhancement on later phases.
   ° May fade in signal intensity and becomes mildly hyperintense compared to the background liver parenchyma on the interstitial phase of contrast enhancement, with no evidence of peripheral or heterogeneous wash-out.

2 **Pattern II.** The classic and most common type of enhancement. Peripheral nodular enhancement with centripedal progression (Figures 5.6–5.8).
   ° Commonly seen in both small and medium sized (usually between 1 and 5 cm) hemangiomas.
   ° The classic enhancement pattern of hemangiomas on dynamic serial postcontrast images on CT and MRI is:
      i. Peripheral nodular or globular.
      ii. Discontinuous.

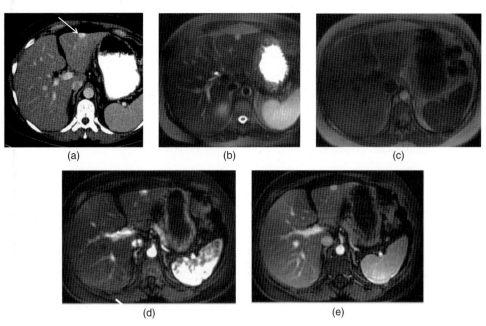

Figure 5.2 *Transverse postcontrast hepatic venous CT image (a), T2-weighted fat-suppressed SS-ETSE (b), T1-weighted 2D-GE (c), T1-weighted postgadolinium 3D-GE hepatic arterial dominant (d) and hepatic venous phase (e) images show a typical small hemangioma (arrow) with type 1 enhancement pattern.* The hemangioma demonstrates its typical markedly high T2 signal (b) and prominent enhancement on postgadolinium images (d, e). The hemangioma shows fast filling with contrast which is seen on the hepatic arterial dominant phase MR image (d). Homogeneous enhancement of the hemangioma is seen on the hepatic venous phase CT image (a). The hemangiomas retain the gadolinium and appear as enhancing lesions on the hepatic venous and interstitial phase images. Due to the radiation concern, CT examinations are usually performed with one phase acquisition, which is usually performed on the hepatic venous phase.

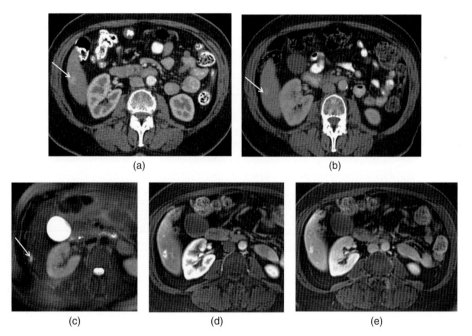

Figure 5.3 *Transverse postcontrast hepatic arterial dominant phase (a), hepatic venous phase (b) CT images, T2-weighted fat-suppressed SS-ETSE (c), T1-weighted postgadolinium 3D-GE hepatic arterial dominant (d) and hepatic venous phase (e) images show a typical small hemangioma (arrows) with type 1 enhancement pattern.* The hemangioma shows fast filling with contrast and homogeneous enhancement on postcontrast hepatic arterial dominant (a, d) and hepatic venous phase (b, e) CT and MR images.

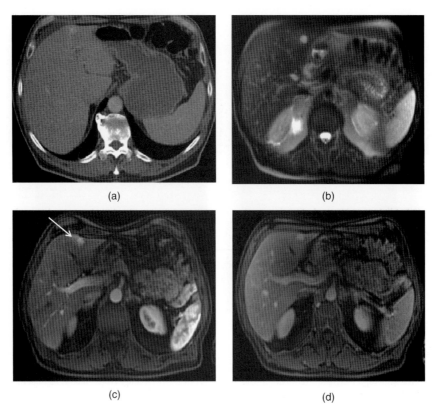

Figure 5.4 *Transverse postcontrast hepatic venous CT image (a), T2-weighted fat-suppressed SS-ETSE (b), T1-weighted fat-suppressed postgadolinium 3D-GE hepatic arterial dominant (c) and hepatic venous phase (d) images show a typical small hemangioma (arrow) with type 1 enhancement pattern.* In addition to the typical features of fast filling hemangioma, note the presence of adjacent increased transient enhancement on the hepatic arterial dominant phase, which develops secondary to shunting (arrow, c) at the adjacent liver parenchyma.

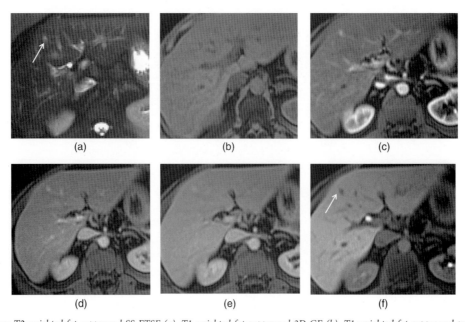

Figure 5.5 *Transverse T2-weighted fat-suppressed SS-ETSE (a), T1-weighted fat-suppressed 3D-GE (b), T1-weighted fat-suppressed postgadolinium 3D-GE hepatic arterial dominant (c) and hepatic venous phase (d), interstitial phase (e) and hepatocyte phase (f) images show a typical small hemangioma (arrow) with type 1 enhancement pattern.* The hepatocyte phase images are acquired with gadoxetic acid at 20 min after the administration of contrast. The hemangioma does not demonstrate the uptake of gadoxetic acid as it does not contain hepatocytes and therefore shows low signal intensity (arrow, f).

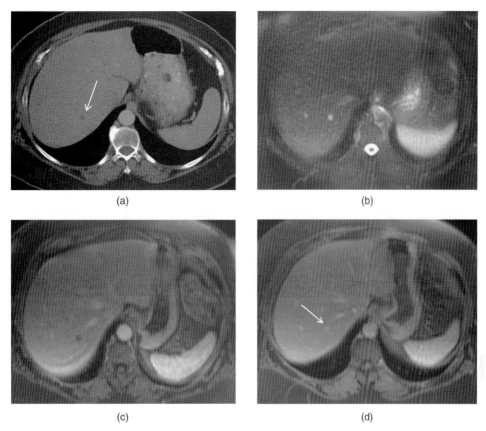

Figure 5.6 *Transverse postcontrast hepatic venous CT image (a), T2-weighted STIR (b), T1-weighted postgadolinium 3D-GE hepatic venous (c) and interstitial phase (d) images show a typical small hemangioma (arrow) with type 2 enhancement pattern showing gradual homogeneous fill with contrast seen on the interstitial phase MR image (arrow, d).* The hemangioma shows a subtle peripheral nodular enhancement on CT image (arrow, a). Due to the radiation concern, CT examinations are usually performed with one phase acquisition, which is usually performed on the hepatic venous phase.

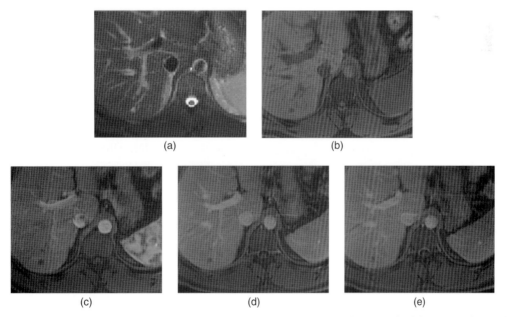

Figure 5.7 *Transverse T2-weighted fat-suppressed SS-ETSE (a), T1-weighted fat-suppressed 3D-GE (b), T1-weighted fat-suppressed postgadolinium 3D-GE hepatic arterial dominant (c) and hepatic venous phase (d), interstitial phase (e) images show a small hemangioma with type 2 enhancement.* The hemangiomas show peripheral nodular enhancement and progressive gradual filling on postgadolinium images (c–e).

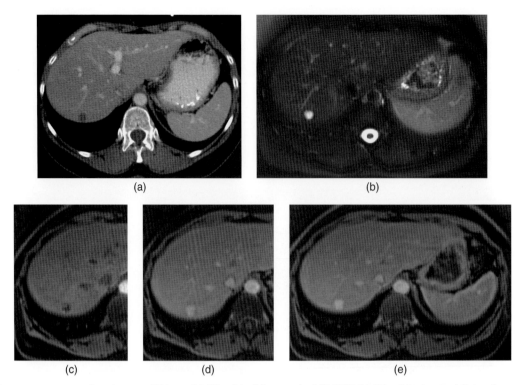

(a)   (b)

(c)   (d)   (e)

Figure 5.8 *Transverse postcontrast hepatic venous CT image (a), T2-weighted fat-suppressed SS-ETSE (b), T1-weighted postgadolinium fat-suppressed 3D-GE hepatic arterial dominant (c), hepatic venous (d) and interstitial phase (e) images show a typical small hemangioma (arrow) with type 2 enhancement pattern.* The lesion appears as a low attenuating lesion on CT and peripheral nodular enhancement pattern is not appreciated. Typical MRI features are demonstrated, including high T2 signal and peripheral discontinuous nodular enhancement with gradual progressive filling by the coalescence of nodules.

iii. Coalesce and slowly progress centripetally to complete or nearly complete fill-in of the entire lesion by 2–10 min.

3 **Pattern III.** Peripheral nodular enhancement with centripetal progression and a persistent nonenhancing central component, that could represent scar/fibrosis, or cystic changes (Figure 5.9).
° Seen mainly in giant hemangiomas (usually larger than 5 cm).

4 **According to the size, hemangiomas may be:**
1 **Small:** <1.0 cm.
- Most commonly demonstrate pattern 2 enhancement.
- Pattern 1 is the second most common enhancement type.
- May fade in signal to background liver (approx 20% of these lesions). But no hemangioma shows wash-out.

2 **Medium:** 1.0–5 cm.
- Exhibit pattern 2 enhancement and represent the classic hemangioma (Figure 5.10).
- Pattern 3 enhancement is the next.
- Pattern 1 enhancement is exceedingly rare.

3 **Large:** 5–10 cm.
4 **Massive:** >10 cm (Figures 5.11 and 5.12).

Large hemangiomas (>5 cm) most frequently have a multi-lobulated appearance with mildly complex high signal intensity on T2-weighted images and demonstrate type 3 enhancement. They usually have substantial central fibrous tissue (Figure 5.9).
- The rapidity of enhancement of type 2 and 3 hemangiomas have been classified depending on postcontrast hepatic venous phase images into:
1 **Slow enhancing hemangiomas:**
- Show minimal early enhancement and often enhance no more than 25% of the entire lesion by 2.5 min.
- The most characteristic type for hemangioma.
- Should be differentiated from avascular and chemotherapy-treated metastasis.

2 **Medium:**
- Show moderate early enhancement and often enhance up to 50% of the lesion by 2.5 min.

3 **Fast:**
- Show substantial early enhancement and often enhance up to 70% of the entire tumor by 2.5 min postcontrast.
- Commonly seen in small type. Although all lesion sizes may display fast enhancement (<20% of large hemangiomas).
- For small lesions, careful differentiation from hypervascular metastasis.

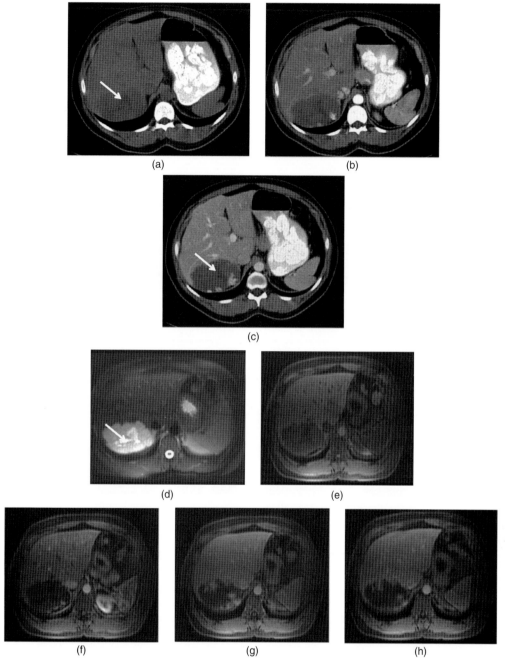

Figure 5.9 *Transverse precontrast (a), postcontrast hepatic arterial dominant (b), hepatic venous phase (c) CT images show a large hemangioma in the posterior segment of the right liver lobe.* The lesion is hypoattenuating and demonstrates peripheral nodular enhancement on the early phase (b) with coalescence of nodules on the later phase (c). Note the central areas of lower attenuation in the lesion, which represent scarring (arrow; a, c). Transverse T2-weighted SS-ETSE (d), T1-weighted fat-suppressed 3D-GE (e), T1-weighted postgadolinium fat-suppressed 3D-GE hepatic arterial dominant (f), hepatic venous (g) and interstitial (h) phase images show the large hemangioma with central scarring (arrow, d). Note the central progressive filling on postgadolinium images (f–h). However, filling of the large hemangiomas with contrast usually takes time and therefore it is not necessary to take delayed images, as they are not diagnostically contributory.

- **Atypical or uncommon appearances of hemangioma**
  - ° Perilesional high signal on T2 and perilesional increased enhancement that likely reflects vascular shunting around hemangiomas (Figure 5.13). Most often seen associated with small capsule-based hemangiomas (Figure 5.4).
  - ° Internal hemorrhage may be seen in giant hemangiomas (Figure 5.12).
  - ° Compression of adjacent portal veins: Uncommonly seen in giant lesions; result in increased signal on T2 of affected liver, and transient segmental increased enhancement on

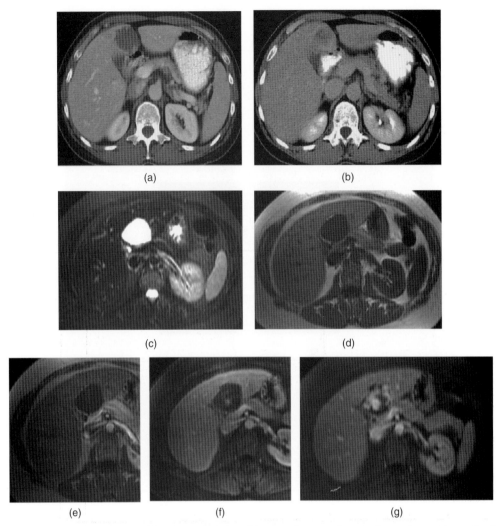

Figure 5.10 *Transverse postcontrast hepatic venous (a) and interstitial phase (b) images show a medium size hemangioma with type II enhancement pattern in the left lobe of the liver.* Transverse T2-weighted STIR (c), T1-weighted 2D-GE (d), T1-weighted postgadolinium hepatic arterial dominant phase (e), fat-suppressed hepatic venous (f) and interstitial phase (g) images. The hemangioma shows typical markedly high T2 signal and the gradual progressive enhancement on postcontrast images (a, b, e–g).

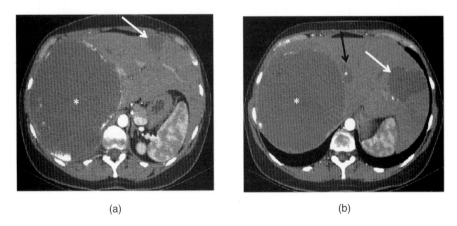

Figure 5.11 *Transverse postcontrast hepatic arterial dominant phase CT images (a, b) show four different hemangiomas including a giant (asteriks, a, b), large (white arrow, b), medium (white arrow, a), and small (black arrow, b) sized hemangiomas with peripheral discontinuous nodular enhancement.*

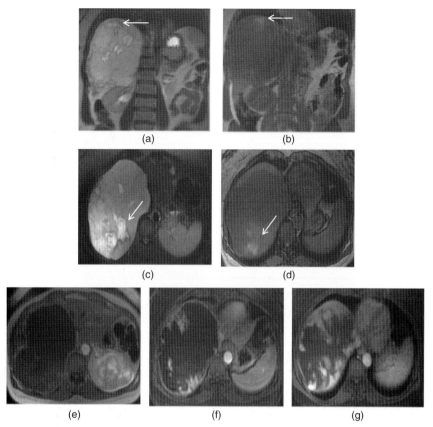

Figure 5.12 *Coronal T2-weighted SS-ETSE (a), T1-weighted 2D-GE (b), transverse T2-weighted SS-ETSE (c), T1-weighted out-of-phase 2D-GE (d), T1-weighted postgadolinium hepatic arterial dominant phase (e), hepatic venous phase (f), and interstitial phase (g) images show a giant hemangioma.* The hemangioma has multifocal T2 hyperintense and T1 hyperintense areas, which represent foci of internal hemorrhage and cystic spaces. The hemangioma shows its typical early peripheral nodular enhancement with progressive filling of the contrast on the later phases.

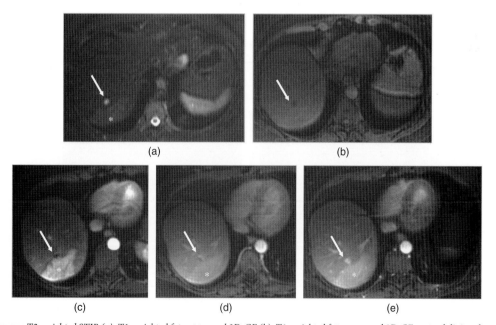

Figure 5.13 *Transverse T2-weighted STIR (a), T1-weighted fat-suppressed 3D-GE (b), T1-weighted fat-suppressed 3D-GE postgadolinium hepatic arterial dominant phase (c), fat-suppressed hepatic venous (d), and interstitial phase (e) images show a small hemangioma (arrows) with type II enhancement pattern, which is associated with the presence of adjacent perfusional abnormality – shunting (asterisk, a–e) in the segment VII.* Note that the perfusional abnormality – shunting in the segment VII demonstrates mildly increased T2 signal (a) and transient increased early enhancement (c), which tends to fade in the later phases (d, e).

immediate postgadolinium images secondary to auto-regulatory increased hepatic arterial supply, with evening of distribution on delayed images.

° Exophytic or pedunculated masses (Figure 5.14).
° Sclerosed types. Fibrous central stroma is seen at the center of lesions and capsular retraction may be present in peripherally located lesions (Figure 5.15). Occasionally these lesions may not be high signal on T2.
° Peripheral continuous enhancing rim (Figure 5.16).
° Non-enhancing hemangioma (Figure 5.17).

• **Hemangiomas in the setting of cirrhosis or chronic liver disease:**
° In subjects with chronic liver disease, the hemangiomas have a size distribution similar to normals, whereas in subjects with cirrhosis lesions are usually <2 cm. Size propensity likely reflects the background vascular milieu.
° Tend to decrease in size with the progression of liver disease.
° Lesions that exhibit fast fill-in must be distinguished from HCC (hemangiomas are bright on T2, HCCs isointense or mildly high in T2 signal).
° On delayed images they retain contrast and do not wash-out; both features distinguish from HCC (Figure 5.18).

• **Differential diagnosis of hemangioma:**
1 **Hypovascular chemotherapy-treated metastases.** Metastases demonstrate mild to moderate high T2 signal while hemangiomas show moderate to markedly high T2 signal. Chemotherapy-treated metastases may show peripheral jagged enhancement; however, these metastases generally show continuous ring enhancement on arterial phase images, whereas hemangiomas show discontinuous nodular enhancement (be careful with fast enhancing hemangiomas). Retention of contrast on delayed images may also be seen in chemotherapy-treated metastases due to the presence of fibrosis. Hemangioma-like lesions that appear too atypical: check for history of a primary tumor and chemotherapy treatment.

2 **Small homogeneously enhancing hypervascular metastasis.** Fast filling hemangiomas most often remain hyperenhanced compared to the background liver on the interstitial phase, while small homogeneously enhancing hypervascular metastases demonstrate wash-out or fading on the interstitial phases. Note that fading may be observed with small hemangiomas, but never wash-out. Additionally, hemangiomas demonstrate moderately high T2 signal, while small metastases generally show mildly high T2 signal.

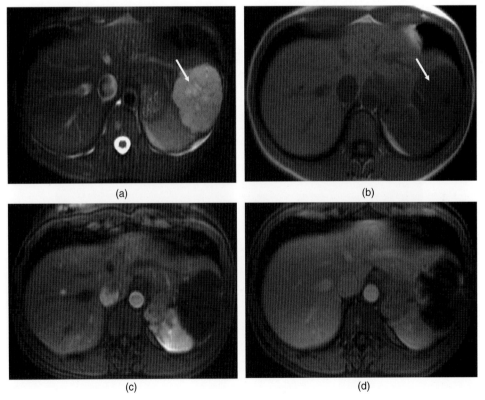

(a) (b)

(c) (d)

Figure 5.14 *Transverse T2-weighted fat-suppressed SS-ETSE (a), T1-weighted 2D-GE (b), postgadolinium T1-weighted 3D-GE fat-suppressed hepatic arterial dominant phase (c), hepatic venous phase (d) images show a large exophytic hemangioma located in the left lobe of the liver adjacent to the spleen. The hemangioma shows typical enhancement features and has a small central scar (arrows, a, b), which is better appreciated on T2- and T1- weighted precontrast images (a, b).*

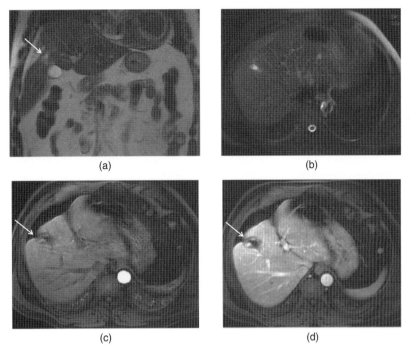

(a)

(b)

(c)

(d)

Figure 5.15 *Coronal T2-weighted SS-ETSE (a), transverse T2-weighted fat-suppressed SS-ETSE (b), T1-weighted postgadolinium hepatic arterial (c) and hepatic venous (d) phase images show a sclerosed hemangioma.* The hemangioma shows markedly high signal with mildly increased peripheral signal, which is also associated with capsular retraction. Early peripheral nodular enhancement (c) with later progression (d) is detected on postgadolinium images (c, d).

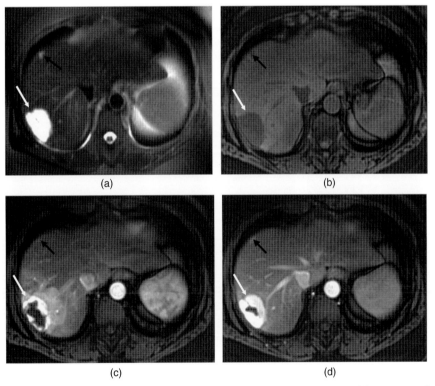

(a)

(b)

(c)

(d)

Figure 5.16 *Transverse T2-weighted fat-suppressed SS-ETSE (a), T1-weighted fat-suppressed 3D-GE (b), postgadolinium T1-weighted 3D-GE fat-suppressed hepatic arterial dominant phase (c), hepatic venous phase (d) images show a large hemangioma (white arrow) and a small hemangioma (black arrow).* Both hemangiomas demonstrate typical markedly high T2 signal (a). The large hemangioma (white arrow) shows atypical enhancement pattern which is characterized by progressive continuous thick peripheral enhancement on postgadolinium images (c, d). Increased transient early enhancement on the hepatic arterial dominant phase (c), which fades on the hepatic venous phase (d) is seen secondary to AV shunting, which is also associated with early filling of the right hepatic vein on the hepatic arterial dominant phase (c). The small hemangioma (black arrow) shows progressive filling with contrast on postgadolinium images (c, d).

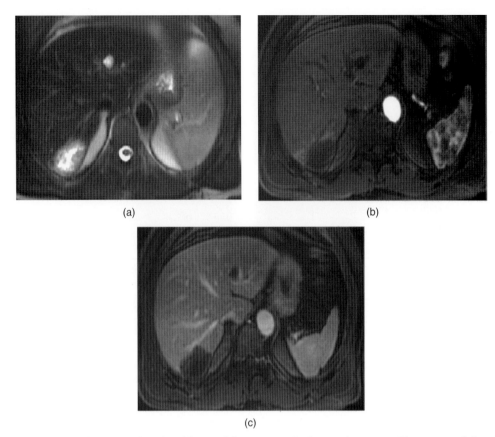

(a)

(b)

(c)

Figure 5.17 *Transverse T2-weighted fat-suppressed SS-ETSE (a), postgadolinium T1-weighted 3D-GE fat-suppressed hepatic arterial phase (b), hepatic venous phase (c) images demonstrate a hemangioma with heterogeneous high T2 signal (a) and no enhancement on postgadolinium images (b, c).* Note the presence of early transient enhancement around the lesion on the arterial phase secondary shunting, which fades on the hepatic venous phase. A few small cysts are also seen in the left lobe of the liver.

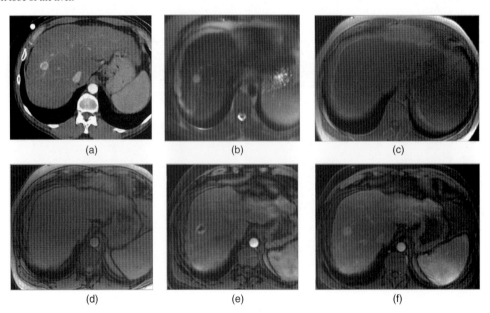

(a)

(b)

(c)

(d)

(e)

(f)

Figure 5.18 *Transverse postcontrast hepatic arterial dominant phase CT image (a), transverse T2-weighted fat-suppressed SS-ETSE (b), T1-weighted 2D-GE in-phase (c) and out-of-phase (d), T1-weighted postgadolinium fat-suppressed 3D-GE hepatic arterial dominant phase (e) and hepatic venous phase (f) images show a hemangioma in a patient with chronic liver disease and cirrhosis.* The hemangioma shows atypical enhancement and demonstrates predominantly thick peripheral enhancement on postcontrast CT image. The hemangioma depicts peripheral relatively thick enhancement on the hepatic arterial dominant phase with progressive enhancement and filling with contrast on the hepatic venous phase.

3 **Small cholangiocarcinomas/epithelioid hemangioendotheliomas.** Lesions can be moderately high signal on T2 and retain contrast on delayed images. See sections below on their characteristic features.

4 **Metastases showing peripheral dominant enhancement with central progression.** They usually have mildly or moderately high T2 signal whereas hemangiomas have markedly high signal. Metastases are usually round whereas hemangiomas usually over 3 cm appear lobulated. Peripheral discontinuous nodular early enhancement is not seen with metastases (Figure 5.19).

5 Be careful when comparing prior CTs to current MR studies. CT may not demonstrate small hemangiomas, and therefore lesions may seem to appear to represent new lesions on MR studies, worrisome for malignancy. This knowledge, and classic appearance as hemangiomas on MR should suggest this circumstance.

Focal nodular hyperplasia (FNH)

- Focal nodular hyperplasia (FNH) is developmental in origin, consisting of a nonneoplastic hyperplastic response of hepatic parenchyma to the increased blood flow related to a preexisting arterial malformation.
- FNH is the second most common benign hepatic tumor after hemangioma and often discovered incidentally (Figure 5.20)

- FNH is seen in 1–5% of the population and has a female predilection (2 : 1). Eighty percent occur in women of child-bearing age.
- Typically occurs in a subcapsular location (Figures 5.21–5.23) and may be exophytic and/or pedunculated (Figures 5.24 and 5.25).
- FNH is considered a non-encapsulated lesion; however, in a small percentage of cases, a partial or complete fibrous pseudocapsule is present.
- FNH does not have malignant potential with a very rare incidence of hemorrhage.
- FNH is more common in women during the third to fifth decade of life.
- FNH is a hypervascular well-circumscribed solid rounded/lobulated benign tumor characterized by a proliferation of hepatocytes, bile ductules, Kupffer's cells, and blood vessels.
- FNH usually has a "central scar" which is a fibrotic central tissue containing arterial vessels and bile ductules (Figures 5.20, 5.22, 5.25–5.27). Additionally, radiating fibrous septa are seen throughout the lesion.
- Necrosis, hemorrhage or fatty change may be very rarely seen.
- FNHs may be seen in the presence of fatty liver (Figure 5.27)
- Although they are usually solitary, multiple FNH may be found as a component of a syndrome which is also associated with the presence of hepatic hemangiomas and vascular liver abnormalities as well as intracranial tumors and vascular

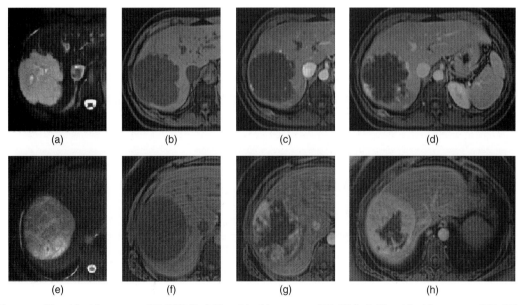

(a) (b) (c) (d)

(e) (f) (g) (h)

Figure 5.19 *Transverse T2-weighted fat-suppressed SS-ETSE (b, e), T1-weighted fat-suppressed 3D-GE (b, f), T1-weighted fat-suppressed 3D-GE hepatic arterial dominant (c, g) and hepatic venous phase (d, h) images.* A giant hemangioma with typical signal, morphologic, and enhancement features is demonstrated on MR images (a–d). A giant leiomyosarcoma metastasis is seen on MR images (e–h). The hemangioma with markedly high signal demonstrates lobulated contours as giant hemangiomas. Central scarring is also present in the hemangioma (a). The metastasis shows heterogeneous moderately high T2 signal (e) and fills with contrast heterogeneously and progressively on postgadolinium images (g, h). The metastasis has rounded contours and heterogeneous T2 signal compared to the hemangioma. Note that the metastasis shows heterogeneous early peripheral dominant progressive enhancement with later central progression, whereas the hemangioma shows early peripheral discontinuous nodular enhancement with later central progression.

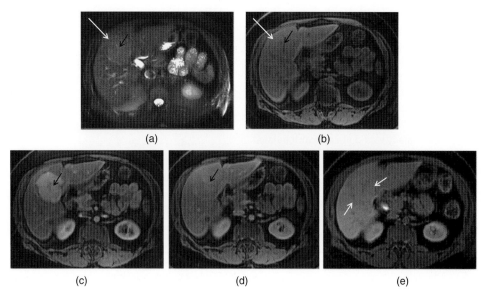

Figure 5.20 *Transverse T2-weighted fat-suppressed SS-ETSE (a), T1-weighted fat-suppressed 3D-GE (b), T1-weighted fat-suppressed 3D-GE postgadolinium hepatic arterial dominant (c), interstitial (d) and hepatocyte phase (e) images show a typical focal nodular hyperplasia (FNH) (white arrows).* The FNH has mildly increased T2 signal (a) and mildly low T1 signal (b) on precontrast images. The lesion shows typical homogeneous early increased enhancement (c) and becomes isointense with the background liver on the later phases (d). Note the central scar of the lesion (black arrows) showing increased T2/decreased T1 signal on precontrast images (a, b) and showing delayed enhancement on the interstitial phase (d). Gadolinium-BOPTA, a hepatocyte specific agent, was used and the hepatocyte phase acquired after 1 h shows the uptake of the agent by the FNH. Due to uptake of the agent, the lesion shows similar signal compared to the liver.

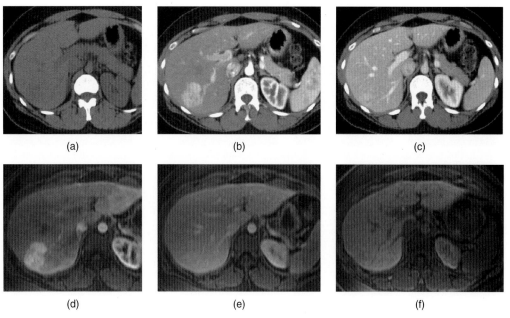

Figure 5.21 *Transverse precontrast (a), hepatic arterial dominant phase (b), hepatic venous phase (c) CT images, transverse hepatic arterial dominant (d), hepatic venous (e) and hepatocyte (f) phase fat-suppressed 3D-GE images show a focal nodular hyperplasia.* The lesion is mildly hypodense on precontrast CT image (a) and shows early relatively homogeneous increased enhancement on the early phase (b, d) and shows similar enhancement to the background liver on hepatic venous phase (c, e). The lesion becomes relatively isointense due to the uptake of gadolinium-BOPTA on the hepatocyte phase acquired 1 h after its administration.

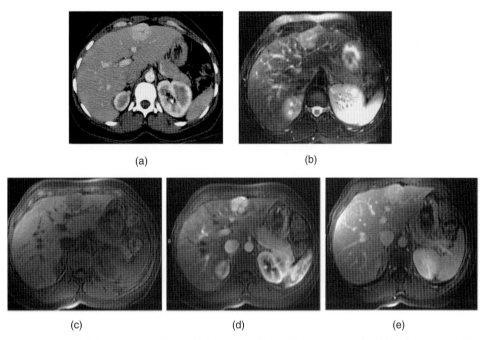

Figure 5.22 *Transverse postcontrast early hepatic venous phase CT (a), transverse T2-weighted fat-suppressed SS-ETSE (b), T1-weighted fat-suppressed 3D-GE (c), T1-weighted postgadolinium fat-suppressed hepatic arterial dominant (d) and interstitial (e) phase 3D-GE images show a medium size focal nodular hyperplasia.* The lesion demonstrates early homogeneous increased enhancement on CT (a) and MR (d) images. Due to radiation concerns, one phase of postcontrast imaging is performed on CT. Note the presence of central scar on CT and MR images, which is enhancing on the interstitial phase MR image (e).

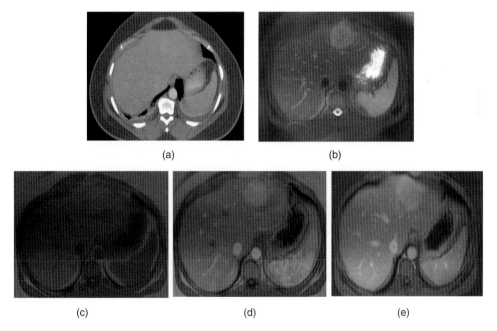

Figure 5.23 *Transverse postcontrast hepatic venous phase CT (a), transverse T2-weighted fat-suppressed SS-ETSE (b), T1-weighted 2D-GE (c), T1-weighted postgadolinium hepatic arterial dominant (d) and fat-suppressed early hepatic venous (e) phase 3D-GE images show a medium size focal nodular hyperplasia.* The lesion shows increased homogeneous enhancement on the hepatic arterial dominant phase (d) and early hepatic venous phase (e) MR images. The lesion shows mildly increased enhancement on the hepatic venous phase CT image as FNHs tend to fade and become isointense with the remaining liver parenchyma on the later phases of enhancement (a).

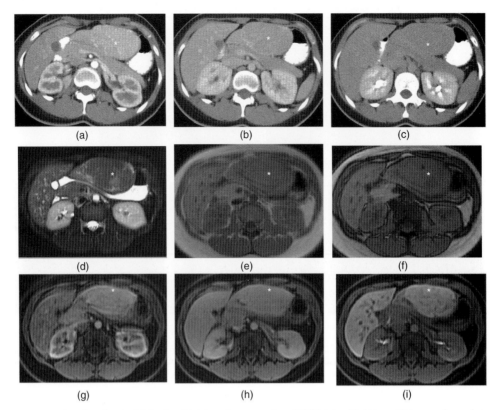

Figure 5.24 *Transverse postcontrast hepatic arterial dominant (a), hepatic venous phase CT (b), interstitial phase CT images show a hypervascular exophytic lesion (asterisk, a–c) arising from the left hepatic lobe.* The lesion shows early increased homogeneous enhancement and becomes isodense to the background liver on the later phases. Transverse T2-weighted fat-suppressed SS-ETSE (d), T1-weighted 2D-GE in-phase (e) and out-of-phase (f), T1-weighted fat-suppressed postgadolinium hepatic arterial dominant (g), interstitial (h) and hepatocyte (i) phase 3D-GE images show an exophytic pedunculated focal nodular hyperplasia (FNH) (asterisk) with atypical features. The lesion shows mildly heterogeneous signal on T2-weighted image and near isointense to the liver on precontrast T1 weighted images without fat content. The lesion shows typical enhancement features, including early homogeneous increased enhancement (g) with fading and similar enhancement to the liver on the interstitial phase (h). The lesion shows mildly increased enhancement on the hepatocyte phase at 20 min after the administration of gadoxetic acid.

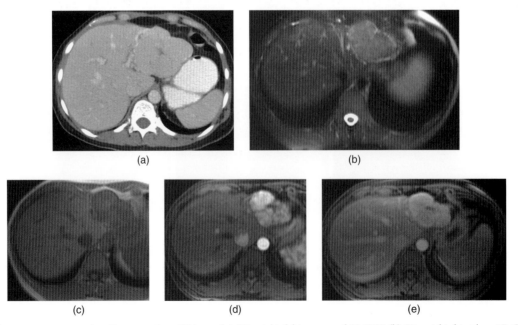

Figure 5.25 *Transverse postcontrast hepatic venous phase CT image (a), T2-weighted fat-suppressed SS-ETSE (b), T1-weighted in-phase 2D-GE (c), hepatic arterial dominant phase (d), hepatic venous phase (e) fat-suppressed 3D-GE images show a large focal nodular hyperplasia located in the atrophic left lobe of the liver.*

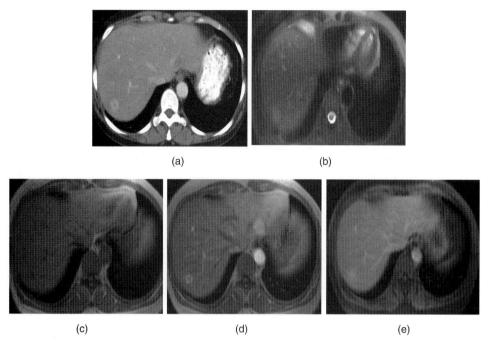

(a)　　　　　　　　　(b)

(c)　　　　　　　　(d)　　　　　　　　(e)

Figure 5.26 *Transverse postcontrast hepatic venous CT image (a) shows, a well-defined, rounded, small enhanced focal nodular hyperplasia, at segment VII with internal non enhancing central stellate scar.* Transverse T2-weighted fat-suppressed SS-ETSE (b), T1-weighted 2D-GE (c), T1-weighted postgadolinium 2D-GE hepatic arterial dominant (d) and fat-suppressed interstitial phase 3D-GE (e) images demonstrate the early enhancing small focal nodular hyperplasia (d) with an enhancing central scar on the interstitial phase (e).

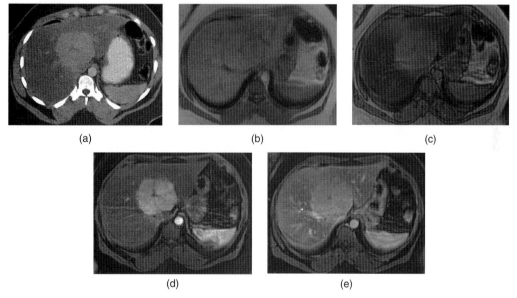

(a)　　　　　　　　　(b)　　　　　　　　　(c)

(d)　　　　　　　　(e)

Figure 5.27 *Transverse precontrast CT (a), transverse T1-weighted in-phase (b) and out-of-phase (c), T1-weighted postgadolinium hepatic arterial dominant phase (d) and hepatic venous phase (e) images show a large focal nodular hyperplasia located in a diffusely fatty liver.*

lesions, including berry aneurysms and telangiectasias of the brain (Figure 5.28)

- FNHs generally begin to involute in the fifth decade in life, and appear as small rounded lesions that may only be seen on the hepatic arterial phase MR images.
- **Imaging Findings**
- **On CT:**

° Homogeneous iso – or slightly hypo-attenuating mass on precontrast images.

° Hypo-attenuating central scar may be detected.

° Marked homogeneous enhancement during the hepatic arterial dominant phase, which fades rapidly and becomes isodense to the liver parenchyma on the later phases.

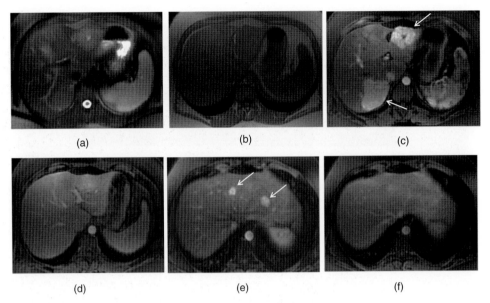

Figure 5.28 *T2-weighted fat-suppressed SS-ETSE (a), T1-weighted in-phase 2D-GE (b), hepatic arterial dominant phase (c, e), hepatic venous phase (d, f) show multiple focal nodular hyperplasias (arrows) in the liver.*

  ° The central scar, which remains hypo-attenuating during the arterial phase, gradually enhances on the later phases (Figure 5.21–5.26)
- **On MRI:**
  1 **On T1 WIs:**
    - Isointense to mildly hypointense.
    - Background fatty liver may be seen in 70% of patients with FNH.
  2 **On T2 WIs:**
    - Isointense to mildly hyperintense.
    - The central scar is hyperintense.
  3 **On postgadolinium T1WIs:**
    - FNH enhances with an intense uniform blush, sparing the central scar, on the hepatic arterial dominant phase, and fades rapidly and becomes isointense with the remaining liver parenchyma on the hepatic venous phase. In the setting of prominent background fatty liver, the lesion may appear to retain contrast as it fades in signal to that of 'normal' liver, which is higher in signal than fatty liver on fat-suppressed images.
    - The central scar of FNH is small in size with sharp angular margins.
    - Figures 5.20–5.33.
  4 **On hepatocyte phase of postgadolinium T1WIs:**
    - FNHs enhance and appear hyperintense or isointense on the hepatocyte phase. Hepatic adenomas do not contain biliary canaluculi, and cannot take up the contrast agent and appear hypointense compared to background liver parenchyma on the hepatocyte phase. This property of contrast uptake relates to cell surface membrane receptors, which are extensive in FNH and minimal in adenomas. Be careful of misdiagnosis of extremely well differentiated HCCs as FNH, especially with gadoxetic acid, as it is a more efficient hepatocyte agent.

- Gadobenate dimeglumine (multihance) and gadoxetic acid disodium (primovist/eovist) have combined early nonspecific extracellular agents with delayed hepatocyte phase. These agents are excreted by the kidneys, but also taken up by the hepatocytes and excreted into bile ducts.
- 5% of gadobenate dimeglumine is eliminated via biliary excretion, while 95% is eliminated by renal excretion. 50% of gadoxetic acid disodium is eliminated via the biliary excretion and 50% by renal excretion.
- On the hepatocyte phase, the liver parenchyma appears moderately enhanced and appears hyperintense compared to the other organs and also hyperintense compared to its appearance on precontrast images. Additionally, since these agents are excreted into the biliary system, the biliary system including the main intrahepatic and extrahepatic ducts appears hyperintense.
- Since gadobenate dimeglumine shows lesser hepatocyte uptake compared to gadoxetic acid disodium, the hepatocyte phase is reached later, at 60 min, compared to 20 min with gadoxetic acid.
- Figures 5.29–5.33
- **Differential diagnosis.**
  ° **Adenoma.** See imaging features below
  ° **Fibrolamellar HCC.** Fibrolamellar HCC contains a large, irregular scar, which is heterogeneous on T2w and postcontrast images.

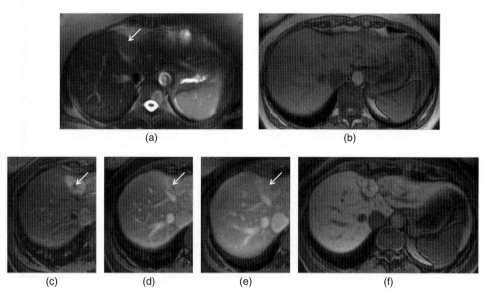

Figure 5.29 *T2-weighted fat-suppressed SS-ETSE (a), T1 out-of-phase 2D-GE (b), hepatic arterial dominant (c), hepatic venous (d), interstitial (e) and 1 h delayed hepatocyte phase (f) postgadolinium fat-suppressed 3D-GE images show a typical focal nodular hyperplasia.* The lesion shows typical mildly high T2 signal (a) and isointense T1 signal (b) with central scar (arrows) showing midly increased T2 signal and late enhancement on the interstitial phase (e). Note that besides its typical enhancement features on postgadolinium images (c–e), the lesion becomes isointense to the liver parenchyma on the hepatocyte phase (f) due to the uptake of gadolinium-BOPTA.

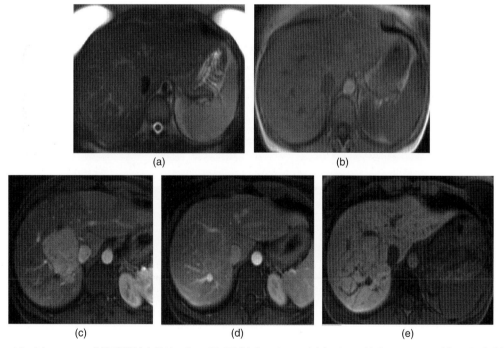

Figure 5.30 *T2-weighted fat-suppressed SS-ETSE (a), T1 in-phase 2D-GE (b), hepatic arterial dominant (c), hepatic venous (d), and 1 h delayed hepatocyte phase (e) postgadolinium fat-suppressed 3D-GE images show atypical focal nodular hyperplasia.* The lesion shows typical precontrast signal characteristics on T1- and T2- weighted images. However, the lesion does not have the central scar but shows early homogeneous enhancement (c) with fading on the hepatic venous phase (d). These features are suggestive of focal nodular hyperplasia or adenoma. However, the uptake of gadolinium-BOPTA at 1 h delayed hepatocyte phase image differentiates focal nodular hyperplasia from adenoma.

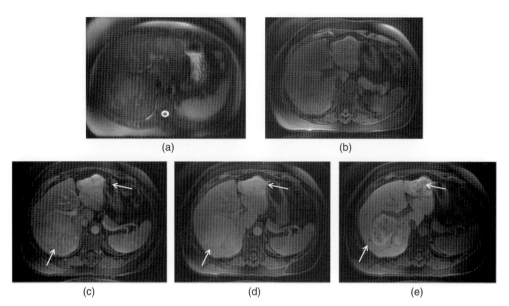

Figure 5.31 *T2-weighted fat-suppressed SS-ETSE (a), T1 fat-suppressed 3D-GE (b), early hepatic venous phase (c), interstitial (d), and 20 min delayed hepatocyte phase (e) postgadolinium fat-suppressed 3D-GE images show two atypical focal nodular hyperplasias.* Note that the lesions show mildly heterogeneous increased enhancement on early hepatic venous phase (c) and interstitial (d) phase images. The differential diagnosis includes adenoma versus focal nodular hyperplasia in a patient with no history of primary malignancy. The hepatocyte phase images show the uptake of gadoxetic acid by the lesions and therefore the lesions demonstrate heterogeneously increased enhancement, especially at the periphery compared to the background liver and are consistent with focal nodular hyperplasias.

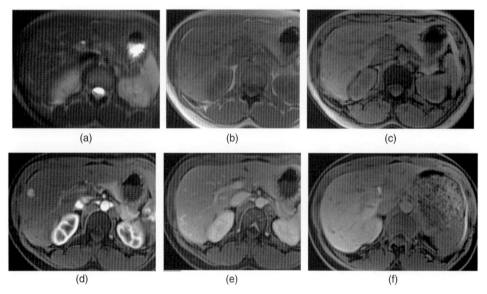

Figure 5.32 *Transverse T2-weighted fat-suppressed SS-ETSE (a), T1-weighted in-phase (b) and out-of-phase (c) 2D-GE, hepatic arterial dominant phase (d), interstitial (e), and 1 h delayed hepatocyte phase (f) fat-suppressed 3D-GE images show a small focal nodular hyperplasia with typical precontrast signal features and delayed uptake on the hepatocyte phase (f).* No central scar is seen in the hepatic arterial dominant phase (d). The lesion shows early homogeneous increased enhancement (d) and fading on the hepatic venous phase (e) on postgadolinium images. The lesion does not demonstrate signal drop on out-of-phase image (c). Peripheral enhancement is seen on the hepatocyte phase (f) due to the uptake of gadolinium-BOPTA suggestive of focal nodular hyperplasia.

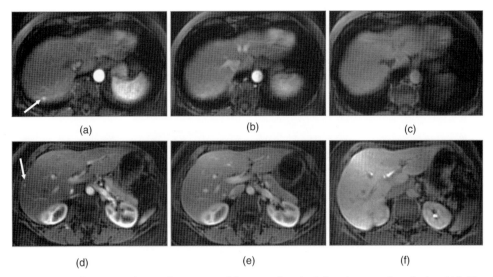

Figure 5.33 *Transverse T1-weighted fat-suppressed 3D-GE hepatic arterial dominant phase (a, d), hepatic venous phase (b, e), and 1 h delayed hepatocyte phase (c, f) images show nodular homogeneously early enhancing lesions (a, d) fading on the hepatic venous phase (b, e) and showing similar enhancement to the background liver on the hepatocyte phase (c, f) due to uptake of gadolinium-BOPTA.*

° **High grade dysplastic nodule.** The presence of chronic liver disease is the key to the distinction for small lesions (as small FNHs may not show a central scar). If there is chronic liver disease, the likelihood of high grade dysplastic nodules is extremely high compared to FNH.

Hepatocellular adenomas

- Are uncommon benign neoplasms, most often observed in women who are taking, or have taken, oral contraceptives.
- Female to male ratio is 10 : 1.
- Most are solitary (80%)
- Approximately 70% are fat-containing (Figure 5.34) (a rare feature in FNH, which is however associated with background fatty liver).
- Associated with:
  ° The use of oral contraceptive pills. Adenomas may involute after the cessation of oral contraceptive use, but involution is usually mild in this setting.
  ° Anabolic steroids, especially in men.
  ° Disorders associated with abnormal carbohydrate metabolism, such as diabetes mellitus, galactosemia, and glycogen storage disease type 1 and 3. Type 1A glycogen storage disease, Von Gierke disease often develop multiple hepatic adenomas at young age.
- Most often asymptomatic. Rarely patients may present with discomfort due to large size of tumor or with acute abdominal pain, related to hemorrhage into the tumor or into the peritoneal cavity.
- Lesions spontaneously begin to involute in women in their 50s, most likely related to hormone changes of menopause.
- Multiple adenoma syndrome is a rare form of this entity.
- Malignant transformation is rare and sporadic and likely related to the underlying genetics of the tumor. Most

cases of apparent malignant transformation may reflect histopathological misinterpretation of the original specimen.

- **Histopathology:**
  ° Sheets of normal-appearing hepatocytes separated by dilated sinusoids but lacking the normal acinar architecture of hepatic parenchyma.
  ° Enclosed by a pseudocapsule.
  ° Do not contain bile ducts, which is the distinguishing feature from FNH. As a result, hepatocyte-specific contrast agents cannot be excreted into nonexistent bile ducts. This process may be related though to cell surface membrane receptors.
  ° Intratumoral fat is common; necrosis, hemorrhage, or large subcapsular vessels are also observed not infrequently.
  ° Solitary tumors appear as a bulging mass with dilated blood vessels traversing the surface, partially or completely enclosed by a pseudocapsule, which is derived from compressed and collapsed hepatic parenchyma.
- The CT and MRI appearances of hepatocellular adenoma are varied, and reflect the quantity of fat, hemorrhage, and necrosis within the tumor.
- **On CT:**
  ° May be hypoattenuating due to the presence of fat, old hemorrhage, or necrosis on noncontrast CT images.
  ° May be hyperattenuating owing to recent hemorrhage or large amounts of glycogen on noncontrast CT images.
  ° May be heterogeneous on noncontrast CT images.
  ° May show increased homogenous enhancement on the hepatic arterial dominant phase. On the hepatic venous phase, they may fade or show wash-out. Heterogeneous enhancement may also be on the hepatic arterial dominant or venous phase, especially if the lesion is large in size, or hemorrhage or necrosis is present.
  ° Figures 5.34 and 5.35.

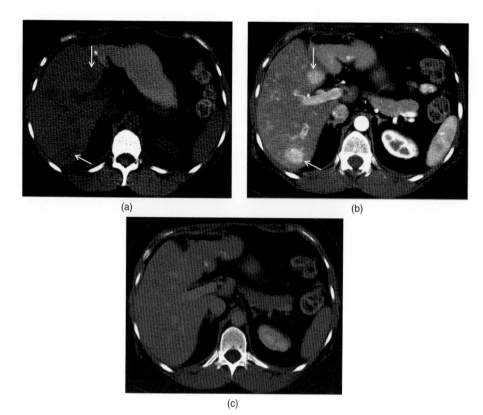

(a)   (b)

(c)

Figure 5.34 *Transverse precontrast CT (a), postcontrast hepatic arterial dominant phase (b) and hepatic venous phase (c) CT images demonstrate several hepatic adenomas (arrows).* They appear as hypoattenuating mass lesions on precontrast CT image (a), show homogeneous prominent enhancement on the hepatic arterial dominant phase (b) and fading on the hepatic venous phase (c). Due to fading, the lesions could not be appreciated on the hepatic venous phase (c).

- **On MRI**
  - **On T1:**
    - Typically homogeneously mildly hypointense or isointense.
    - May be hyperintense on in-phase with homogeneously decreased signal intensity on out-of-phase or fat-suppressed images due to their fat content, which is commonly uniform (in contrast to HCC, which is usually heterogeneous).
    - May be hyperintense on in-phase that does not show drop of signal on out-of-phase, due to the presence of sub-acute hemorrhage.
    - Heterogeneous signal, due to hemorrhage in varying stages of maturation +/− necrosis.
  - **On T2:**
    - Typically homogeneously mildly hyperintense or isointense.
    - Heterogeneous signal pattern if hemorrhage or necrosis is present.
  - **With contrast:**
    - Typically transient homogeneous enhancement on the hepatic arterial dominant phase. Heterogeneous enhancement may also be seen, depending on the presence of hemorrhage or necrosis.
    - Homogeneous enhancement may either show:

(a) Uniform fading to isointensity with liver parenchyma on the hepatic venous phase, which is the most common late enhancement pattern.

(b) Wash-out on venous phase images, that may be early or late. Adenoma is the only benign tumor that can show wash-out. The differentiation between HCC and adenoma may need to be based on the clinical circumstance. HCC should be diagnosed in patients with underlying chronic liver disease or cirrhosis, whereas in women with ongoing or a history of oral contraceptive use and no history or lab findings of chronic liver disease adenoma should be considered in the differential diagnosis. Follow-up MRI may be essential to assess for interval change.

- May be differentiated from FNHs on the hepatocyte phase as FNHs show uptake of the hepatocyte specific agent. However, except FNHs and well differentiated HCCs, all lesions which do not contain hepatocytes appear as hypointense lesions compared to the background liver on the hepatocyte phase. Therefore, clinical history and morphologic signal characteristics of the lesions and their enhancement features on the hepatic arterial dominant, hepatic venous, and interstitial phase images are critical.
- Figures 5.34 – 5.43.

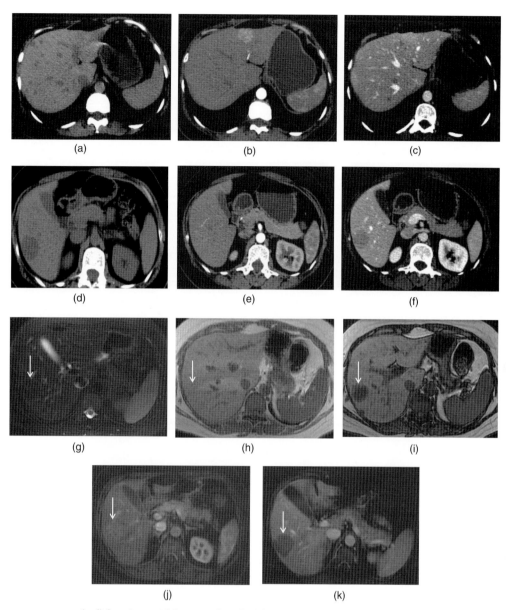

Figure 5.35 *Transverse precontrast (a, d), hepatic arterial dominant phase (b, e), hepatic venous phase (c, f) CT images show a focal nodular hyperplasia in the segment IVA and an adenoma in the segment VI.* The focal nodular hyperplasia shows early increased enhancement on the hepatic arterial dominant phase (b) and becomes isodense on the hepatic venous phase (c). The adenoma shows early homogeneous increased enhancement on the hepatic arterial dominant phase (e) and wash-out on the hepatic venous phase (f). Transverse T2-weighted SS-ETSE (g), T1-weighted in-phase 2D-GE (h) and out-of-phase (i), T1-weighted postgadolinium hepatic arterial dominant (j) and hepatic venous phase (k) 3D-GE images the adenoma in the same patient. The adenoma shows near isointense signal on T2 and in-phase T1-weighted images. MRI images demonstrate fat content of the adenoma which is characterized by the signal drop on out-of-phase images compared to in-phase image. The adenoma demonstrates early mild increased enhancement (j) and wash-out on the hepatic venous phase (k).

- **Differential Diagnosis.**
  - ° **HCC** (see Chapter 7 for imaging features)
  - ° **FNH**
  - ° **Focal fat.** Focal fat should show arterial enhancement comparable to background liver whereas fatty lesions (e.g., adenoma) most often show arterial phase hyperenhancement.

Liver adenomatosis

- Is an uncommon form of liver adenoma
  - ° Characterized by numerous adenomas (>5), most often varying in size from <1 cm to large tumors in the same individual.

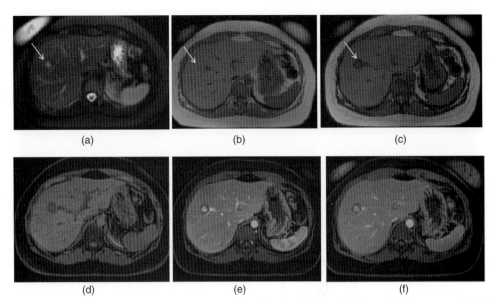

Figure 5.36 *Transverse T2-weighted SS-ETSE (a), T1-weighted in-phase 2D-GE (b) and out-of-phase (c), T1-weighted fat suppressed 3D-GE (d), T1-weighted postgadolinium early hepatic venous phase (e) and hepatic venous phase (f) 3D-GE images show a small adenoma.* The adenoma demonstrates mildly increased T2 signal (a) and decreased peripheral signal on out-of-phase image (c) compared to in-phase image (b). The lesion shows central homogeneous enhancement on postgadolinium images (e, f).

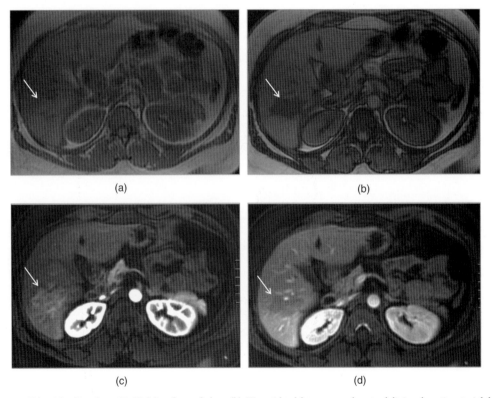

Figure 5.37 *Transverse T1-weighted in-phase 2D-GE (a) and out-of-phase (b), T1-weighted fat suppressed postgadolinium hepatic arterial dominant phase (c) and hepatic venous phase 3D-GE (d) images demonstrate an adenoma.* The lesion shows signal drop on out-of-phase image (b) compared to in-phase image (a). The lesion demonstrates early increased enhancement (c) and wash-out on the later phase (d).

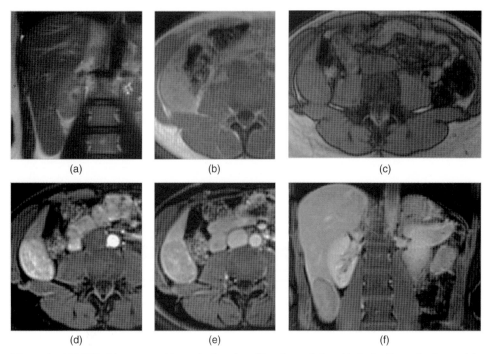

Figure 5.38 *Coronal T2-weighted SS-ETSE (a), transverse T1-weighted in-phase (b) and out-of-phase (c) 2D-GE, T1-weighted postgadolinium hepatic arterial dominant phase (d), hepatic venous phase (e) and coronal interstitial phase 3D-GE images demonstrate a fat containing adenoma in the segment VI. The lesion shows signal drop on out-of-phase image (c) due to its fat content, early enhancement (d) and late wash-out (e, f).*

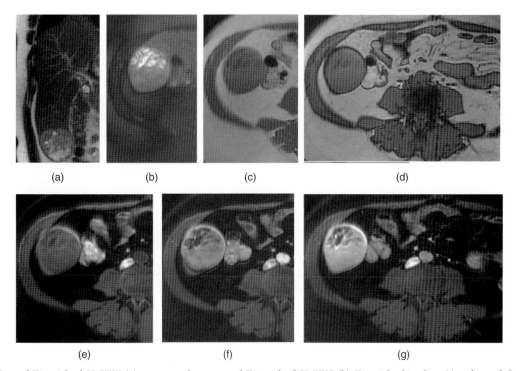

Figure 5.39 *Coronal T2-weighted SS-ETSE (a), transverse fat-suppressed T2-weighted SS-ETSE (b), T1-weighted in-phase (c) and out-of-phase (d) 2D-GE, T1-weighted postgadolinium hepatic arterial dominant phase (e), hepatic venous phase (f) and interstitial phase (g) 3D-GE images show an oval mass with heterogeneous precontrast signal and heterogeneous enhancement. The lesion shows cystic necrotic changes without evidence of fat content. The lesion histopathologically is consistent with adenoma.*

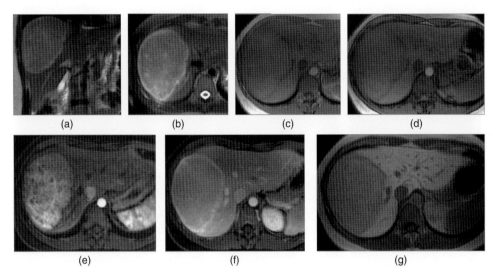

Figure 5.40 *Coronal T2-weighted SS-ETSE (a), transverse fat-suppressed T2-weighted SS-ETSE (b), T1-weighted in-phase (c) and out-of-phase (d) 2D-GE, T1-weighted postgadolinium hepatic arterial dominant phase (e), hepatic venous phase (f) and hepatocyte phase (g) 3D-GE images show a large heterogeneous adenoma without evidence of fat content.* The lesion shows early heterogeneous enhancement (e) with late wash-out and capsular enhancement (f). As the adenoma does not show uptake of gadolinium-BOPTA, it depicts decreased signal compared to the background liver on the hepatocyte phase (g).

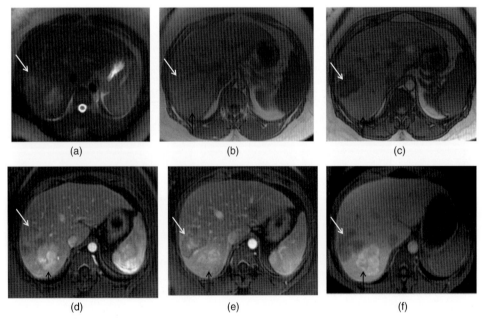

Figure 5.41 *Transverse T2-weighted SS-ETSE (a), T1-weighted in-phase 2D-GE (b) and out-of-phase (c), T1-weighted fat suppressed postgadolinium hepatic arterial dominant phase (d), hepatic venous phase (e) and hepatocyte phase (f) 3D-GE images demonstrate an adenoma (white arrows) and focal nodular hyperplasia (black arrows) in the right lobe of the liver.* The adenoma shows signal drop on out-of-phase image (white arrow, c) compared to in-phase image (b) due to its fat content. The adenoma shows decreased signal on the hepatocyte phase (f) compared to the background liver as it does not show uptake of gadoxetic acid. The focal nodular hyperplasia shows increased enhancement compared to the background liver on the hepatocyte phase due to the uptake of gadoxetic acid.

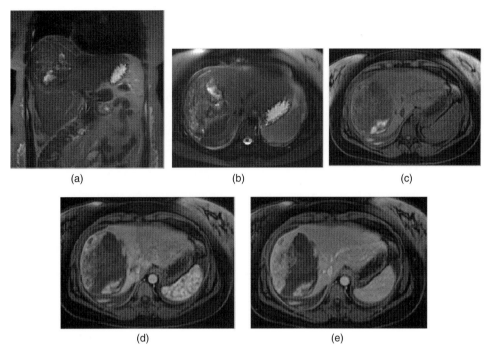

Figure 5.42 *Coronal T2-weighted SS-ETSE (a), transverse fat-suppressed T2-weighted SS-ETSE (b), T1-weighted fat suppressed 3D-GE (c), postgadolinium hepatic arterial dominant phase (d), hepatic venous phase (e) fat-suppressed 3D-GE images show a large enhancing heterogeneous mass with hemorrhage in the right lobe, which is consistent with a hemorrhagic adenoma.* The lesion has layering blood products posteriorly, which show increased T1 signal (c). Transient early increased enhancement is noted around the lesion due to the compression of the right portal vein and inflammatory response.

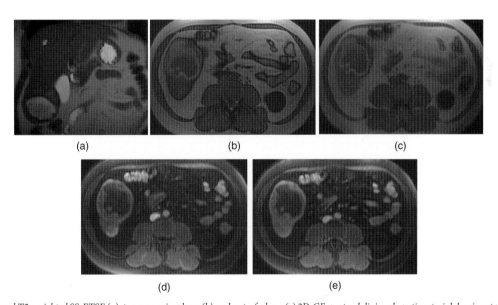

Figure 5.43 *Coronal T2-weighted SS-ETSE (a), transverse in-phase (b) and out-of-phase (c) 2D-GE, postgadolinium hepatic arterial dominant phase (d), hepatic venous phase (e) fat-suppressed 3D-GE images show a heterogeneous mass consistent with hemorrhagic adenoma.* The lesion shows peripheral increased T1 signal on in-phase and out-of-phase images and central cystic changes (b, c) due to hemorrhage. The lesion shows heterogeneously increased enhancement. Source: Semelka 2010. Reproduced with permission of Wiley.

∘ Although historically considered not related to oral contraceptive use, about 50% of patients have taken oral contraceptives.

∘ More common in women, but the ratio is less than for solitary adenomas, perhaps 5 to 1.

∘ May have abnormal liver function tests, which may be related to background fatty liver, which is common for multiple adenoma syndrome, but relatively uncommon in solitary adenoma.

∘ Hemorrhage may be seen.

∘ Adenomas may contain fat, but with a lesser frequency than is observed in solitary adenoma.

∘ Enhancement patterns are similar to solitary adenomas, although there is a lesser tendency for early intense arterial enhancement.

∘ Figures 5.44 – 5.46.

Peliosis hepatis

- Rare benign vascular lesion, characterized by the presence of grossly visible cystic blood-filled spaces and sinusoidal dilatation in the liver, that lacks an endothelial lining.
- Commonly this histology co-exists with adenomas.
- Peliosis hepatis occurs most commonly in the liver, but can occasionally occur in other parts of the reticuloendothelial system, including the spleen or bone marrow.
- Risk factors:
  ∘ No risk factors are most commonly found.
  ∘ Numerous risk factors though have been described, including infectious diseases; cancer; transplantations; drugs such as androgenenic anabolic steroids and oral contraceptives; diabetes; sprue; necrotizing vasculitis; and exposure to polyvinyl chloride and arsenic.
- **Imaging:**
- **CT:**
- Lesions are frequently multiple. They are usually hypodense on precontrast images. Areas of hemorrhage may be seen as hyperdense areas on precontrast examinations. Moderate, usually homogeneous, enhancement is present.
- **MRI:** Multiple lesions are usually present and may be extensive. Variable signal intensity on T1-weighted images is observed, reflecting various stage of hemorrhage, but the majority are isointense or hypointense. Hyperintense signal may be observed on T1-weighted images due to hemorrhage.
- Variable signal intensity on T2-weighted images, but most lesions show moderately high T2 signal.
- Following contrast administration, the lesions may show relatively intense arterial phase enhancement, which engenders considerable alarm in the interpreting radiologist. The enhancement though varies among the population of lesions, and lesions may mildy to moderately fade or show variable late enhancement, including generally progressive enhancement of the lesions with time.
- Figures 5.47 and 5.48.

Angiomyolipoma and lipoma

- Angiomyolipoma is an uncommon benign mesenchymal tumor composed of smooth muscle, blood vessels, and variable amounts of adipose tissue.
- Although there is an association with tuberous sclerosis, they are more commonly sporadic.
- They are well-defined, sharply marginated masses with high fat content. Lesions most often have high fat content.
- Lesions may appear as two forms (based on fat content):
  1 With high fat content:
  - High signal intensity on T1, phase cancellation on out-of-phase, fat signal on T2, and low signal on fat-suppression (either T1 or T2 weighted fat suppressed images). Minimal enhancement is usually seen on postgadolinium images. The lesions show negative HU values on precontrast CT due to their fat content.

  2 With low fat content:
  - Intermediate signal on T1, variable signal drop on out-of-phase (reflecting fat content, mild to moderately high signal on T2, minimal fat suppression. The extent of enhancement is variable and reflects the extent of vascular component.
- Figures 5.49 and 5.50
  Differential Diagnosis
  - Adenoma. Adenomas are more common and have a much lesser fat content.
  - HCC. Angiomyolipomas with low fat content have a more organized pattern of vascular enhancement on the arterial phase than HCC, and will not show late wash-out and capsule enhancement.
- Lipomas are rarer than angiomyolipomas.
- Lipomas show pure or abundant fat content without appreciable enhancement on both CT and MRI.

Inflammatory myofibroblastic tumor (inflammatory pseudotumor)

- Inflammatory myofibroblastic tumors (IMTs) are characterized by proliferation of nonneoplastic myofibroblastic spindle cells. IMTs are rare lesions of uncertain etiology that may arise in many organs in the body including the liver.

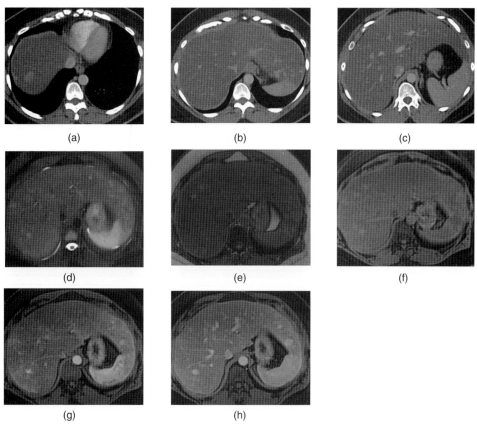

Figure 5.44 *Transverse postcontrast CT images (a-c), T2-weighted fat-suppressed SS-ETSE (d), T1-weighted out-of-phase images (e), fat-suppressed 3D-GE images (f), early hepatic venous phase (g) and hepatic venous phase (h) images show multiple oval lesions which demonstrate homogeneous enhancement on postcontrast images.* These lesions represent multiple adenomotosis in the liver. Note that the liver is fatty.

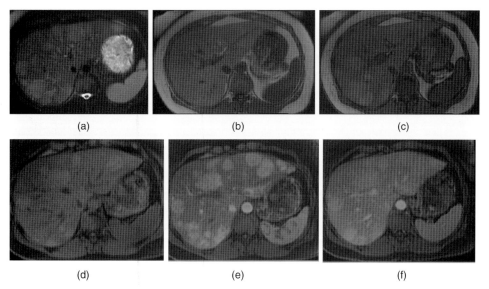

Figure 5.45 *Transverse T2-weighted SS-ETSE (a), T1-weighted in-phase 2D-GE (b) and out-of-phase (c), T1-weighted fat suppressed 3D-GE (d), postgadolinium hepatic arterial dominant phase (e), hepatic venous phase (f) images show multiple homogeneously enhancing adenomas in the fatty liver.*

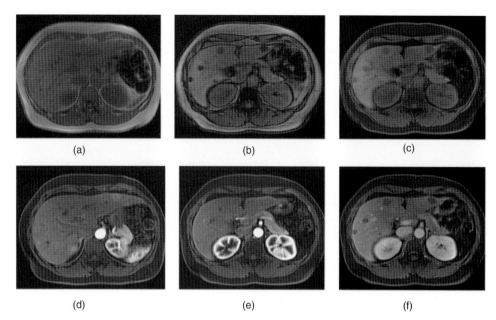

Figure 5.46 *Transverse T1-weighted in-phase (a) and out-of-phase (b) 2D-GE, T1-weighted fat suppressed 3D-GE (c), postgadolinium hepatic arterial dominant phase (d, e), hepatic venous phase (f) 3D-GE images show multiple fat-containing adenomas in the liver.* The lesions show signal drop on out-of-phase image (b) compared to in-phase image (a). The lesions show homogeneously early increased enhancement (d, e) and wash-out on the later phase (f).

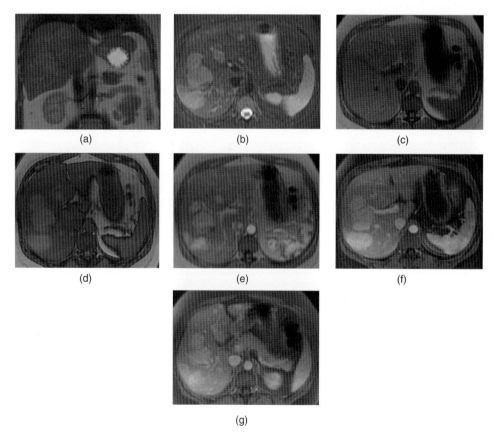

Figure 5.47 *Coronal T2-weighted SS-ETSE (a), transverse T2-weighted STIR (b), transverse T1-weighted in-phase (c) and out-of-phase 2D-GE (d), T1-weighted postgadolinium hepatic arterial dominant phase 2D-GE (e), hepatic venous phase fat-suppressed 3D-GE (f, g) images demonstrate multiple hypervascular lesions consistent with peliosis hepatis.* The lesions show moderately high T2 signal on T2-weighted STIR image (b) while they are isointense on T1-weighted in-phase image (c). As diffuse fat deposition is seen in the liver, the lesions appear as hyperintense lesions on out-of-phase image (d). Due to their hypervascular nature, the lesions show early homogeneously increased enhancement in the hepatic arterial dominant phase (e) and maintain their enhancements in the later phases (f, g).

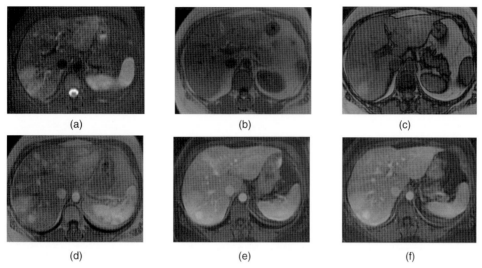

Figure 5.48 *Transverse T2-weighted STIR (a), T1-weighted in-phase (b) and out-of-phase (c) 2D-GE, T1-weighted early hepatic arterial dominant phase 2D-GE (d), hepatic venous phase fat-suppressed 3D-GE (e, f) images show multiple hypervascular lesions consistent with peliosis hepatis.* The lesions show mild to moderately high signal on T2-weighted image (a) and high T1-signal on in-phase and out-of-phase images (b, c) due to the presence of hemorrhage/blood products in the lesions. The lesions demonstrate increased early enhancement on the hepatic arterial dominant phase (d) and maintain their enhancement in the later phases (e, f).

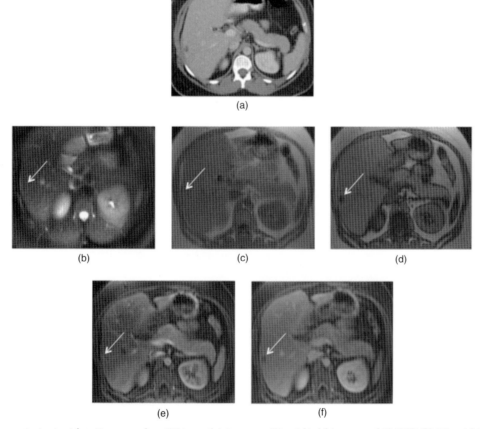

Figure 5.49 *Transverse postcontrast hepatic venous phase CT image (a), transverse T2-weighted fat-suppressed SS-ETSE (b), T1-weighted in-phase (c) and out-of-phase (d) 2D-GE, T1-weighted postgadolinium fat-suppressed hepatic arterial dominant phase (e) and hepatic venous phase (f) 3D-GE images show a small angiomyolipoma (arrows) in the right lobe of the liver.* The lesion appears as a hypoattenuating fat-containing lesion with negative HU values on CT. The lesion drops in signal due to its fat content on out-of-phase image (d). The lesion shows mild enhancement on postgadolinium images (e, f). The lesion appears as an enhancing hyperintense lesion on the hepatic arterial dominant phase (e) because the background liver does not show prominent enhancement as the lesion does. On the hepatic venous phase (f), the lesion appears hypointense compared to the background liver as the liver now shows prominent and more enhancement compared to the lesion.

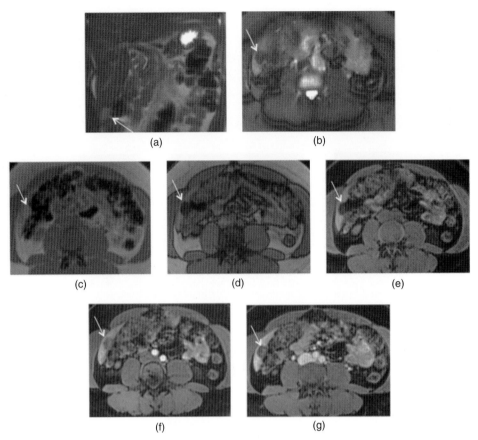

Figure 5.50 *Coronal T2-weighted SS-ETSE (a), transverse T2-weighted fat-suppressed SS-ETSE (b), T1-weighted in-phase (c) and out-of-phase (d) 2D-GE, fat-suppressed 3D-GE (e), postgadolinium hepatic arterial dominant phase (f) and hepatic venous phase (g) 3D-GE images show an oval fat-containing lesion (arrows) with mild enhancement.* The lesion contains abundant amount of fat and is consistent with an angiomyolipoma.

- The liver is the second most common organ involved following the lungs.
- The etiology of IMTs is unknown. Traumas, surgical procedures, immune – autoimmune mechanisms and infectious causes have been implicated. Implicated infectious causes include Epstein-Barr virus, actinomycetes, nocardiae, and mycoplasma.
- **Microscopically:**
  - They contain cells associated with acute and chronic inflammation, including lymphocytes, plasma cells, myofibroblastic spindle cells, macrophages, and histiocytes.
  - Prominent fibrosis and collagen content are characteristic features.
  - Areas of necrosis and obliteration of blood vessels may be noted.
- **Clinically:**
  - Most frequently seen in Asia and more common in men and young adults.
  - They may be associated with systemic symptoms, including fever, weight loss, malaise, right upper quadrant pain, biliary obstruction, or portal hypertension.
  - Although the disease often responds to steroid administration and the prognosis is usually good, fatal outcome has also been reported.
- **Imaging:**
  - Commonly present as single masses, although multifocal masses are not uncommon.
  - Ill-defined or well-defined tumor-like lesions within the parenchyma or periportal soft tissue mass involving the hilum.
  - Central necrosis may be seen. Capsular retraction may be detected due to its fibrotic content.
- **CT:**
  - Hypoattenuated lesions on unenhanced CT images. The lesions may also contain cystic areas.
  - Various patterns of enhancement are seen on postcontrast CT images, including progressive heterogeneous enhancement, homogeneous enhancement, and peripheral enhancement with progressive centripedal enhancement. Additionally, enhancement of septa in multiloculated cystic lesions is seen.

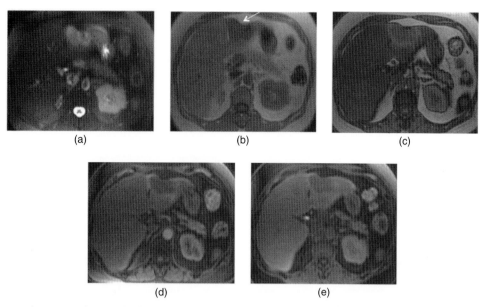

Figure 5.51 *Transverse fat-suppressed T2-weighted SS-ETSE (a), T1-weighted in-phase (b) and out-of-phase (c) 2D-GE, T1-weighted postgadolinium fat-suppressed hepatic arterial dominant phase (d) and hepatocyte phase (e) 3D-GE images demonstrate an inflammatory myofibroblastic tumor which shows capsular retraction (arrow, b) due to its fibrous content.* The lesion is located in the left lobe of the liver and demonstrates moderately high T2 signal (a) and low T1 signal (b) on precontrast sequences. The background liver is fatty and the compressed liver parenchyma around the lesion appears as a hyperintense rim due to its inability to deposit fat. The lesion does not show prominent enhancement on the hepatic arterial dominant phase due to its fibrous content and appears as a hypointense lesion due to the lack of hepatocytes on the hepatocyte phase.

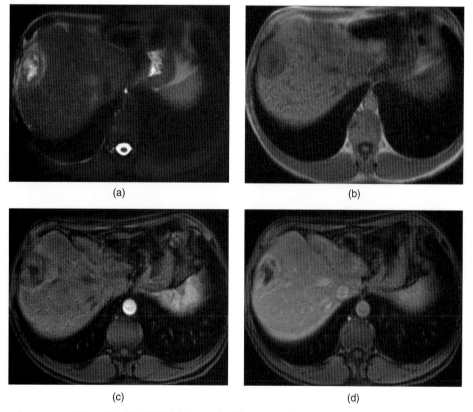

Figure 5.52 *Transverse fat-suppressed T2-weighted SS-ETSE (a), T1-weighted fat-suppressed 3D-GE (b), T1-weighted postgadolinium fat-suppressed hepatic arterial dominant phase (c) and hepatic venous phase (d) 3D-GE images show an inflammatory myofibroblastic tumor located in segment VIII of the right lobe of the liver.* This complex lesion has a central cystic – necrotic component demonstrating markedly high T2 signal. Early peripheral transient increased enhancement, which is consistent with inflammation, is seen around the lesion on the hepatic arterial dominant phase. The lesion shows progressive enhancement on the hepatic venous phase. Postcontrast hepatic venous phase CT (e) and postgadolinium hepatic arterial dominant phase (f) images show the progressive prominent decrease in size of the lesion after the treatment. The lesion (arrow) is hardly visible and appears as a tiny enhancing focus on the last postgadolinium image (f). Source: Semelka 2010. Reproduced with permission of Wiley.

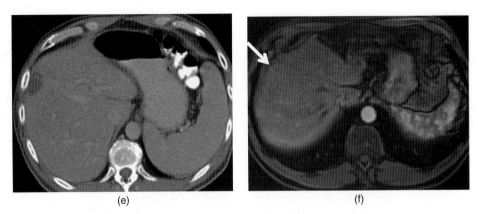

(e)   (f)

Figure 5.52 *(Continued.)*

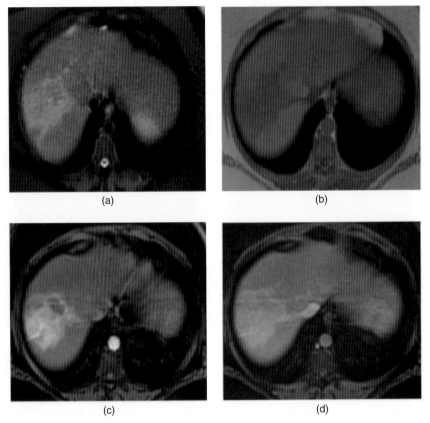

(a)   (b)

(c)   (d)

Figure 5.53 *Transverse fat-suppressed T2-weighted SS-ETSE (a), T1-weighted in-phase (b) 2D-GE, T1-weighted postgadolinium fat-suppressed hepatic arterial dominant phase (c) and hepatic venous phase (d) 3D-GE images demonstrate an irregular infiltrative lesion located in segment VIII. The lesion shows moderately high T2 signal (a) and prominent early enhancement on the hepatic arterial dominant phase (c) which fades on the hepatic venous phase (d).*

- **MRI:**
  - Mild to moderately high signal on T2-weighted images. Cystic components and central necrosis may show moderate to markedly high signal.
  - Mild to moderately low signal on T1-weighted images.
  - May be cystic and multiloculated, and may contain septa.
  - Various enhancement patterns can be seen, including homogeneous moderate to intense enhancement on the hepatic arterial dominant phase and fading on later phases; progressive heterogeneous enhancement; early peripheral enhancement with progressive centripedal enhancement on later phases. Delayed enhancement may be seen

prominently due to fibrotic component on the interstitial phase. Septa of multiloculated cystic lesions demonstrate enhancement. Enhancement extent likely corresponds with the age of the lesion.

° Lesions of recent onset enhance more vigorously, and can simulate malignant disease. A critical observation is that lesions fade in signal. This appearance is similar to chronic eosinophilic infiltrate, which also has a propensity to involve Asians. As lesions age, they progressively adopt a less aggressive appearance, and the appearance resembles that of progressively more mature fibrotic tissue. At later stages, the lesions have irregular angular margins with minimal early enhancement and progressive late enhancement, which is the appearance of a focus of fibrosis from any underlying cause. Lesions may also eventually spontaneously resolve.

° The lesions may respond to treatment (steroids) or spontaneously regress and disappear. Spontaneous regression of an aggressive looking lesion, without therapy, over a six month period, is supportive of the diagnosis. However, areas of residual fibrosis may remain after the regression of the lesions and may demonstrate mildly low signal on T2- and T1-weighted images and exhibit negligible enhancement.

° Figures 5.51–5.53.

• **Differential diagnosis:**
   ° HCC. HCCs wash out whereas IMTs do not show wash-out and may fade on late postcontrast images.

° Abscess
° Lymphoma
° Cholangiocarcinoma

References

1 Ramalho, M., Altun, E., Heredia, V. *et al.* (2007) Liver imaging: 1.5 T versus 3 T. Magn Reson Imaging Clin N Am, 15, 321–347.

2 Sousa MS, Ramalho M, Heredia V, et al. (2014) Perilesional enhancement of liver cavernous hemangiomas in magnetic resonance imaging. Abdom Imaging, 39, 722–730.

3 Anderson, S.W., Kruskal, J.B., and Kane, R.A. (2009) Benign hepatic tumors and iatrogenic pseudotumors. Radiographics, 29, 211–229.

4 Hussain, S.M., Zondervan, P.E., Ijerzermans, J.N. *et al.* (2002) Benign versus malignant hepatic nodules: MR imaging findings with pathologic correlation. Radiographics, 22, 1023–1039.

5 Horton, K.M., Bluemke, D.A., Hruban, R.H. *et al.* (1999) CT and MR imaging of benign hepatic and biliary tumors. Radiographics, 19, 431–451.

6 Grazioli, L., Morana, G., Kirchin, M.A., and Scheneider, G. (2005) Accurate differentiation of focal nodular hyperplasia from hepatic adenoma at gadobenate dimeglumine-enhanced MR imaging: prospective study. Radiology, 236, 166–177.

7 Gandhi, S.N., Brown, M., Wong, J.G. *et al.* (2006) MR contrast agents for liver imaging: what, when, how. Radiographics, 26 (6), 1621–1636.

8 Venkataraman, S., Semelka, R.C., Braga, L. *et al.* (2003) Inflammatory myofibroblastic tumor of the hepatobiliary system: report of MR imaging appearance in four patients. Radiology, 227, 758–763.

CHAPTER 6

Liver metastases

Ersan Altun[1], Mohamed El-Azzazi[1,2,3,4], Richard C. Semelka[1], and Miguel Ramalho[1,5],

[1] The University of North Carolina at Chapel Hill, Department of Radiology, Chapel Hill, NC, USA
[2] University of Dammam, Department of Radiology, Dammam, Saudi Arabia
[3] King Fahd Hospital of the University, Department of Radiology, Khobar, Saudi Arabia
[4] University of Al Azhar, Department of Radiology, Cairo, Egypt
[5] Hospital Garcia de Orta, Department of Radiology, Almada, Portugal

- Metastases are the most common malignant tumors of the liver.
- The liver, lungs, and bones are the most common sites of metastases in the body.
- Liver metastases usually appear as multiple nodules, but may also appear as a solitary nodule (colon cancer is the primary that has the greatest tendency to result in a solitary metastasis). Multiple nodules may form confluent masses. The presence of diffuse nodular metastases may mimic cirrhotic liver. Isolated infiltrative parenchymal metastatic lesions are also occasionally seen. Isolated infiltrative metastatic lesions may also be seen along the portal tracts and in the porta hepatis.
- Metastasis may be complicated by hemorrhage, central necrosis, or cystic change. Metastases may also contain calcifications, which are most frequently associated with mucinous adenocarcinomas of the colon and ovary, and medullary thyroid carcinoma.
- The presence of diffuse nodular metastases may mimic cirrhotic liver, especially following response to chemotherapy (an appearance most often seen with breast cancer).
- **CT features of liver metastases on precontrast images**
  - Usually seen as hypoattenuating lesions (Figure 6.1)
  - May be seen as hyperattenuating lesions if they contain hemorrhage or high protein such as mucin as in hemorrhagic metastases, or mucinous tumors such as ovarian mucinous tumors or mucinous colon carcinoma.
  - Calcifications may be seen in the metastases of mucinous adenocarcinoma of the colon and ovary, and medullary thyroid cancer.
- **MR features of liver metastases on precontrast sequences**
  - Mild to moderately high in signal intensity on T2-WIs (Figure 6.2).

  - Moderately low in signal intensity on T1-WIs (Figure 6.2).
  - High signal intensity on T1-WIs may be seen in various metastatic lesions due to the presence of paramagnetic substances, including extracellular methemoglobin (hemorrhagic metastases), melanin (malignant melanoma) (Figure 6.3), protein (ovarian adenocarcinoma, multiple myeloma, and pancreatic mucinous cystic tumors) (Figure 6.4), and coagulative necrosis (colon adenocarcinoma).
- **Target sign**
  - A central area of high signal intensity on T2-WIs and low signal intensity on T1-WIs corresponds to central liquefactive necrosis (Figures 6.2 and 6.5).
  - Peripheral rim of tissue with relatively lower signal on T2-WI and relatively higher signal on T1-WI corresponds to viable tumor (Figure 6.5).
- **Halo sign**
  - A central area of lower signal intensity relative to the higher intensity tumor periphery on T2-WI (Figure 6.6) and a central higher signal intensity relative to lower signal intensity on T1-WI.
  - The central area corresponds to coagulative necrosis, fibrin, and mucin, while the tumor periphery corresponds to viable tumor cells.
  - Seen not uncommonly (approximately 25%), metastases from colorectal carcinoma.
- **Enhancement of metastases on CT and MRI**
  - Enhancement characteristics of metastases are better defined on MRI than CT, reflecting that MRI is more sensitive to gadolinium contrast than CT to iodine contrast, and MRI is generally performed multiphase, whereas CT

Liver Imaging: MRI with CT Correlation, First Edition. Edited by Ersan Altun, Mohamed El-Azzazi and Richard C. Semelka.

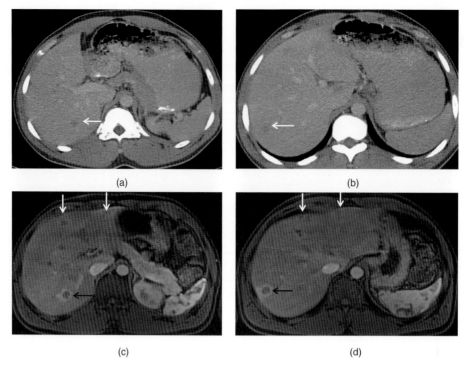

Figure 6.1 *Transverse postcontrast hepatic venous phase images (a, b) demonstrate small, ill-defined hypodense enhancing lesions (arrows) in the right hepatic lobe in a patient with colon adenocarcinoma.* Transverse postgadolinium hepatic arterial dominant phase T1-weighted fat-suppressed 3D-GE images (c, d) demonstrate the lesions (black arrows) detected in the right hepatic lobe seen on CT. These lesions demonstrate typical peripheral enhancement and are consistent with liver metastases secondary to colon adenocarcinoma. Please note that peripheral prominent enhancement is very well seen on MR images compared to CT. Additional smaller lesions (white arrows; c, d) showing peripheral enhancement are also noted on MRI. Associated wedge-shaped and circumferential parenchymal enhancement are also detected around the lesions on MRI.

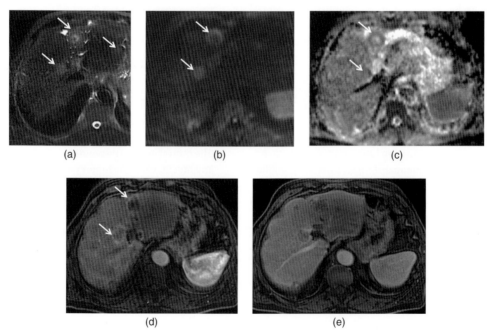

Figure 6.2 *Transverse T2-weighted fat-suppressed SS-ETSE (a), diffusion weighted image (DWI) (b), ADC map (c), T1-weighted postgadolinium hepatic arterial dominant phase (d) and hepatic venous phase (e) fat-suppressed 3D-GE images demonstrate multiple hypovascular colon adenocarcinoma metastases (arrows).* The lesions show mildly high T2 signal on T2-weighted image (a). Some of these lesions show diffusion restriction on DWI image (b) and ADC map (c). The lesions show peripheral diffusion restriction which is characterized by peripheral high signal on DWI (b) and low signal on ADC map (c). The center of these lesions show necrosis, which does not show diffusion restriction. These lesions show early peripheral enhancement (d) with progressive enhancement in the later phases (e).

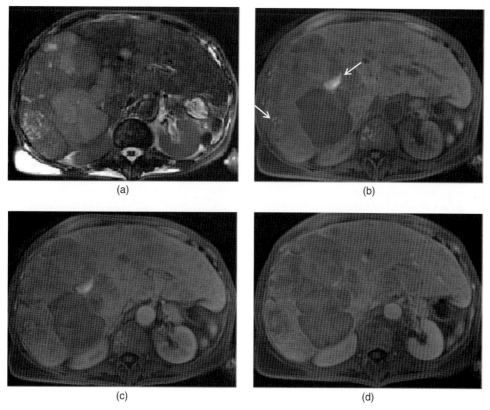

Figure 6.3 *Transverse T2-weighted fat-suppressed SS-ETSE (a), T1-weighted fat-suppressed 3D-GE (b), T1-weighted postgadolinium hepatic arterial dominant phase (c) and hepatic venous phase (d) fat-suppressed 3D-GE images demonstrate multiple metastases secondary to ocular malignant melanoma.* Multiple lesions showing heterogeneous precontrast signal and enhancement are seen in the liver. Some of these lesions (arrows, b) show precontrast high T1 signal due to the presence of melanin.

with only 1 postcontrast phase, or with fewer phases than MRI, because of radiation concerns.

° The enhancement of metastatic lesions is frequently peripheral (ring type of enhancement) and limited to the outer margins of the lesion (Figure 6.7).

° **Perilesional Enhancement**

° However, perilesional enhancement may also be seen not uncommonly. The enhancement occurs beyond the margins of the lesion delineated on precontrast images. This is observed most frequently in colon cancer and pancreatic ductal adneocarcinoma.

° Perilesional enhancement may develop due to hepatic parenchyma compression, associated peripheral desmoplastic reaction, inflammatory infiltrates, and neovascularization.

° More common in hypovascular metastases and uncommon in hypervascular metastases.

° **Perilesional enhancement** may be

  1 **Circumferential:**

  - May be observed in colon adenocarcinoma metastases (Figures 6.8 and 6.9).

2 **Wedge-shaped:**

  - May be seen in metastases from pancreatic ductal adenocarcinoma (Figures 6.9 and 6.10).

- **The pattern of lesional enhancement of liver metastases has a strong association with the size of the lesion.**

1 **Ring enhancement:**

  - Is the most characteristic appearance of liver metastases.
  - Usually seen when the lesion is > 1.5 cm.
  - On hepatic arterial dominant phase images, the outer margin of the metastasis (the most vascularized portion) enhances prominently and the inner portion has negligible enhancement (Figures 6.1, 6.2, 6.4–6.8).
  - On interstitial phase images, there is an equilibration of enhancement as the contrast gradually reaches the less vascularized central tumor and its interstitial compartment (Figures 6.2 and 6.6).
  - The outer margin demonstrates a decrease in the degree of enhancement that may appear as heterogeneous fading to near isointensity (isodensity on CT) or wash-out, and the inner area shows an increase in the degree of enhancement in later phases (Figure 6.11).
  - The centripetal enhancement with the wash-out of the outer margin observed in the interstitial phase is highly

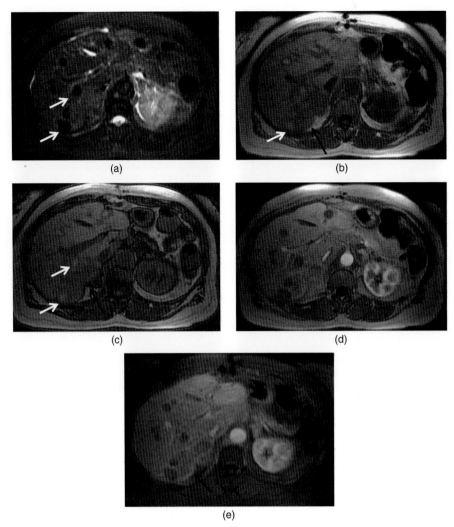

(a)   (b)

(c)   (d)

(e)

Figure 6.4 *Transverse fat-suppressed T2-weighted SS-ETSE (a), T1-weighted in-phase (b), out-of-phase (c) 2D-GE, postgadolinium T1-weighted hepatic arterial dominant phase 2D-GE (d) and fat-suppressed 3D-GE (e) images demonstrate multiple mucinous adenocarcinoma metastases in the liver.* The lesions (white arrows) demonstrate low T2 signal and high T1 signal on precontrast images due to high protein content. Mild enhancement is also noted in these lesions. Please note that additional heterogeneously enhancing metastases (black arrows), which do not have high protein content, are also detected in the posterior segment of the liver.

suggestive of malignancy, and most typical of hypervascular metastases such as carcinoid and neuroendocrine tumors such as gastrinoma (Figure 6.12).

2 Homogeneous enhancement:

- Usually when the lesion is <1.5-cm (Figures 6.13–6.15).

3 Heterogeneous:

- Uncommon.
- Usually when the lesion is >1.5 cm (Figure 6.16).
- Usually reflects necrosis or hemorrhage within the metastases.

- *Association between vascularity of liver metastases and degree of enhancement*

   I Avascular:

- Lack of lesional enhancement is usually seen on both hepatic arterial dominant and interstitial phase images.
- A thin lesional or perilesional enhancement may alternatively be seen in the margin, especially in the interstitial phase (Figures 6.17 and 6.18).
- Appear as completely cystic or necrotic metastases.
- Cystic metastases, most commonly from ovarian cancer, may be seen as avascular metastases.
- Metastases, which undergo treatment such as chemotherapy, chemoembolization, ablation treatments including radiofrequency, microwave, and cryoablation, may appear as avascular metastases.

   II Isovascular:

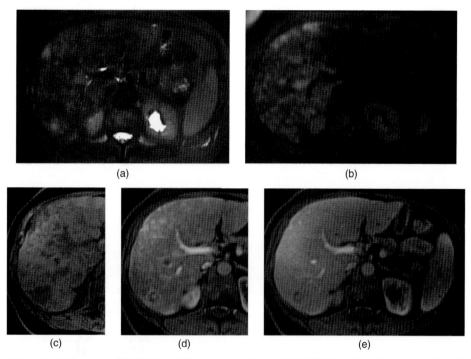

(a)

(b)

(c)

(d)

(e)

Figure 6.5 *Transverse T2-weighted fat-suppressed SS-ETSE (a), diffusion weighted image (DWI) (b), T1-weighted fat-suppressed 3D-GE (c), T1-weighted post-gadolinium hepatic arterial dominant phase (d) and hepatic venous phase (e) fat-suppressed 3D-GE images demonstrate multiple hypervascular metastases secondary to breast cancer.* The lesions show mildly high signal on T2-weighted image (a) and high signal on DWI (b). The lesions demonstrate progressive enhancement on postgadolinium images and most of them appear isointense to the liver parenchyma on the hepatic venous phase.

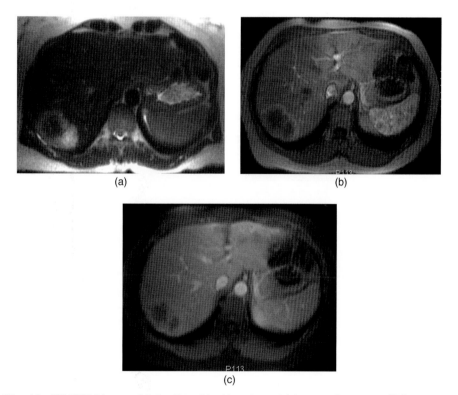

(a)

(b)

(c)

Figure 6.6 *Transverse T2-weighted SS-ETSE (a), postgadolinium T1-weighted hepatic arterial dominant phase 2D-GE (b), hepatic venous phase fat-suppressed 3D-GE (c) images show a single metastasis from colon adenocarcinoma.* The lesion shows halo sign on T2-weighted image with central low signal and peripheral high signal. The lesion shows typical cauliflower shape and predominant peripheral enhancement, with progressive stromal enhancement on postgadolinium images. Source: Semelka 2010. Reproduced with permission of Wiley.

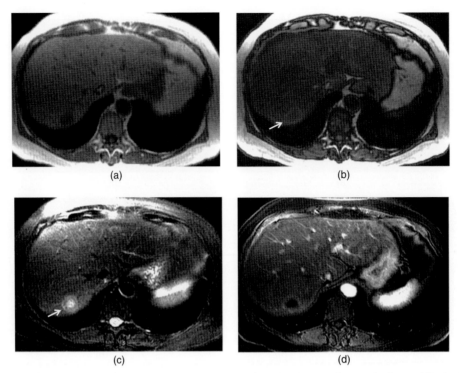

Figure 6.7 *Transverse T1-weighted in-phase (a) and out-of-phase (b) 2D-GE, T2-weighted SS-ETSE (c) and T1-weighted postgadolinium (d) images demonstrate a solitary metastasis from breast cancer.* The lesion shows target sign on T2-weighted image with a central high T2 signal and peripheral low signal intensity. However, please note that an outer high signal intensity layer is also present around this lesion on T2-weighted image, representing the compressed liver parenchyma. This compressed liver parenchyma appears as a hyperintense halo surrounding the hypointense lesion on out-of-phase image. Although the liver is fatty, the compressed liver parenchyma around the lesion appears as hyperintense halo as it is not capable of depositing fat.

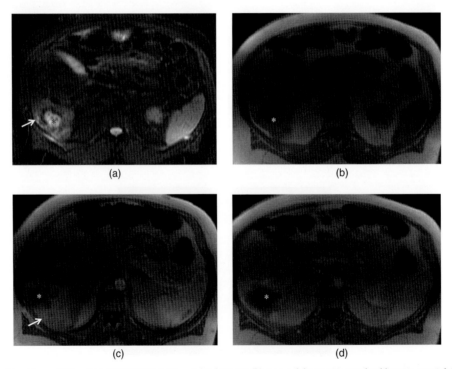

Figure 6.8 *Transverse fat-suppressed T2-weighted SS-ETSE (a), T1-weighted 2D-GE (b), postgadolinium T1-weighted hepatic arterial dominant phase (c) and hepatic venous phase (d) images show a liver metastasis (*) from colon adenocarcinoma.* The lesion shows target sign on T2 (a) and T1-weighted (b) precontrast images. Perilesional edema (arrow, a) is also noted around the lesion on T2-weighted image. Circumferential parenchymal enhancement (arrow, c) is also seen around the lesion on postgadolinium images.

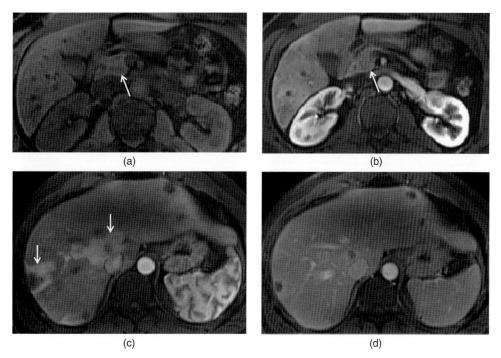

(a)   (b)

(c)   (d)

Figure 6.9 *Transverse T1-weighted fat-suppressed 3D-GE (a), postgadolinium hepatic arterial dominant (b, c) and hepatic venous phase (d) images demonstrate a small pancreatic adenocarcinoma (arrows; a, b) and multiple liver metastases (c, d).* The pancreatic adenocarcinoma is located in the pancreatic head (arrows; a, b). Circumferential and wedge-shaped transient perilesional enhancements are noted around the hypointense metastases on the hepatic arterial dominant phase (c).

- Lesions demonstrate similar enhancement as the background parenchyma on the hepatic arterial dominant phase (See Figure 2.27).
- These lesions (i) may either become isointense (isodense on CT) relative to the background liver in the interstitial phase or (ii) may become hypointense (hypodense on CT) by showing wash-out or (iii) may become hyperintense (hyperdense on CT) by showing progressive homogeneous enhancement in the interstitial phases.
- Metastases from colon adenocarcinoma, thyroid carcinoma, and breast cancer may appear as isovascular metastases.
- Metastases, which undergo treatment such as chemotherapy or chemoembolization, may become isovascular following treatment.

III Hypovascular:

- (i) Lesions demonstrate lesser enhancement compared to background liver parenchyma in the hepatic arterial dominant phase and later phases (Figure 6.20).
- (ii) Lesions may alternatively demonstrate thin rim of peripherally increased enhancement in the hepatic arterial dominant phase compared to background parenchyma.
- Lesions demonstrate progressive increased enhancement in the interstitial phase although they appear relatively hypointense (hypodense on CT) compared to background liver parenchyma.
- Colon adenocarcinoma, urothelial cell carcinoma, pancreatic ductal adenocarcinoma, small bowel adenocarcinoma, lung carcinoma, bladder carcinoma, and prostate carcinoma usually appear as hypovascular metastases.

IV Hypervascular:

- (i) Lesions demonstrate intense peripheral thick ring-like enhancement on the hepatic arterial dominant phase images followed by progressive centripetal enhancement with peripheral wash-out on interstitial phase (Figure 6.12).
- (ii) Lesions may also alternatively demonstrate intense uniform enhancement on the hepatic arterial dominant phase images followed by later wash-out or fading in the interstitial phase (Figures 6.21 and 6.22).
- Breast cancer, renal cell carcinoma, carcinoid tumor, neuroendocrine tumors (Figures 6.23 and 6.24), islet cell tumor, thyroid carcinoma, sarcomas, and malignant melanoma usually appear as hypervascular metastases. The most common consistently hypervascular metastases are generally neuroendocrine tumors.

- **Metastases from colon cancer:**
  ° Are commonly hypovascular (90%).

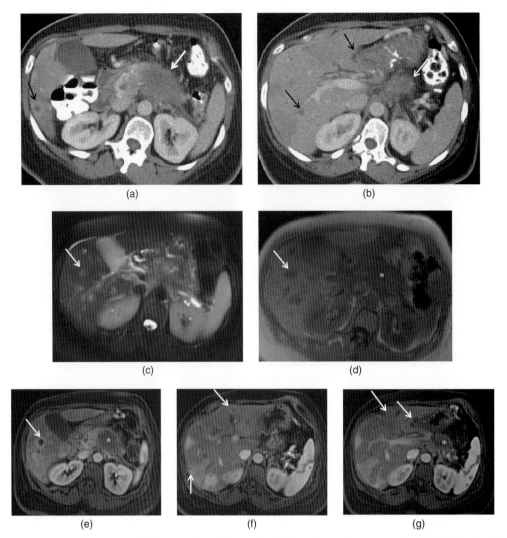

(a)

(b)

(c)

(d)

(e)

(f)

(g)

Figure 6.10 *Transverse postcontrast hepatic arterial dominant phase CT images (a, b) show a large adenocarcinoma involving the body of the pancreas (white arrows; a, b) and multiple liver metastases (black arrows; a, b).* Transverse fat-suppressed T2-weighted SS-ETSE (c), T1-weighted 2D-GE (d), postgadolinium T1-weighted fat-suppressed hepatic arterial dominant phase 3D-GE images (e – g) demonstrate multiple liver metastases (arrows) showing peripheral enhancement and associated wedge-shaped and circumferential enhancement. The pancreatic body adenocarcinoma (*) is seen (d, e, g).

° Thin peripheral ring enhancement is seen in the hepatic arterial dominant phase, which remains enhanced on the interstitial phase images. The remaining central portion of lesions show progressive enhancement (Figures 6.25 and 6.26).

° When tumors exceed 3-cm in diameter, they typically become lobulated and develop a cauliflower-type appearance (Figure 6.27).

° Small subcapsular metastases are observed in approximately 1/3 of patients (Figure 6.28).

° Circumferential perilesional enhancement may be seen around the lesions, especially in the hepatic arterial dominant phase.

- **Metastases from breast cancer:**
  ° Are commonly hypervascular (90%).

° Present commonly as round masses.

° Thick ring-like peripheral enhancement in the hepatic arterial dominant phase with progressive enhancement in later phases is commonly seen (Figure 6.29).

° Small lesions (<1 cm) may show homogeneously increased enhancement in the hepatic arterial dominant phase.

° Large lesions may show heterogeneous enhancement.

° Chemotherapy-treated metastases may show minimal early enhancement with progressively intense enhancement of a peripheral rim on delayed images, reflecting good response.

° The presence of diffuse nodular metastases may mimic cirrhotic liver, especially following response to chemotherapy.

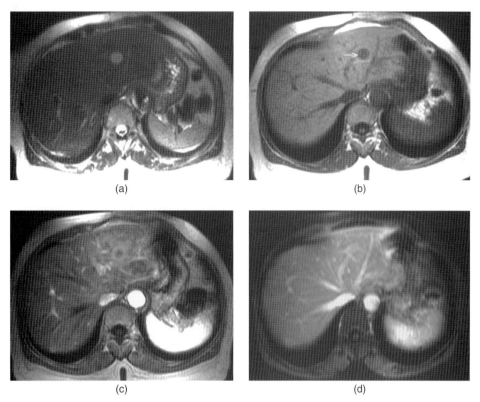

(a) (b)

(c) (d)

Figure 6.11 *Transverse T2-weighted SS-ETSE (a), T1-weighted 2D-GE (b), postgadolinium T1-weighted hepatic arterial dominant phase (c) and hepatic venous phase (d) images show a liver metastasis from colon adenocarcinoma.* Note that the peripheral thick rim enhancement of the lesion seen on the hepatic arterial dominant phase image (c) fades on the hepatic venous phase (d) and the inner part of the lesion shows progressive enhancement on the hepatic venous phase image (d).

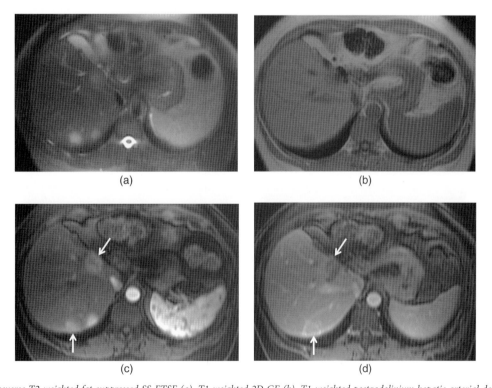

(a) (b)

(c) (d)

Figure 6.12 *Transverse T2-weighted fat-suppressed SS-ETSE (a), T1-weighted 2D-GE (b), T1-weighted postgadolinium hepatic arterial dominant phase (c) and hepatic venous phase (d) fat-suppressed 3D-GE images demonstrate multiple hypervascular metastases secondary to pancreatic neuroendocrine tumor.* The lesions show mild to moderately high signal on T2-weighted image (a). The lesions (arrows) show prominent enhancement in the hepatic arterial dominant phase (c) and wash-out on the hepatic venous phase (d).

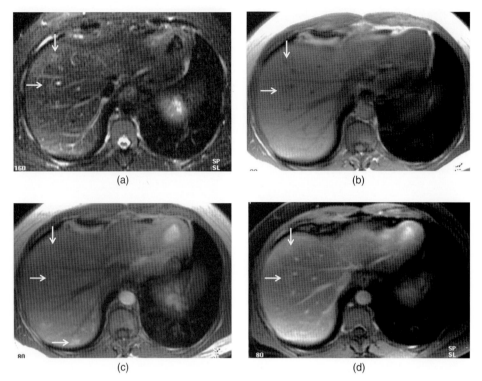

Figure 6.13 *Transverse T2-weighted fat-suppressed SS-ETSE (a), T1-weighted 2D-GE (b), T1-weighted postgadolinium hepatic arterial dominant phase 2D-GE (c) and fat-suppressed hepatic venous phase 3D-GE (d) images show multiple hypervascular metastases (arrows).* The lesions show mild T2 and T1 signal on precontrast images. The lesions show mild homogeneous enhancement on the hepatic arterial dominant phase (c) and maintain their enhancement on the hepatic venous phase image (d).

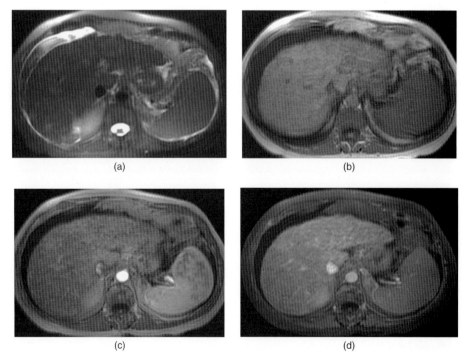

Figure 6.14 *Transverse T2-weighted fat-suppressed SS-ETSE (a), T1-weighted 2D-GE (b), T1-weighted postgadolinium hepatic arterial dominant phase 2D-GE, hepatic venous phase fat-suppressed 3D-GE images show multiple diffuse small and miliary metastases in the liver showing homogeneous increased enhancement in the hepatic arterial dominant phase (c).* Some of these lesions show fading on the hepatic venous phase (d).

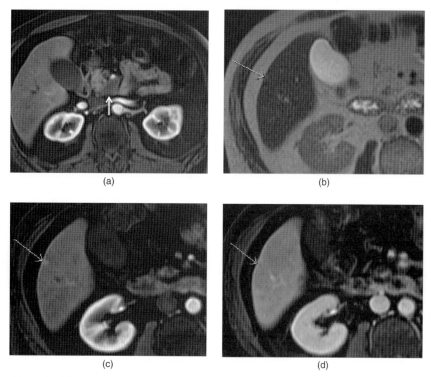

(a) (b)

(c) (d)

Figure 6.15 *Postgadolinium T1-weighted fat-suppressed image (a) demonstrates a small hypointense pancreatic adenocarcinoma (arrow) in the uncinate process. A small subcapsular hypervascular metastasis is seen in the right lobe of the liver showing midly high signal on T2-weighted image (b), homogeneously increased signal on the hepatic arterial dominant phase (c) and slight wash-out on the hepatic venous phase (d) images.*

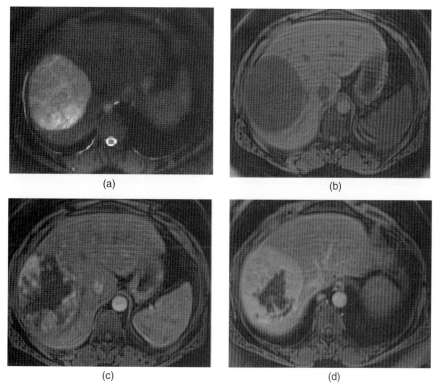

(a) (b)

(c) (d)

Figure 6.16 *Transverse T2-weighted fat-suppressed SS-ETSE (a), T1-weighted fat-suppressed 3D-GE (b), postgadolinium fat-suppressed T1-weighted hepatic arterial dominant phase (c) and hepatic venous phase (d) images show a heterogeneous large metastasis from leiomyosarcoma. The lesion shows moderately increased high signal on T2-weighted image (a) and heterogeneous progressive enhancement on postgadolinium images (c, d).*

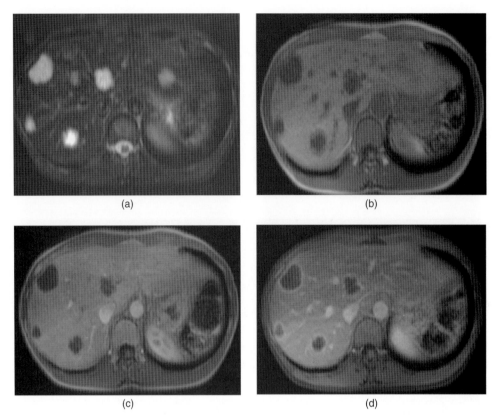

Figure 6.17 *Transverse T2-weighted fat-suppressed SS-ETSE (a), T1-weighted 2D-GE in-phase (b) and out-of-phase (c), postgadolinium T1-weighted hepatic arterial dominant phase 2D-GE (d) and fat-suppressed hepatic venous phase 3D-GE (e) images demonstrate multiple avascular cystic metastases from ovarian cancer.* These cystic metastases show wall enhancement but no stromal enhancement.

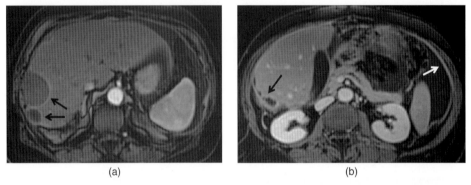

Figure 6.18 *Transverse postgadolinium fat-suppressed T1-weighted hepatic arterial dominant phase (a) and hepatic venous phase (b) images show subcapsular avascular cystic metastases (black arrow; a, b) from ovarian cancer.* The subcapsular cystic lesions do not show internal stromal enhancement but mild to moderate wall enhancement. Please note the moderate amount of free fluid and enhancing peritoneal thickening (white arrow, b) in the abdomen.

- **Metastases from melanoma:**
  - ° Melanin content is better evaluated with MRI compared to CT.
    - (a) Melanocytic type: They represent well-differentiated type of malignant melanoma. Typically, they show high signal intensity on T1-WI (Figure 6.30) and low signal intensity on T2-WI because of the paramagnetic property of melanin. A mixture of high and low signal intensity on T1- and T2-WI are common.
    - (b) Amelanocytic type: They represent poorly differentiated type of malignant melanoma. Do not contain melanin and therefore will not produce the paramagnetic effect, and will appear mildly hyperintense on T2-weighted images and mildly to moderately hypointense on T1-weighted images.

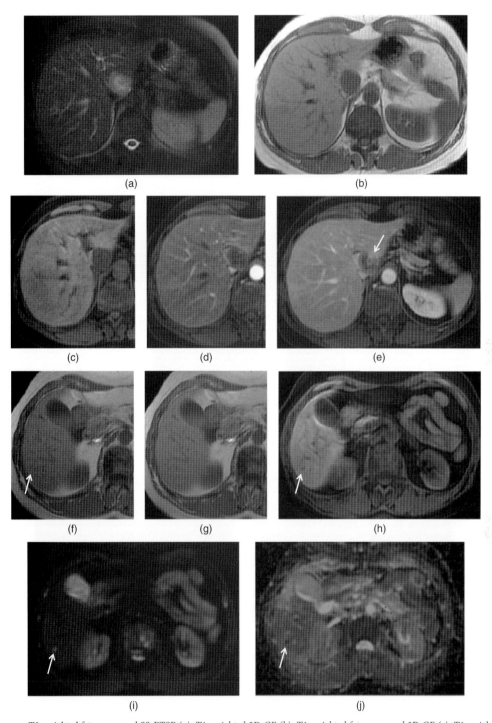

Figure 6.19 *Transverse T2-weighted fat-suppressed SS-ETSE (a), T1-weighted 2D-GE (b), T1-weighted fat-suppressed 3D-GE (c), T1-weighted fat-suppressed postgadolinium hepatic arterial dominant phase (d) and hepatic venous phase (e) demonstrate an enhancing metastasis (arrow) in the caudate lobe secondary to breast cancer.* The lesion predominantly shows peripheral enhancement. Transverse T2-weighted fat-suppressed SS-ETSE (f), T1-weighted 2D-GE (g), T1-weighted fat-suppressed 3D-GE (h), diffusion weighted image (i) and ADC map (j) demonstrate a tiny metastasis showing diffusion restriction in the same patient with breast cancer.

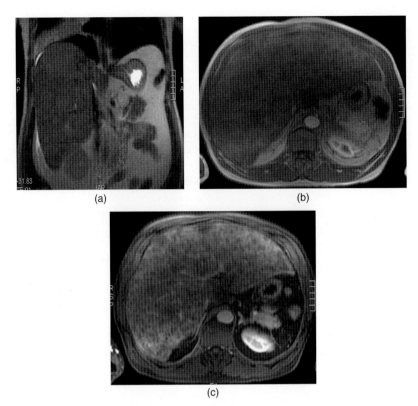

Figure 6.20 *Coronal T2-weighted SS-ETSE (a), transverse T1-weighted postgadolinium 2D-GE (b) and postgadolinium T1-weighted hepatic venous phase (c) fat-suppressed 3D-GE image demonstrates multiple hypovascular metastases in the liver secondary to lung cancer.* The metastases show decreased enhancement compared to the background liver parenchyma (c). Note that there is an atelectasis in the right lung base on coronal T2-weighted image (a).

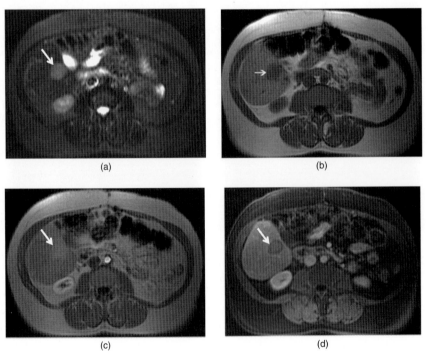

Figure 6.21 *Transverse T2-weighted fat-suppressed SS-ETSE (a), T1-weighted 2D-GE (b), T1-weighted postgadolinium hepatic arterial dominant phase 2D-GE (c), hepatic venous phase 3D-GE (d) images show a hepatic hypervascular metastasis (arrows) from carcinoid tumor.* The tumor shows moderately high signal on T2-weighted image (a) and prominent enhancement on the early postgadolinium image (c) with later wash-out (d).

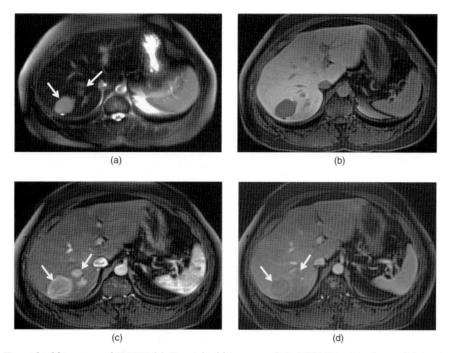

Figure 6.22 *Transverse T2-weighted fat-suppressed SS-ETSE (a), T1-weighted fat-suppressed 3D-GE (b), T1-weighted postgadolinium hepatic arterial dominant phase 3D-GE (c), hepatic venous phase 3D-GE (d) images show hypervascular metastases secondary to multiple myeloma.* These metastases demonstrate markedly high signal on T2-weighted image and show prominently increased enhancement with late central wash-out and peripheral rim enhancement. Source: Semelka 2010. Reproduced with permission of Wiley.

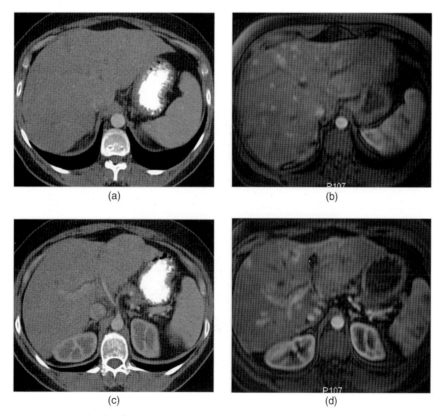

Figure 6.23 *Transverse postcontrast images (a, c) and transverse postgadolinium hepatic arterial dominant phase (b, d) images show multiple hypervascular metastases from neuroendocrine tumor.* The lesions appear as hypodense and enhancing hyperdense lesions on CT. Note that MRI shows more lesions compared to CT. Source: Semelka 2010. Reproduced with permission of Wiley.

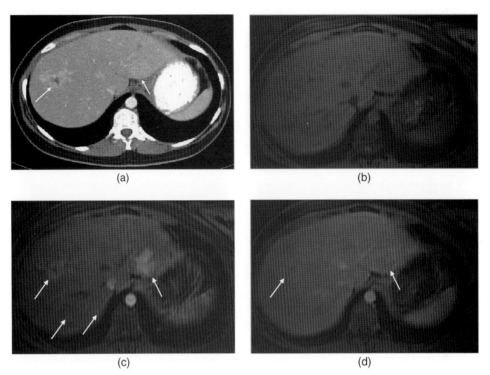

Figure 6.24 *Transverse postcontrast hepatic venous phase CT image (a), T1-weighted fat-suppressed 3D-GE (b), T1-weighted postgadolinium hepatic arterial dominant phase (c) and hepatic venous phase (d) 3D-GE images show several hypervascular metastases from neuroendocrine tumor.* The metastases demonstrate prominent enhancement in the hepatic arterial dominant phase (c) and wash-out on the hepatic venous phase (d).

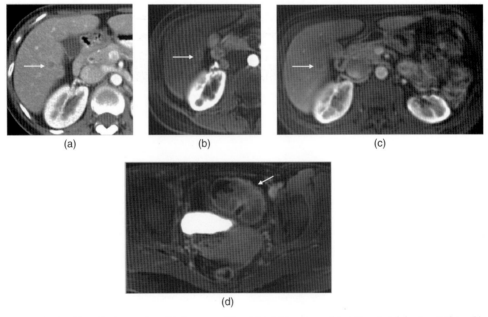

Figure 6.25 *Transverse postcontrast hepatic venous phase (a), transverse T1-weighted fat-suppressed hepatic arterial dominant phase (b) and hepatic venous phase (c) 3D-GE images show a small hypovascular liver metastasis (arrows, a–c) secondary to colon cancer.* The lesion shows typical peripheral ring enhancement (a–c). An enhancing tumor (arrow, d) is noted in the sigmoid colon in the pelvis on transverse pelvic fat-suppressed 3D-GE image (d).

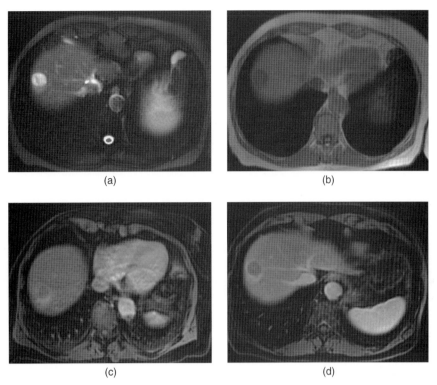

Figure 6.26 *Transverse T2-weighted fat-suppressed SS-ETSE (a), T1-weighted 2D-GE (b), T1-weighted fat-suppressed postgadolinium 3D-GE (c, d) images show a colon cancer liver metastasis with moderately high T2 signal and peripheral dominant progressive enhancement.*

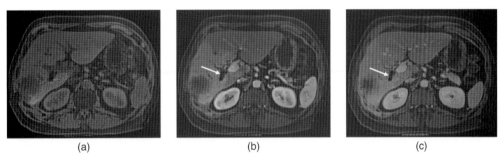

Figure 6.27 *Transverse fat-suppressed T1-weighted 3D-GE pregadolinium (a), postgadolinium hepatic arterial dominant phase (b) and hepatic venous phase (c) images show a hypovascular metastasis from colon adenocarcinoma.* The lesion shows typical cauliflower shape (a) and peripherally dominant progressive enhancement (b, c). Note the presence of associated bland thrombus in the right portal vein and its branches (arrows; b, c). The right lobe of the liver shows transient increased enhancement on the hepatic arterial dominant phase secondary to compensatory increased hepatic arterial flow. Increased enhancement of the right hepatic lobe fades in the hepatic venous phase.

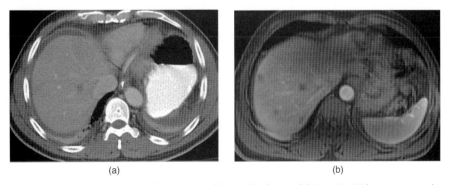

Figure 6.28 *Transverse postcontrast hepatic venous phase CT image (a) and T1-weighted postgadolinium 3D-GE hepatic venous phase (b) images show hypovascular liver metastases secondary to colon adenocarcinoma.* Note that the lesions are more conspicuous on MR compared to CT and increased number of lesions are detected on MR. Some of these metastases are subcapsular and peripheral.

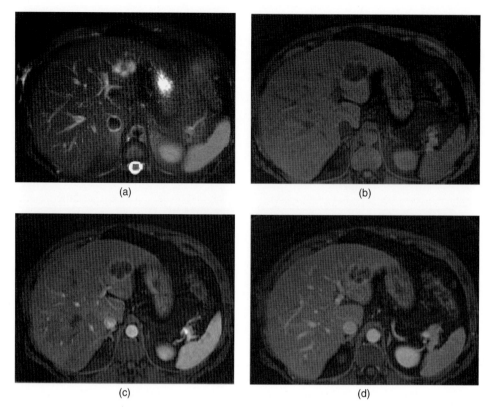

(a)

(b)

(c)

(d)

Figure 6.29 *Transverse T2-weighted fat-suppressed SS-ETSE (a), T1-weighted fat-suppressed pregadolinium (b), postgadolinium hepatic arterial dominant phase (c) and hepatic venous phase (c, d) 3D-GE images show a lobulated mass showing a breast cancer metastasis in the liver.* The lesion shows peripheral thick ring-like enhancement in the hepatic arterial dominant phase with progressive stromal enhancement in the hepatic venous phase.

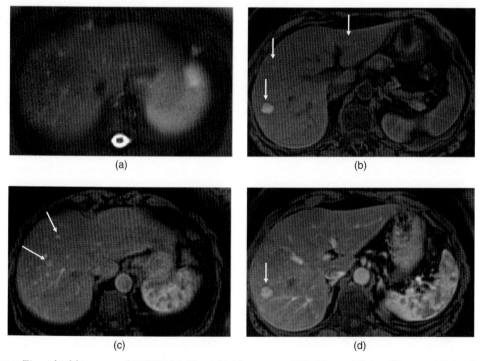

(a)

(b)

(c)

(d)

Figure 6.30 *Transverse T2-weighted fat-suppressed SS-ETSE (a), T1-weighted fat-suppressed 3D-GE pregadolinium (b), postgadolinium hepatic arterial dominant phase 3D-GE images (c, d) show hypervascular metastases from malignant melanoma.* Malignant melanoma metastases demonstrate increased signal on T1-weighted precontrast image (b) due to paramagnetic effect of melanin. These lesions (arrows; c, d) show increased enhancement on postgadolinium images.

Differential diagnosis

Hypervascular small metastases versus small fast filling hemangiomas

- Hypervascular small metastases usually demonstrate mild to moderately high signal on T2-WI while small fast-filling hemangiomas show moderate to markedly high signal on T2-WI.
- Small (<1.0 cm) hypervascular metastases often enhance in an intense homogeneous fashion on the hepatic arterial dominant phase images and tend to wash-out or fade relative to the background liver parenchyma in later phases (Figure 6.31).
- Small fast-filling hemangiomas may enhance in similar fashion on the hepatic arterial dominant phase images; however, tend to retain contrast and appear hyperintense (hyperdense on CT) compared to the background parenchyma on later phases (Figure 6.31). Note that small hemangiomas can fade in signal over time, but will never wash out on delayed images.

Chemotherapy-treated metastases versus hemangiomas

- Metastases usually demonstrate mildly high signal on T2-WI while hemangiomas show moderate to markedly high signal on T2-WI (Figure 6.32).
- Chemotherapy-treated metastases may show peripheral nodular enhancement on the hepatic arterial dominant phase and progressive enhancement on later phases (Figure 6.32). However, they do not show typical enhancement pattern of hemangiomas, which is characterized by discontinuous peripheral nodular enhancement on the hepatic arterial dominant phase, followed by coalescence of nodules on later phases.

Hypervascular small metastases versus FNH and Hepatocellular Adenoma

- The history of primary malignancy should be questioned.
- The history of oral contraceptive use should be questioned.
- Small hypervascular metastases show mild to moderately high T2 signal and mild to moderately low T1 signal.
- Focal nodular hyperplasia (FNH) (Figure 6.33) and adenomas (Figure 6.34) are isointense or mildly hyperintense on T2-WI and isointense or mildly hypointense on T1-WI.
- Hepatocellular adenomas may contain fat while metastases do not.
- Small FNHs which generally do not have central scars show homogeneous increased enhancement in the hepatic arterial dominant phase and tend to become isointense with the remaining liver parenchyma in later phases (Figure 6.33).
- Hepatocellular adenomas show similar enhancement pattern to small FNHs (Figure 6.34)

- FNHs show uptake of hepatocyte-specific gadolinium agents while metastases and adenomas do not (Figures 6.33 and 6.34).

Hypervascular small metastases versus vascular shunts/anomalies

- Vascular anomalies including collaterals, shunts, and fistula demonstrate structural enhancing vascular abnormalities that show communication and continuation with hepatic arteries, hepatic veins, and portal veins.
- Areas showing transient vascular enhancement (Figure 6.35) do not show precontrast T1-WI or T2-WI, or DWI correlations.
- Metastases tend to be rounded and shunts tend to be linear-shaped or wedge-shaped.

Hypovascular metastases versus abscesses

- The history of fever and right upper quadrant pain should be questioned.
- The history of immunosuppression should be questioned.
- The history of primary malignancy should be questioned.
- Precontrast imaging characteristics are similar.
- Transient increased perilesional enhancement in the hepatic arterial dominant phase is more common in abscesses (almost always present with bacterial abscesses) compared to metastases but present commonly in colon cancer metastases. Caution: timing must be exact in the hepatic arterial dominant phase to observe perilesional enhancement.
- Both show peripheral increased enhancement in the hepatic arterial dominant phase.
- The septa of abscesses demonstrate progressive increased enhancement while the internal stroma of metastases show progressive enhancement.
- The presence of air is suggestive of abscess.
- Metastases may also be occasionally infected (Figure 6.36).

Hypervascular metastases versus high grade dysplastic nodules and hepatocellular carcinomas (HCCs)

- The history and findings of chronic liver disease and cirrhosis are particularly important as dysplastic nodules and HCCs are very common in patients with chronic liver disease and cirrhosis and extremely rare in patients without chronic liver disease and cirrhosis.
- Additionally, metastases rarely develop in patients with cirrhosis. However, metastases may develop in patients with chronic active hepatitis. This reflects that metastases require a relatively fertile vascular ground in order to take root in the liver, which is poor in cirrhosis but may be not too dissimilar from normals in the setting of chronic active hepatitis.

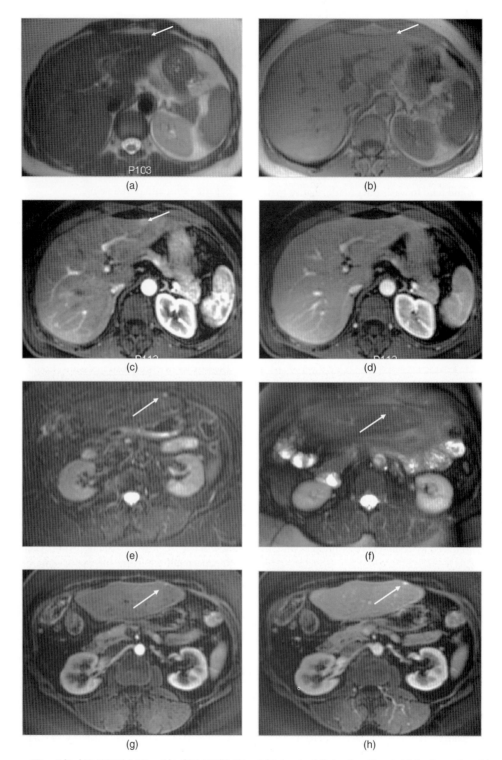

(a)

(b)

(c)

(d)

(e)

(f)

(g)

(h)

Figure 6.31 *Transverse T2-weighted SS-ETSE (a), T1-weighted 2D-GE (b), T1-weighted postgadolinium hepatic arterial dominant phase (c) and hepatic venous phase (d) 3D-GE images demonstrate a small hypervascular metastasis from carcinoid tumor.* The lesion shows very mild T2 and T1 signal on precontrast (a, b) images and prominent enhancement on the hepatic arterial dominant phase (c) and fading on the hepatic venous phase (d). Transverse T2-weighted STIR (e), SS-ETSE (f), T1-weighted postgadolinium hepatic arterial dominant phase (g) and hepatic venous phase (h) 3D-GE images demonstrate a small fast-filling hemangioma showing moderately high signal and prominent enhancement. The hemangioma retains its high signal on the hepatic venous phase (d).

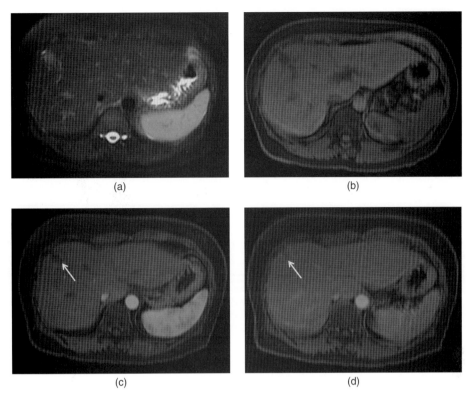

Figure 6.32 *Transverse T2-weighted fat-suppressed SS-ETSE (a), T1-weighted fat-suppressed 3D-GE (b), T1-weighted postgadolinium fat-suppressed hepatic arterial dominant phase (c) and hepatic venous phase (d) images demonstrate a colon adenocarcinoma metastasis (arrows) mimicking a hemangioma.* The lesion shows mild to moderate T2 signal (a) and peripheral nodular enhancement (arrow, c) on the hepatic arterial dominant phase (c) with central progression in the hepatic venous phase (d).

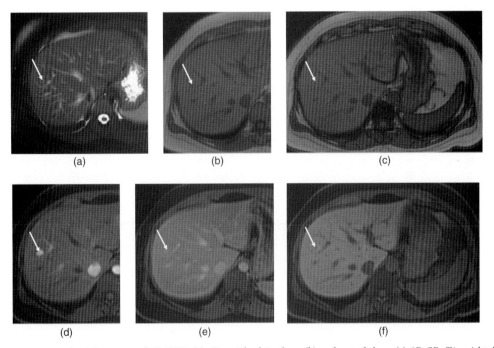

Figure 6.33 *Transverse T2-weighted fat-suppressed SS-ETSE (a), T1-weighted in-phase (b) and out-of-phase (c) 2D-GE, T1-weighted postgadolinium fat-suppressed 3D-GE hepatic arterial dominant phase (d), hepatic venous phase (e) and hepatocyte phase (f) images show a small focal nodular hyperplasia (arrows) (FNH).* The lesion does not show any signal change on out-of-phase image, which is suggestive of the lack of fat content. Prominent enhancement in the hepatic arterial dominant phase with fading on the hepatic venous phase is seen. The lesion shows enhancement in the hepatocyte phase, which is typical for FNH.

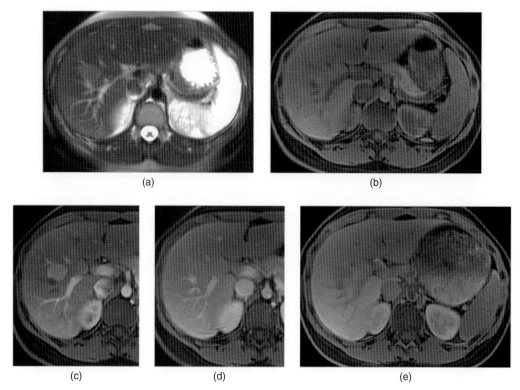

Figure 6.34 *Transverse T2-weighted fat-suppressed SS-ETSE (a), T1-weighted fat-suppressed 3D-GE (b), T1-weighted postgadolinium fat-suppressed 3D-GE hepatic arterial dominant phase (c), hepatic venous phase (d) and hepatocyte phase (e) images demonstrate a hepatic adenoma with mildly high T2 signal.* Prominent enhancement on the hepatic arterial dominant phase (c) with fading on the hepatic venous phase (d) is seen. The lesion appears hypointense compared to the background liver, which is suggestive of adenoma.

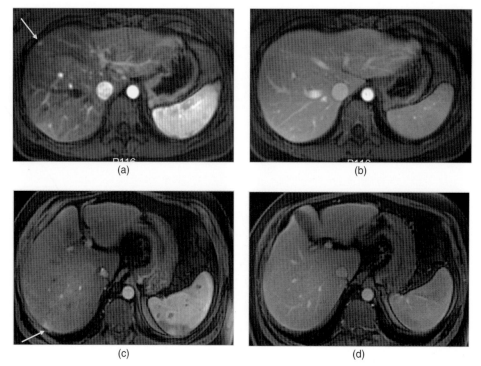

Figure 6.35 *Transverse T1-weighted fat-suppressed hepatic arterial dominant phase (a, c) and hepatic venous phase (b, d) images show vascular shunts/perfusion abnormalities in two different patients.* Vascular shunts/perfusion abnormalities are usually located peripherally (arrows, a – c) and fade in the venous phases (b, d).

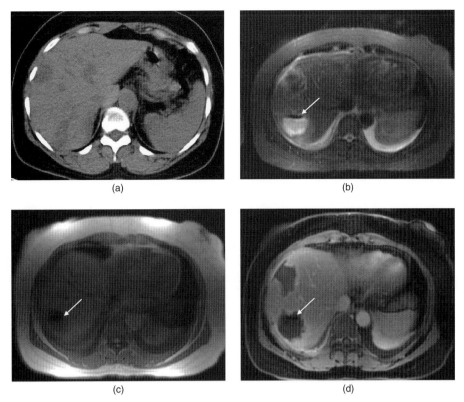

(a)

(b)

(c)

(d)

Figure 6.36 *Transverse precontrast CT (a), transverse T2-weighted fat-suppressed SS-ETSE (b), T1-weighted precontrast 2D-GE (c) and postgadolinium fat-suppressed 3D-GE (d) images show infected metastases in the liver.* The posteriorly located lesion (arrow, b-d) shows air–fluid level due to infection. The lesions demonstrate peripheral enhancement on postgadolinium image (d). Note bilateral pleural effusions.

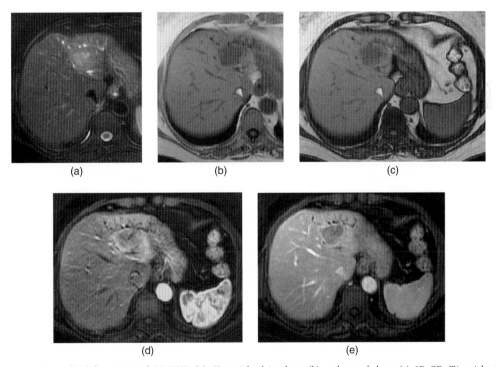

(a)

(b)

(c)

(d)

(e)

Figure 6.37 *Transverse T2-weighted fat-suppressed SS-ETSE (a), T1-weighted in-phase (b) and out-of-phase (c) 2D-GE, T1-weighted postgadolinium fat-suppressed 3D-GE hepatic arterial dominant phase (d), hepatic venous phase (e) images show a mass lesion in the left hepatic lobe associated with peripheral ductal dilatation in a patient with endometrial cancer.* The lesion shows mildly increased T2 signal and heterogeneous enhancement on postgadolinium images (d, e). The left lobe of the liver demonstrates edema and increased transient enhancement in the hepatic arterial dominant phase secondary to compressive effects of the lesion. Although bile duct dilatation is more frequent with cholangiocarcinoma, MRI features of this lesion are not specific. The histopathological diagnosis was consistent with cholangiocarcinoma.

Single hypovascular metastases versus mass forming cholangiocarcinomas

- The history of primary malignancy should be questioned.
- Cholangiocarcinomas demonstrate mild peripheral enhancement in the hepatic arterial dominant phase and progressive enhancement in later phases, which is more prominent in the interstitial phase. However, subtle early diffuse heterogeneous enhancement may be observable. Additionally, chemotherapy- treated metastases show prominent delayed enhancement on the interstitial phase.
- The enhancement pattern is similar to hypovascular metastases and therefore it is difficult to differentiate these two entities by evaluating morphologic features (Figure 6.37), although typically, cholangiocarcinomas show more enhancement on the interstitial phase due to their abundant fibrotic stroma.
- Colon cancer metastases, which are the most common type of hypovascular metastases, should have a more cauliflower-type morphology, whereas capsular retraction is more common in cholangiocarcinomas. However, capsular retraction may also be seen with colon carcinoma metastases, particularly when they are treated with chemotherapy and local ablation therapy.

References

1 Ku, Y.M., Shin, S.S., Lee, C.H., and Semelka, R.C. (2009) Magnetic resonance imaging of cystic and endocrine pancreatic neoplasms. Top Magn Reson Imaging, 20, 8–11.

2 Khandani, A.H. and Semelka, R.C. (2005) Can the relation between gadopentate dimeglumine and FDG uptake in colorectal liver metastases be used clinically? Radiology, 237, 1–2.

3 Braga, L., Semelka, R.C., Pietrobon, R. et al. (2004) Does hypervascularity of liver metastasesas detected on MRI predict disease progression in breast cancer patients? AJR, 182, 1207–1213.

4 Danet, I.M., Semelka, R.C., Leonardou, P. et al. (2003) Spectrum of MRI appearances of untreated metastases of the liver. AJR, 181, 809–817.

5 Danet, I.M., Semelka, R.C., Nagase, L.L. et al. (2003) Liver metastases from pancreatic adenocarcinoma: MR imaging characteristics. J Magn Reson Imaging, 18, 181–188.

6 Pedro, M.S., Semelka, R.C., and Braga, L. (2002) MR imaging of hepatic metastases. Magn Reson Imaging Clin N Am, 10, 15–29.

7 Braga, L., Semelka, R.C., Pedro, M.S., and Barros, N. (2002) Post-treatment malignant liver lesions. MR imaging. Magn Reson Imaging Clin N Am, 10, 15–29.

8 Bader, T.R., Semelka, R.C., Chiu, V.C. et al. (2001) MRI of the carcinoid tumors: spectrum of appearances in the gastrointestinal tract and liver. J Magn Reson Imaging, 14, 261–269.

9 Balci, N.C. and Semelka, R.C. (2001) Radiologic diagnosis and staging of pancreatic ductal adenocarcinoma. Eur J Radiol, 38, 105–112.

10 Namasivayam, S., Martin, D.R., and Saini, S. (2007) Imaging of liver metastases: MRI. Cancer Imaging, 7, 2–9.

11 Sica, G.T., Hoon, J., and Ros, P.R. (2000) CT and MR imaging of hepatic metastases. AJR, 174, 691–698.

12 Oliva, M.R. and Saini, S. (2004) Liver cancer imaging: role of CT, MRI, US and PET. Cancer Imaging, 4, S42–S46.

CHAPTER 7
Hepatocellular carcinoma

Ersan Altun[1], Mohamed El-Azzazi[1,2,3,4], Richard C. Semelka[1], and Mamdoh AlObaidy[1,5]
[1] The University of North Carolina at Chapel Hill, Department of Radiology, Chapel Hill, NC, USA
[2] University of Dammam, Department of Radiology, Dammam, Saudi Arabia
[3] King Fahd Hospital of the University, Department of Radiology, Khobar, Saudi Arabia
[4] University of Al Azhar, Department of Radiology, Cairo, Egypt
[5] King Faisal Specialist Hospital & Research Center, Department of Radiology, Riyadh, Saudi Arabia

- Hepatocellular carcinoma (HCC) is the most common primary malignancy of the liver.
- Age-standardized incidence rates vary from 2.1/100.000 in North America to 80/100.000 in China. There is a male preponderance among all ethnic groups.
- HCCs commonly develop in patients with chronic liver disease and cirrhosis.
- Chronic hepatitis C and B are recognized as the major risk factors. The incidence of HCC in patients with chronic hepatitis is 0.5%. Chronic hepatitis C and B account for 75–85% of HCCs. Hepatitis C has 3–4 times increased risk compared to Hepatitis B for the development of HCC. Other risk factors include alcohol consumption and nonalcoholic fatty liver disease, especially nonalcoholic steatohepatitis. The annual rate of developing HCC in patients with cirrhosis is 1–6%.
- The great majority of HCCs occur in patients with cirrhosis (>80%), but they can occur in patients with chronic hepatitis (20%). Note that the term *non-cirrhotic liver* also refers to *chronic hepatitis livers*, and should not be confused with a nondiseased (e.g., normal) liver. HCC in a normal liver is extremely rare, and may be observed in < 1 in 5000 HCC cases.
- HCC most commonly arises from preexisting dysplastic nodules (DNs), described as stepwise carcinogenesis. HCC occurring de novo is rare.
- Stepwise carcinogenesis is considered a linear process, progressing from regenerative nodules (RNs), to DNs, to HCC.
- Hepatocyte injury from chronic liver disease, including viral hepatitis, alcohol consumption, and nonalcoholic fatty liver disease leads to the formation of RNs, as a repair mechanism to replace the damaged hepatocytes and hepatic tissue. RNs are benign hyperplastic tissue. Some hepatocytes in RNs may show atypical features and become dysplastic. Dsyplastic cells increase in number and form DNs, which are pre-malignant. HCCs develop within DNs, initially as a small focus, which increases in size. DNs develop neovascularity, which originates from hepatic arterial branches, which perpetuates the growth of DNs, and facilitates development into HCCs.

- **Histopathologically HCC is characterized by:**
  ° Soft, hemorrhagic, occasionally bile-stained, nodules or masses with a propensity for necrosis.
  ° Spontaneous hemorrhage may be present.
  ° Central scar may be seen.
  ° Fatty infiltration (tends to be more heterogenous, unlike that of adenoma, which tends to be homogenous) may be seen.

- **HCC may arise as:**
  ° Solitary (50%)
  ° Multifocal (40%)
  ° Diffuse (10%)

- **Solitary and Multifocal HCCs**
- Solitary and multifocal HCCs usually appear as encapsulated well-defined rounded tumors.
- HCC is generally a hypervascular tumor (90%) that receives its blood supply from hepatic arterial branches. The most sensitive phase of enhancement for detecting small HCCs is hepatic arterial dominant phase imaging because HCCs demonstrate prominent enhancement in this phase.
- HCCs have a tendency to invade vascular structures, including the portal vein and hepatic veins. The branches of the portal vein are more commonly affected compared to the branches of hepatic veins. This is rare for well-differentiated solitary tumors, and in general is uncommon in solitary and multifocal tumors, but invariably occurs in diffuse HCC.
- On CT
- CT has 80–90% sensitivity, 90% specificity for the detection of HCCs.

Liver Imaging: MRI with CT Correlation, First Edition. Edited by Ersan Altun, Mohamed El-Azzazi and Richard C. Semelka.
© 2015 John Wiley & Sons, Inc. Published 2015 by John Wiley & Sons, Inc.

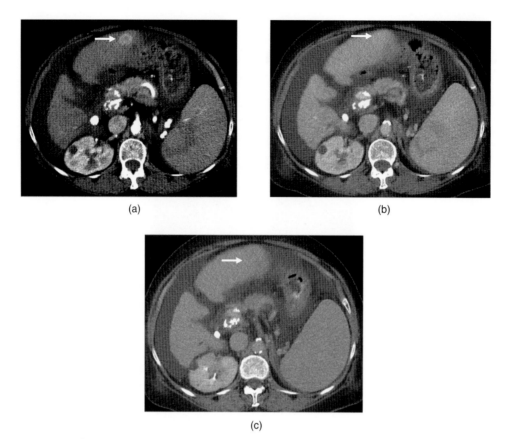

(a)   (b)

(c)

Figure 7.1 *Transverse postcontrast hepatic arterial dominant (a), hepatic venous (b) and interstitial (c) phase images show a small hypervascular lesion, which is consistent with HCC, in a cirrhotic patient.* The lesion shows prominent enhancement in the hepatic arterial dominant phase (a), fading in the hepatic venous phase (b) and subtle wash-out in the interstitial phase (c). The lesion appears mildly hypodense compared to the other phases due to wash-out. Note the presence of ascites and splenomegaly, suggestive of portal hypertension.

- On Pre-contrast CT images
  - HCCs are usually hypoattenuated, especially if they are larger than 3 cm.
  - HCCs may also be isoattenuated to liver parenchyma, especially if they are less than 3 cm. However, indirect signs can be identified on unenhanced images by
    - A hypoattenuated rim, which represents the tumor capsule.
    - Focal bulging in the contour of the liver.
    - Exophytic mass-like structure.
  - Areas of necrosis or fatty infiltration appear as hypoattenuated foci within the mass.
  - Recent hemorrhage appears as hyperattenuated foci within the mass.
  - Calcifications may occasionally be seen.
- On dynamic contrast-enhanced CT images
- The tumor enhancement characteristics are:
- Hypervascular enhancement is the most common pattern.
- Enhancement characteristics of hypervascular HCCs are as follows:
  1 In the hepatic arterial dominant phase: HCCs show prominent enhancement. Enhancement is usually homogeneous if lesion size is smaller than 3 cm, and heterogeneous if the lesion is larger than 3 cm. The capsule of the tumor may appear as a hypoattenuated rim (Figures 7.1 and 7.2).
  2 In the hepatic venous phase: HCCs typically demonstrate wash-out and become hypoattenuated compared to background liver parenchyma (Figures 7.1 and 7.2). Tumor capsule shows enhancement in this phase. HCCs may also occasionally become isoattenuated in this phase.
  3 In the interstitial phase: Areas of fibrosis, including the capsule (Figure 7.2) and septa, usually demonstrate prolonged enhancement.
- On MRI
- MRI has 90–95% sensitivity and 90–95% specificity for the detection of HCCs.
- The absence of motion artifacts and the optimal timing of postgadolinium imaging in the early phase of enhancement, which is the hepatic arterial dominant phase, are critical factors for the diagnosis of HCCs (Figures 7.3 and 7.4).
- On T2-weighted images:
  - HCCs usually show mild hyperintense signal (Figure 7.5) on T2-weighted images, especially if they are larger than 3 cm.

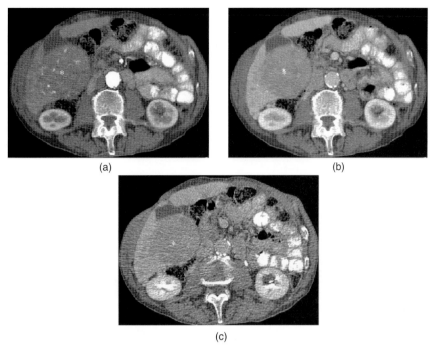

Figure 7.2 *Transverse postcontrast hepatic arterial dominant (a), hepatic venous (b) and interstitial (c) phase images demonstrate a large exophytic HCC in a cirrhotic patient.* The lesion shows enhancement on the hepatic arterial dominant phase (a) and wash-out on the hepatic venous (b) and interstitial (c) phase images. The lesion appears isodense or slightly hypodense compared to the liver on the hepatic arterial dominant phase (a). The lesion appears markedly hypodense on the hepatic venous (b) and interstitial phase (c) images due to wash-out. Slight capsular enhancement is noted in the interstitial phase (c).

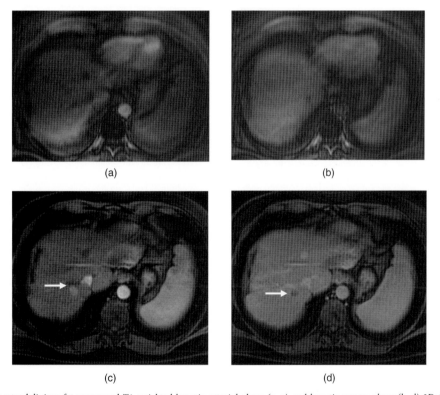

Figure 7.3 *Transverse postgadolinium fat-suppressed T1-weighted hepatic arterial phase (a, c) and hepatic venous phase (b, d) 3D-GE images illustrate the importance of breath holding.* In the first set of postgadolinium images (a, b), blurring due to motion artifacts are very prominent. In the second set of images (c, d), the same patient shows a hypervascular mass (arrows; c, d) demonstrating early enhancement in the arterial phase (c) and wash-out on the venous phase (d). The diagnosis is HCC in this patient with chronic liver disease. The HCC is not visualized in the first images due to motion artifacts.

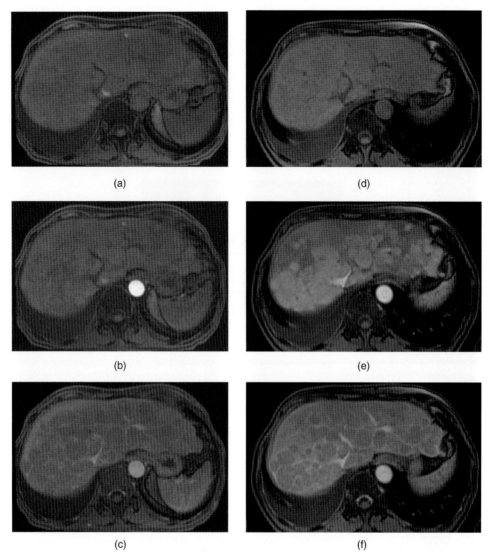

Figure 7.4 *Transverse T1-weighted fat-suppressed 3D-GE (a, d), postgadolinium fat-suppressed early hepatic arterial phase (b), hepatic arterial dominant phase (e), hepatic venous phase (e, f) 3D-GE images illustrate the importance of correct timing on postgadolinium images (b–f).* The first set of images (a–c) were acquired 1 month before the second set of images (d–f). The timing is suboptimal on postgadolinium images in the first set of images and optimal on postgadolinium images in the second set of images. Multiple nodular enhancing lesions replacing the majority of normal liver parenchyma are well seen in the hepatic arterial dominant phase of the second set of images. Although the nodular lesions are visualized on precontrast (a) and early arterial phase (b) images of the first set, the lesions do not show enhancement due to suboptimal timing. The prominent enhancement of nodular lesions are better visualized in the hepatic arterial dominant phase (e) image of the second set compared to the early hepatic arterial phase (b) of the first set of images. The nodular lesions show wash-out and capsular enhancement on the hepatic venous phase images (c, f). These nodular lesions are consistent with multifocal HCC.

- ° Small HCCs (<3 cm) are frequently isointense on T2-weighted images, although they may also show mildly low or high signal (Figures 7.6–7.8).
- ° Isointensity on T2-weighted images may correlate with a more favorable histology for well-differentiated HCC.
- • On T1-weighted images:
  - ° HCCs are usually isointense on T1-weighted images if they are smaller than 3 cm although they may be hypointense or hyperintense (Figures 7.6–7.8). Larger tumors (>3 cm) usually show low heterogeneous signal on T1-weighted images (Figure 7.5).
  - ° Small tumors less than 3 cm may occasionally demonstrate high signal on T1-weighted images. The hyperintensity on T1-weighted images may be due to
  - ° Protein deposition: More common (Figure 7.9).
  - ° Fatty infiltration: Identified by drop of signal on out-of-phase images (Figures 7.10 and 7.11). The signal decrease on out-of-phase imaging is generally more heterogeneous compared to hepatic adenomas.
  - ° Hemorrhage (Figure 7.12).

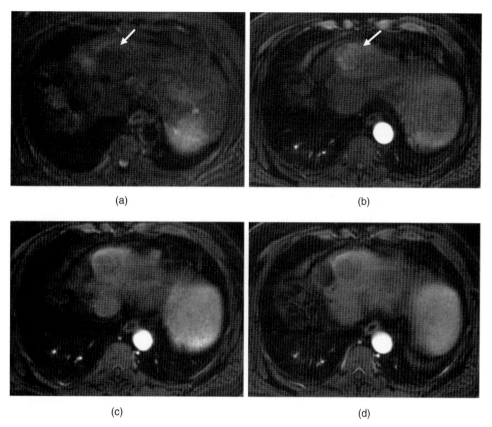

(a) (b)

(c) (d)

Figure 7.5 *Transverse T2-weighted fat-suppressed SS-ETSE (a), T1-weighted fat-suppressed postgadolinium hepatic arterial dominant phase (b), consecutive hepatic venous phase (c, d) 3D-GE images show a medium-sized hypervascular HCC (arrows) located at the dome of the liver, demonstrating typical early homogeneous enhancement (b) and later wash-out with capsular enhancement (c, d). Note that the lesion is mildly hypointense on T2-weighted image.*

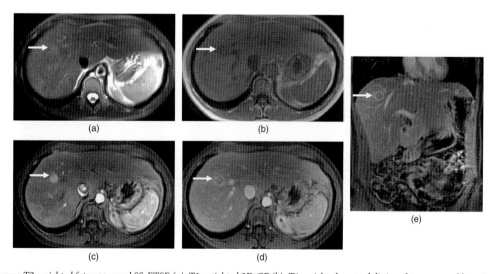

(a) (b)

(c) (d) (e)

Figure 7.6 *Transverse T2-weighted fat-suppressed SS-ETSE (a), T1-weighted 2D-GE (b), T1-weighted postgadolinium fat-suppressed hepatic arterial dominant phase (c), hepatic venous phase (d) and coronal hepatic venous phase 3D-GE images show a small typical hypervascular HCC (arrows) in a patient with chronic hepatitis. The lesion shows mildly high T2 signal (a) and moderately low T1 signal (b) on precontrast images. The lesion shows prominent homogeneous enhancement due to its hypervascular nature in the hepatic arterial dominant phase (c) and typical washout with capsular enhancement in the hepatic venous phase (d, e).*

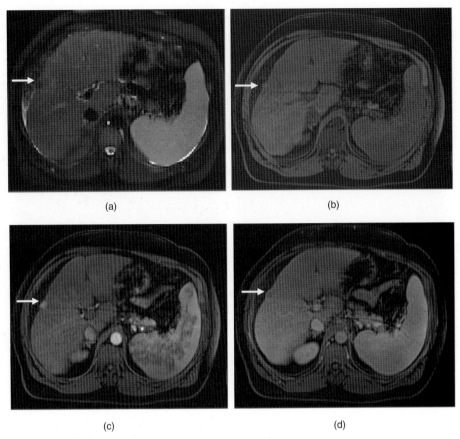

Figure 7.7 *Transverse T2-weighted fat-suppressed SS-ETSE (a), T1-weighted fat-suppressed 3D-GE (b), T1-weighted fat-suppressed postgadolinium hepatic arterial dominant phase (c) and hepatic venous (d) phase 3D-GE images show a small hypervascular exophytic HCC (arrows) in the cirrhotic liver.* The lesion is hypointense on T2-weighted image (a) and isointense on T1-weighted image (b). The lesion shows typical early homogeneous enhancement (c) and later wash-out with capsular enhancement (d).

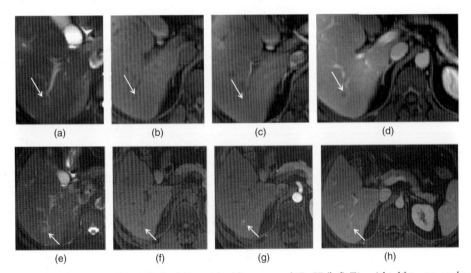

Figure 7.8 *Transverse T2-weighted fat-suppressed SS-ETSE (a, e), T1-weighted fat-suppressed 3D-GE (b, f), T1-weighted fat-suppressed postgadolinium hepatic arterial dominant phase (c, g) and hepatic venous phase (d, h) 3D-GE images show a very small hypervascular HCC (arrows) in a patient with chronic hepatitis.* The second set of images (e–h) were acquired 3 months after the first set of images (a–d). Although the lesion is very small, homogeneous early enhancement (c) and later wash-out (d) are noted on the first set of images, which are concerning for a small HCC. The followup examination (e–h) performed 3 months later demonstrated the interval enlargement of the HCC.

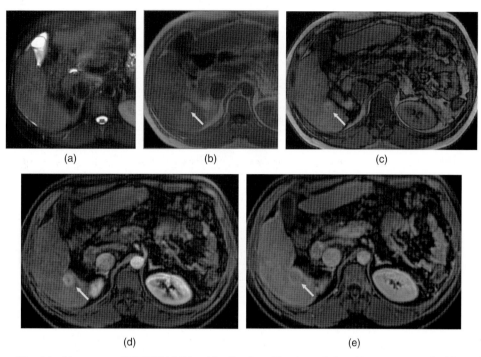

Figure 7.9 *Transverse T2-weighted fat-suppressed SS-ETSE (a), T1-weighted in-phase (b) and out-of-phase (c) 2D-GE, T1-weighted fat-suppressed postgadolinium hepatic arterial dominant phase (d) and hepatic venous phase (e) 3D-GE images demonstrate a small HCC with high protein content.* The lesion shows high signal on T1-weighted in-phase (b) and out-of-phase (c) images due to high protein content. The lesion has a small central scar. The lesion shows moderate enhancement in the hepatic arterial dominant phase (d) and wash-out with capsular enhancement on the hepatic venous phase (e).

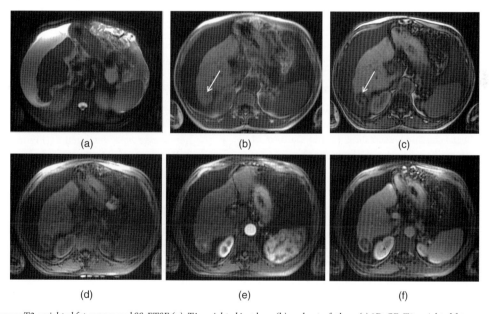

Figure 7.10 *Transverse T2-weighted fat-suppressed SS-ETSE (a), T1-weighted in-phase (b) and out-of-phase (c) 2D-GE, T1-weighted fat-suppressed postgadolinium hepatic arterial dominant phase (d) and hepatic venous phase (e) and interstitial phase (f) 3D-GE images show a fat-containing hypovascular HCC (b, c) in the cirrhotic liver.* The lesion shows prominent signal decrease on out-of-phase image (c) due to its fat content. The lesion shows mild peripheral and central enhancement on postgadolinium images (e, f).

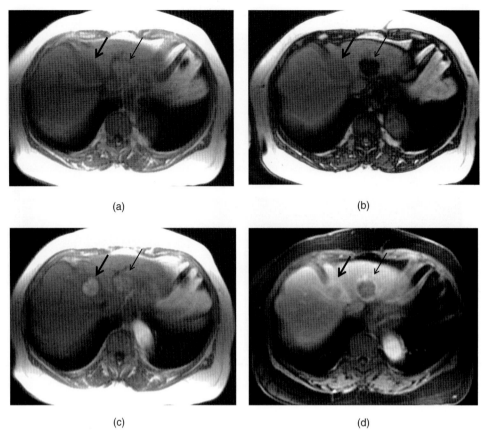

(a)

(b)

(c)

(d)

Figure 7.11 *Transverse T1-weighted in-phase (a) and out-of-phase (b) 2D-GE, T1-weighted postgadolinium hepatic arterial dominant phase (c) and fat-suppressed hepatic venous phase (d) 3D-GE images show two HCCs side by side in the left lobe of the liver.* A fat- containing hypovascular HCC (thin arrow) shows a prominent signal drop in out-of- phase image (b) compared to in-phase image (a). This fat-containing HCC is hypovascular and does not show prominent enhancement in the hepatic arterial dominant phase (c) compared to precontrast T1-weighted image (a). This fat-containing HCC appears hypointense in the hepatic venous phase (d) due to fat-suppression effect and shows prominent capsular enhancement. Note that the hypointense appearance of the lesion on the hepatic venous phase is not due to wash-out but fat-suppression effect. The other HCC (thick arrow) is hypervascular and does not contain fat. This non-fat-containing HCC appears hypointense on both in-phase and out-of-phase images (a, b) and shows significant early homogeneous enhancement (c) and wash-out in the later phase (d). Source: Semelka 2010. Reproduced with permission of Wiley.

- On post-gadolinium T1-weighted fat-suppressed 3D-GE images:
  - HCCs have been classified according to the pattern of enhancement in the hepatic arterial dominant phase:
    1 Hypervascular:
    - The most common type (90%)
    - The majority of small tumors (<3 cm) will enhance prominently on the hepatic arterial dominant phase. This is the most sensitive finding for the detection of small HCCs. Larger HCCs show heterogeneous prominent enhancement.
    - Later wash-out and enhancement of the surrounding capsule are seen on the hepatic venous and interstitial phases. This is the most specific finding.
    - Figures 7.5–7.9.
    - Greater and heterogeneous contrast enhancement is usually associated with higher grade tumors (Figures 7.12–7.14).

- HCCs usually appear as hypointense lesions on the hepatocyte phase following the administration of hepatocyte specific agents (Figure 7.15). However, well-differentiated HCCs may show some uptake on the hepatocyte phase.

2 Isovascular:

- The tumor shows similar enhancement characteristics to the background liver on the hepatic arterial dominant phase.
- The tumor displays wash-out below the signal intensity of background parenchyma, and capsule enhancement on the later phases. It is critical to study venous phase images in order to identify masses that show development of a well-defined enhanced capsule to establish this diagnosis. Note that fading of RNs and DNs with interval progression of enhancement of surrounding fibrous tissue can simulate the appearance of an

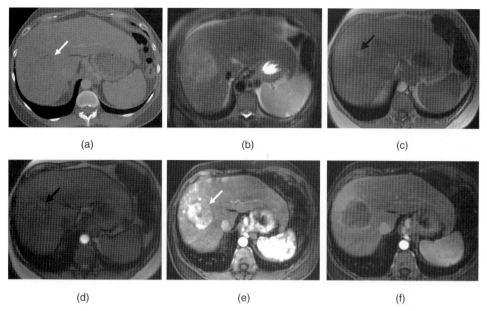

(a) (b) (c)

(d) (e) (f)

Figure 7.12 *Transverse postcontrast hepatic venous phase (a), transverse T2-weighted fat-suppressed SS-ETSE (b), T1-weighted in-phase (c) and out-of-phase (d) 2D-GE, T1-weighted postgadolinium fat-suppressed hepatic arterial dominant phase (e), hepatic venous phase (f) 3D-GE images show a large hypervascular HCC (white arrows) in the right lobe of the liver.* The lesion appears as a mildly hypodense lesion on the hepatic venous phase CT image (a) due to its wash-out, and the early enhancement characteristics were not visualized as CT examination was performed on the hepatic venous phase only, due to radiation concerns. Focal hyperintense hemorrhagic foci (black arrows; c, d) are also noted in the lesion on in-phase and out-of-phase images (c, d). Note the typical prominent early enhancement (e) and later wash-out with capsular enhancement (f). Large gastroesophageal varices are also seen.

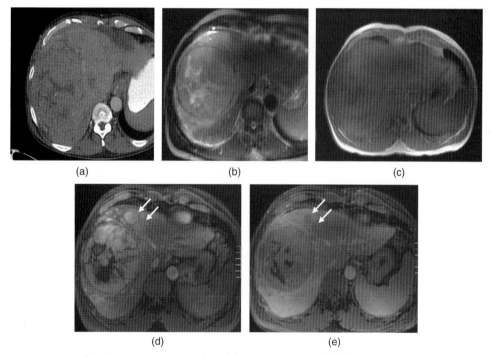

(a) (b) (c)

(d) (e)

Figure 7.13 *Transverse postcontrast hepatic arterial dominant phase (a), transverse T2-weighted fat-suppressed SS-ETSE (b), T1-weighted 2D-GE (c), T1-weighted postgadolinium fat-suppressed hepatic arterial dominant phase (d), hepatic venous phase (e) 3D-GE images show a large hypervascular heterogeneous HCC with central necrosis in the cirrhotic liver.* The lesion appears isodense to the liver on the CT image (a). The lesion appears mildly hyperintense on T1-weighted image due to its high protein content. In addition to the large lesion, multiple satellite lesions (arrows) showing early enhancement and later wash-out with capsular enhancement are noted. Note that the enhancement of lesions is well visualized on MRI compared to CT.

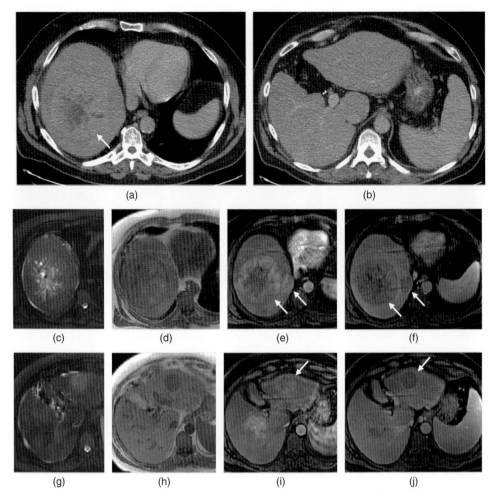

Figure 7.14 *Transverse postcontrast hepatic venous phase CT (a, b), transverse T2-weighted fat-suppressed SS-ETSE (c, g), T1-weighted 2D-GE (d, h), T1-weighted postgadolinium fat-suppressed hepatic arterial dominant phase (e, i), hepatic venous phase (f, j) 3D-GE images demonstrate three hypervascular HCCs (arrows).* The largest lesion contains central necrosis (asterisk, c). Note that the lesions are better visualized on MRI compared to CT due to its higher soft tissue contrast and high sensitivity to gadolinium. The smaller lesions are isodense and not well seen on CT images (a, b).

isovascular HCC. If uncertain, recommend 3-month follow-up.

- These tumors are usually well-differentiated and usually isointense on pre-contrast T1 and T2-weighted images.
- Figures 7.16 and 7.17.

3 Hypovascular:

- The tumor shows minimal increased enhancement in the hepatic arterial dominant phase and appears as a hypointense lesion compared to background liver.
- Minimal enhancement is seen in the later phases and the tumor also appears as a hypointense lesion on later phases. The appearance of an enhanced well-defined rounded capsule facilitates the recognition of this as a cancer.

- These tumors are usually well-differentiated and usually isointense on pre-contrast T1 and T2-weighted images.
- Figures 7.10, 7.11, 7.18, and 7.19.
- The typical signal intensity of a capsule:
  - Isointense to hypointense on T2-weighted images.
  - Isointense to hypointense on T1-weighted images.
  - No enhancement to negligible mild enhancement on the hepatic arterial dominant phase images that becomes more intense on later phase images.
- "Nodule-within-nodule" appearance
  - Is a feature suggestive of stepwise carcinogenesis and represents the development of a small focus of HCC in a DN.
  - On T2-weighted images, the nodule – within – nodule appears as a hyperintense focus within a hypointense nodule.

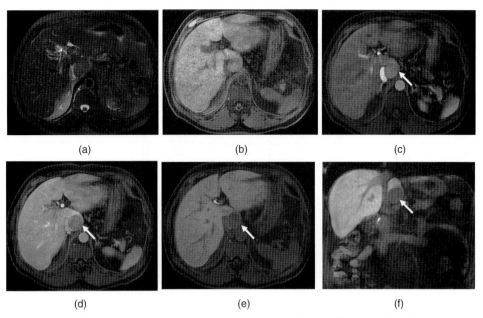

(a)   (b)   (c)

(d)   (e)   (f)

Figure 7.15 *Transverse T2-weighted fat-suppressed SS-ETSE (a), T1-weighted fat-suppressed 3D-GE (b), T1-weighted fat-suppressed postgadolinium hepatic arterial dominant phase (c), hepatic venous phase (d) and hepatocyte phase (e, f) 3D-GE images show a hypervascular HCC (arrows) located in the caudate lobe with typical early enhancement (c) and late wash-out (d). Note that the lesion does not show enhancement on the hepatocyte phase (e, f) acquired 20 min after the administration of gadoxetic acid.*

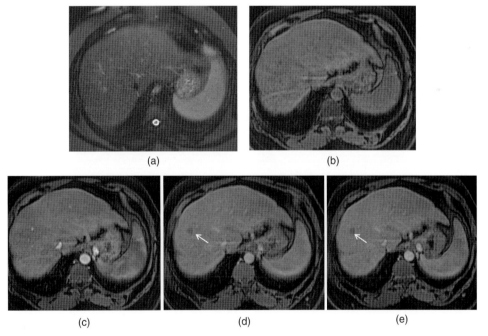

(a)   (b)

(c)   (d)   (e)

Figure 7.16 *Transverse T2-weighted fat-suppressed SS-ETSE (a), T1-weighted fat-suppressed 3D-GE (b), T1-weighted fat-suppressed postgadolinium hepatic arterial dominant phase (c) and consecutive hepatic venous phase (d, e) 3D-GE images show a small isovascular HCC in a cirrhotic liver. The isovascular HCC is isointense to the background liver on precontrast images (a, b). The lesion is also isointense to the background liver in the hepatic arterial dominant phase (c). However, the lesion shows wash-out on the hepatic venous phase (d, e).*

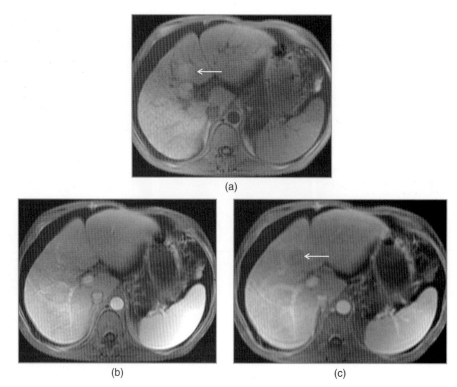

(a)

(b)   (c)

Figure 7.17 *Transverse T1-weighted fat-suppressed 3D-GE (a), T1-weighted fat-suppressed postgadolinium consecutive hepatic venous phase (b, c) 3D-GE images show an isovascular HCC (arrows).* The HCC demonstrates mildly increased T1 signal (a). The lesion appears isointense on the earlier hepatic venous phase image (b) but shows wash-out on the later hepatic venous phase image (c).

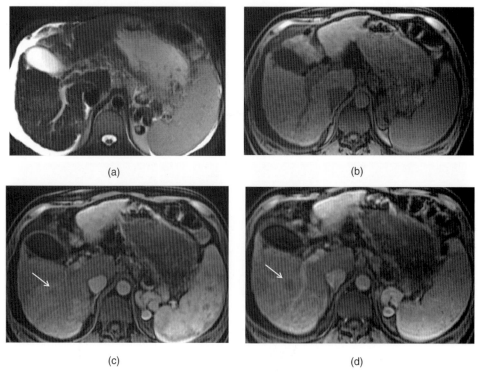

(a)   (b)

(c)   (d)

Figure 7.18 *Transverse T2-weighted fat-suppressed SS-ETSE (a), T1-weighted fat-suppressed 3D-GE (b), T1-weighted fat-suppressed postgadolinium hepatic arterial dominant phase (c) and hepatic venous phase (d) 3D-GE images show a hypovascular HCC (arrows).* The lesion is isointense on precontrast images (a, b). The lesion appears hypointense on postgadolinium images (c, d). Note that the lesion becomes more apparent in the later phase (d).

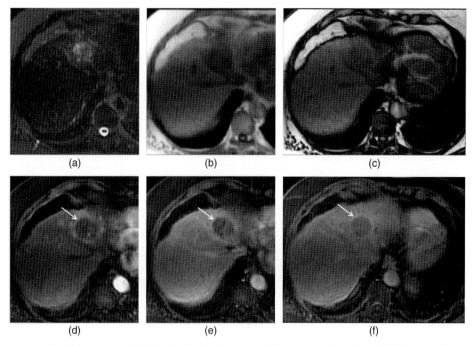

Figure 7.19 *Transverse T2-weighted fat-suppressed SS-ETSE (a), T1-weighted in-phase (b) and out-of-phase (c) 2D-GE, T1-weighted fat-suppressed postgadolinium hepatic arterial dominant phase (d) and hepatic venous phase (e) and interstitial phase (f) 3D-GE images show a hypovascular HCC located in the segment IVA. The lesion shows subtle enhancement in the hepatic arterial dominant phase (d). The lesion shows mild enhancement with prominent capsular enhancement in the later phases (e, f). Transient early increased enhancement is also noted around the lesion in the hepatic arterial dominant phase, which represents inflammation/shunting.*

° On postgadolinium T1-weighted images, the nodule – within – nodule appears as a smaller nodular focus in a larger DN, which shows more prominent enhancement or similar enhancement compared to the DN on the hepatic arterial dominant phase. The focus of HCC shows wash-out on later phases, and the remaining portions of the DN fade to isointensity with the background liver parenchyma.

- Imaging features of solitary and multifocal HCCs associated with poor prognosis:
  ° Increased number of HCC foci in the liver (Figures 7.4 and 7.20)
  ° Thick ring enhancement on the hepatic arterial dominant phase (Figure 7.21)
  ° Presence of venous thrombosis
  ° Presence of hemorrhage
  ° Large size
  ° Prominent increase in size within a short time interval
  ° Mild to moderately high T2 signal (as opposed to isointensity)
  ° Presence of metastases Special note should be given to mild-moderately high T2 signal of a nodule as this is in keeping with HCC (as opposed to other nodules such as RN and DN), suggests the lesion may grow somewhat rapidly, and is a common finding. Arterial phase thick ring enhancement (Figure 7.21) is also important to recognize.

Ring enhancement is rare for HCC (as opposed to metastases where this is the hallmark enhancement pattern). The finding suggests that the tumor is so aggressive that it conscripts and induces a greater number of vessels that simulate the growth characteristics of a liver metastasis. This appearance is seen most often in patients with Hepatitis C virus. Tumor growth can be explosive, so if there is uncertainty whether this pattern is present, a 2-month follow-up is recommended rather than the usual 3- month, for a suspected small HCC.

- **Diffuse HCCs**
- Characterized by an infiltrative ill-defined mass.
- Associated with very high serum alpha fetoprotein (AFP) levels, but 1/3 of cases can have normal AFP.
- Invariably associated with venous thrombosis.
- On T2-weighted images:
  ° Amorphous, wedge-shaped or segmental, mild to moderate high signal intensity
- On T1-weighted images:
  ° Isointense, or amorphous, wedge-shaped or segmental, mild to moderately low signal.
- On post-gadolinium fat-suppressed T1-weighted images:
- Patchy heterogeneous enhancement in the hepatic arterial dominant phase with heterogeneous wash-out on the later phases. Wash-out is irregular but present, and portions of late enhancing capsules are also evident.

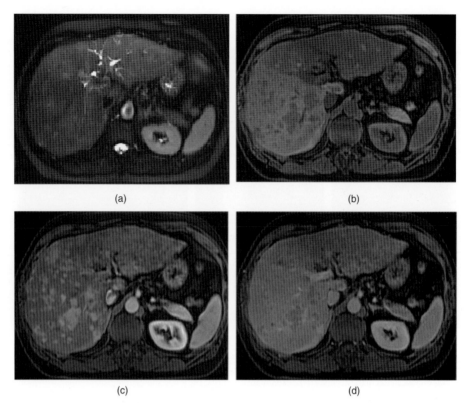

(a) (b)

(c) (d)

Figure 7.20 *Transverse T2-weighted fat-suppressed SS-ETSE (a), T1-weighted fat-suppressed 3D-GE (b), T1-weighted fat-suppressed postgadolinium hepatic arterial dominant phase (c) and hepatic venous phase (d) 3D-GE images show numerous foci of hypervascular HCCs in the liver.* Note that there is no tumor thrombus in the portal vein and its branches. These findings are consistent with multifocal HCC. The lesions in the left lobe of the liver coalesce with each other. The lesions show early prominent enhancement (c) with later washout (d).

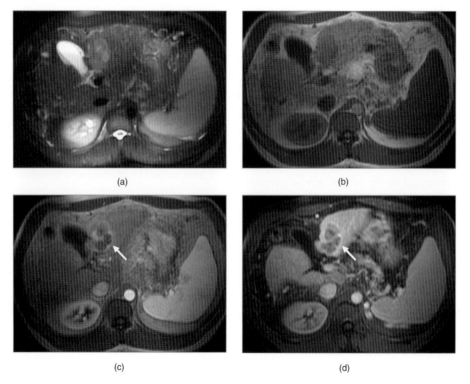

(a) (b)

(c) (d)

Figure 7.21 *Transverse T2-weighted fat-suppressed SS-ETSE (a), T1-weighted 2D-GE (b), T1-weighted postgadolinium hepatic arterial dominant phase 2D-GE (c), hepatic venous phase fat-suppressed 3D-GE (d) images show a HCC (arrows) with peripheral rim enhancement on postgadolinium images (c, d) in a patient with cirrhotic liver.*

- Tumor thrombosis almost always involves the portal vein branches. Hepatic venous branches are occasionally involved, sometimes alone, but most often in combination with portal vein thrombus.
- Figures 7.22 and 7.23
- **Portal or hepatic vein tumor thrombus characteristics:**
  ○ Tumor thrombus expands the vascular lumen.
  ○ Tumor thrombus shows mild-moderate high signal intensity on T2-weighted images and mild-moderate high signal intensity on T1-weighted images.
  ○ Tumor thrombus shows enhancement on the hepatic arterial dominant phase and wash-out in the hepatic venous and interstitial phases. The enhancement is usually heterogeneous.
  ○ The presence of enhancement distinguishes it from bland thrombus.
  ○ Because of the greater sensitivity for MR for contrast enhancement, this feature is much better observed on MR than on CT.
  ○ Increased transient enhancement of the segmental or lobar hepatic parenchyma supplied by the thrombosed portal vein in the hepatic arterial dominant phase may be observed due to compensatory increased arterial flow. This abnormally increased-enhancement liver parenchyma is often larger in size than the actual tumor as it represents increased enhancement of the entire segmental hepatic parenchyma and not just the tumor.
  ○ Figures 7.22 and 7.23.
- **Signs of arterioportal shunting:**
  ○ Arterioportal shunting may be associated with HCCs.
  ○ Early or prolonged enhancement of the portal vein may be seen.
  ○ Transient segmental, lobar or wedge-shaped, increased enhancement peripheral to the tumor is seen in the hepatic arterial dominant phase (Figure 7.19).
- **Elevated AFP with no tumor observed on imaging studies in a cirrhotic patient**
- Patients without HCC generally show progressive decrease in AFP over time.
- In contrast, patients with HCC most often show progressive increase in AFP. Tumors eventually become apparent on MR studies. Critical to perform serial 3-month follow-up MRI studies in patients with AFP > 300 (especially if AFP continues to rise) in order to detect these tumors when they are still small and treatable.
- **Metastases to the liver, regional lymph nodes, adrenal gland, peritoneum, lung, pleura, and bones may be seen.**
  ○ Figures 7.24 – 7.26
- **Differential Diagnosis**
- *High grade dysplastic nodules*
  ○ High-grade DNs usually display isointense signal on T2-weighted and T1-weighted images, and moderately intense enhancement on early postgadolinium images that fade to isointensity on late postgadolinium images.

○ Factors favoring the diagnosis of HCC include
  - Small hypervascular lesions seen together with a preexisting larger HCC, even if lacking wash-out in later phases, have a high likelihood of representing small HCCs.
  - Interval growth of nodule by greater than 30% in a 3-month interval.
  - Size of nodule > 2 cm.
○ Factors favoring the diagnosis of DNs:
  - Stability of lesion size over a one-year period, which is the most reliable feature.
  - Regression of lesion on follow-up studies is suggestive of DN, vascular shunts, or inflammation.
  - Size of nodule < 1.5 cm, fading, and no capsule
- *Mixed HCC – Cholangiocarcinoma*
- Mixed HCC – cholangiocarcinoma shows enhancement characteristics of both tumors. Depending on the proportions of tumor components, the tumor shows variable enhancement patterns. If the tumor is HCC-dominant, it shows early enhancement and later wash-out. If the tumor is cholangiocarcinoma dominant, it shows peripheral and progressive delayed enhancement. If both tumors coexist in substantial proportions, heterogeneous enhancement including both types of enhancement pattern is seen.
- *Metastasis*
  ○ The presence of underlying chronic hepatic disease or cirrhosis is the supportive feature of HCC.
  ○ HCCs typically and usually demonstrate enhancement throughout the entire tumor in the hepatic arterial dominant phase, whereas metastases typically show ring enhancement.
  ○ Aggressive HCCs may rarely show ring-enhancement in the hepatic arterial dominant phase. The history/imaging features of chronic liver disease, presence of wash-out and late capsular enhancement, and absence of a history of a primary extrahepatic tumor, are helpful clues to the diagnosis.
  ○ Small hypervascular metastases (<1.5 – 2 cm) may show prominent homogeneous enhancement on the hepatic arterial dominant phase, similar to the enhancement of small HCCs. Both entities show wash-out in later phases, although the majority of metastases fade in signal. The absence of a history of chronic liver disease, absence of late capsular enhancement, and greater occurrence of fading are the helpful clues for the diagnosis of metastases. Note that carcinoid tumor metastases can simulate the appearance of HCCs: hypervascular enhancement and wash-out with late capsule enhancement; the important clue is that the patient should have carcinoid symptomatology and may have existing histologic evidence of this malignancy.
  ○ Infiltrative metastases such as breast cancer may mimic diffuse HCCs; however, infiltrative metastases are rarely associated with tumor thrombosis. Additionally, there is generally a history of primary malignancy and infiltrative

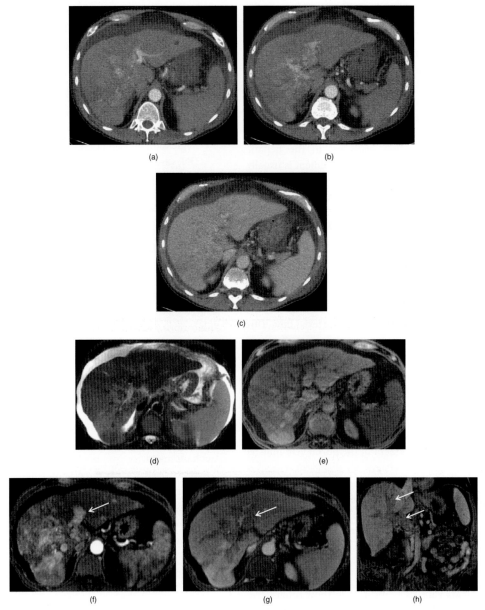

Figure 7.22 *Transverse postcontrast hepatic arterial dominant phase (a, b) and hepatic venous phase (c) CT images show heterogeneous infiltrative lesion showing early enhancement (a, b) with subtle wash-out on the later phase (c).* The branches of right portal vein are not seen due to tumor infiltration. Transverse T2-weighted fat-suppressed SS-ETSE (d), T1-weighted fat-suppressed 3D-GE (e), T1-weighted fat-suppressed postgadolinium hepatic arterial dominant phase (f), hepatic venous phase (g) and coronal 3D-GE interstitial phase (h) images show an infiltrative heterogeneous lesion consistent with diffuse HCC. Interval enlargement of the tumor is noted on MR images compared to CT images. The tumor appears mildly hyperintense on T2-weighted image (d) and mildly hypointense on T1-weighted image (e). The HCC involving most of the right hepatic lobe shows heterogeneous prominently increased enhancement on the hepatic arterial dominant phase (f). Some parts of the lesion show wash-out and appear hypointense on the hepatic venous phase (g). Note the presence of expansile enhancing tumor thrombus in the left portal vein (arrow, f) and its wash-out on the hepatic venous phase (arrow, g). The coronal postgadolinium image shows the tumor thrombus in the main portal vein and its intrahepatic branches (arrows, h). Diffuse HCCs are almost invariably associated with tumor thrombus in the portal veins. Note the presence of increased secondary compensatory arterial enhancement in the right lobe of the liver in the hepatic arterial dominant phase (f).

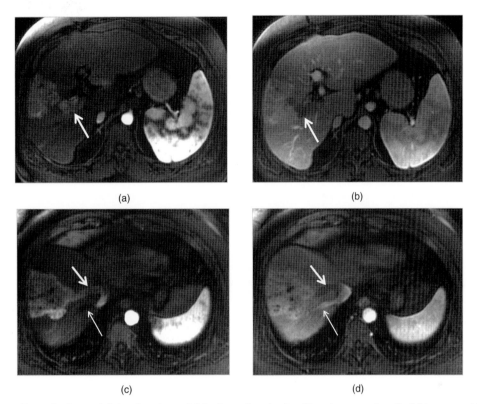

(a)

(b)

(c)

(d)

Figure 7.23 *Transverse T1-weighted postgadolinium hepatic arterial dominant phase (a, c) and hepatic venous phase (b, d) fat-suppressed 3D-GE images show segmental diffuse HCC located at segments VIII and V, invading the right portal vein and right hepatic vein.* The tumor thrombus (thick arrows) shows early enhancement (a, c) and later wash-out (b, d). Note that the diffuse HCC also shows early mildly heterogeneous enhancement (a, c) with small areas of wash-out in the later phases (b, d). There is a right accessory hepatic vein (thin arrow; c, d).

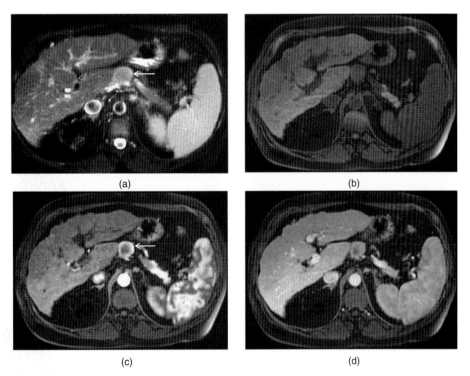

(a)

(b)

(c)

(d)

Figure 7.24 *Transverse T2-weighted fat-suppressed SS-ETSE (a), T1-weighted fat-suppressed 3D-GE (b), T1-weighted fat-suppressed postgadolinium hepatic arterial dominant phase (c), hepatic venous phase (d) 3D-GE images show an enlarged lymph node (arrows; a, b) adjacent to the caudate lobe.* The HCC is not shown.

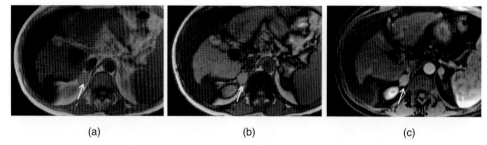

(a)   (b)   (c)

Figure 7.25 *Transverse T1-weighted in-phase (a) 2D-GE, out-of-phase (b) 2D-GE and postgadolinium hepatic arterial dominant phase fat-suppressed 3D-GE images show a right adrenal gland metastasis secondary to HCC. The lesion contains fat on MR images.*

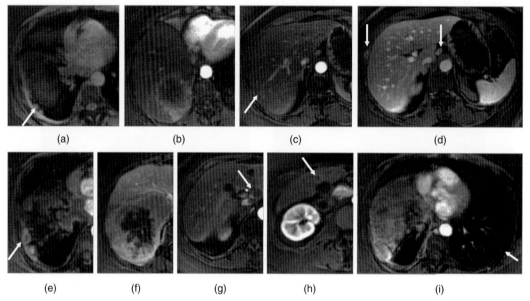

(a)   (b)   (c)   (d)

(e)   (f)   (g)   (h)   (i)

Figure 7.26 *Transverse postgadolinium T1-weighted fat-suppressed 3D-GE images show multiple metastases (arrows) secondary to a large necrotic HCC (b, f), multiple right-sided pleural nodules (a, e), liver metastases (c, h), lymph node metastases (d, g), bone metastasis (d) and lung metastasis (i).*

metastases usually demonstrate progressive enhancement on dynamic postcontrast imaging rather than wash-out.

- *Acute-on-chronic hepatitis, transient perfusion abnormalities, confluent fibrosis*
  - Acute-on-chronic hepatitis may show mildly increased T2 signal, but is usually isointense. Acute-on-chronic hepatitis shows focal increased transient enhancement in the hepatic arterial dominant phase, but critically, this abnormal increased enhancement fades in later phases. Fading often occurs rapidly. No late wash-out is observed with acute-on-chronic hepatitis.
  - No T2 correlation is generally detected for transient perfusion abnormalities. Transient perfusion abnormalities are characterized by focal or segmental increased transient enhancement in the hepatic arterial dominant phase, which fade in later phases. No wash-out is seen. They may be wedge-shaped or segmental-subsegmental, although they are usually linear and subcapsular.

  - Confluent fibrosis shows mildly increased T2 signal and progressive enhancement on dynamic postcontrast imaging. It occurs most often in segment VIII.
- **Fibrolamellar HCC**
- Distinct morphologic subtype of HCC. Not associated with hepatitis or cirrhosis.
- Fibrolamellar HCC is rare and accounts for <1% of all HCCs.
- Occurs in young adults (second and third decade of life) without sex predominance.
- No specific risk factors have been identified.
- Fibrolamellar HCC often exhibits slow growth and is associated with a favorable prognosis, but may be relatively aggressive.
- Not associated with high AFP levels. Hemorrhage and necrosis are rarely seen. Vascular invasion is uncommon.
- Regional adenopathy is common in advanced large tumors. Distant metastases are rare.
- Macroscopically, at initial presentation the tumor usually appears as a single, large, well-demarcated mass. The tumor has a lobular architecture with intervening fibrous septa,

which may coalesce to form a central stellate scar. The central scar is usually present and may contain calcifications. The scar is usually large and irregular on all imaging sequences. This is unlike the scar of FNH, which is small and regular. Although there is no capsule, pseudocapsule may be present.

- On CT:
- The tumor appears as a hypoattenuated heterogeneous mass on precontrast images. Calcifications (30–70%), central scar (70%), and pseudocapsule may be detected on CT. The tumor shows heterogeneous increased enhancement on the hepatic arterial dominant phase and wash-out on later phases with heterogeneous enhancement of central scar, fibrous septa, and pseudocapsule.
- On MRI:
- On T2-weighted images:
- At presentation, it is usually a large, solitary, heterogeneous tumor with moderately high T2 signal. The central scar typically shows heterogeneous T2 signal due to the presence of fibrosis admixed with prominent vascular tissue and tissue with high fluid content.
- On T1-weighted images:
- Heterogeneous and moderately low in signal intensity.
- On postgadolinium fat-suppressed T1-weighted images:
- Diffuse heterogeneous enhancement on the hepatic arterial dominant phase images with wash-out in later phases. The large and irregular central scar, with radiating septa, is present and enhances heterogeneously on delayed phase images. An enhancing pseudocapsule may be present.
- **Differential Diagnosis:**
  - *FNH*
  - FNH is isointense, or mildly hyperintense, or hypointense on precontrast T2-weighed or T1-weighted images,

respectively. The central scar of FNH is small and regular and is usually homogeneous, and often shows high T2 signal.
- FNH shows homogeneous enhancement in the hepatic arterial dominant phase, and fades in the later phases and becomes isointense to the background liver parenchyma, except the small scar, which usually shows prominent enhancement in the interstitial phase, but is almost always regular in enhancement.

References

1 Ramalho, M., Altun, E., Heredia, V. *et al.* (2007) Liver MR imaging: 1.5 T versus 3T Magn Reson Imaging Clin N Am, 15, 321–347.

2 Kierans, A.S., Leonardou, P., Hayshi, P. *et al.* (2010) MRI findings of rapidly progressive hepatocellular carcinoma. Magn Reson Imaging, 28, 790–796.

3 Kim, B.S., Hayashi, P.H., Kim, S.H. *et al.* (2013) Outcomes of patients with elevated alpha fetoprotein level and initial negative findings at MR imaging. Radiology, 268, 109–119.

4 de Campos, R.O., Semelka, R.C., Azevedo, R.M. *et al.* (2012) Combined hepatocellular carcinoma-cholangiocarcinoma: report of MR appearance in eleven patients. J Magn Reson Imaging, 36, 1139–1147.

5 Lee, C.H., Brubaker, L.M., Gerber, D.A. *et al.* (2011) MRI findings of recurrent hepatocellular carcinoma after liver transplantation: preliminary results. J Magn Reson Imaging, 33, 1399–1405.

6 Kanematsu, M., Semelka, R.C., Leonardou, P. *et al.* (2003) Hepatocellular carcinoma of diffuse type: MR imaging findings and clinical manifestations. J Magn Reson Imaging, 18, 189–195.

7 Karadeniz-Bilgili, M.Y., Braga, L., Birchard, K.R. *et al.* (2006) Hepatocellular carcinoma missed on gadolinium enhanced MR imaging, discovered in liver explants: retrospective evaluation. J Magn Reson Imaging, 23, 210–215.

CHAPTER 8

Rare primary and secondary tumors of the liver

Ersan Altun[1], Mohamed El-Azzazi[1,2,3,4] and Richard C. Semelka[1]

[1] The University of North Carolina at Chapel Hill, Department of Radiology, Chapel Hill, NC, USA
[2] University of Dammam, Department of Radiology, Dammam, Saudi Arabia
[3] King Fahd Hospital of the University, Department of Radiology, Khobar, Saudi Arabia
[4] University of Al Azhar, Department of Radiology, Cairo, Egypt

Lymphoma

- Primary and secondary involvement may occur.
- **Primary Liver Lymphoma**
- Primary hepatic lymphoma is an extremely rare primary liver tumor.
- Imaging features of primary lymphoma are nonspecific and may mimic imaging features of adenocarcinoma or cholangiocarcinoma. They usually present as solitary masses (Figure 8.1) although multiple foci may sometimes be seen (Figure 8.2)
- They show mildly high signal on T2-WI and moderate to markedly low signal on T1-WI. Central necrosis, which shows increased moderate to markedly high signal on T2-WI, may be seen (Figure 8.1).
- They are hypovascular tumors and usually show progressive heterogeneous enhancement (Figure 8.1). Peripheral thick ring-like soft tissue with or without central necrosis may be present. Early peripheral enhancement with central progressive enhancement on later phases may also be seen. Perilesional enhancement may also be present.
- **Secondary Liver Lymphoma**
- Secondary involvement of the liver by lymphoma is more common.
- Hodgkin and non-Hodgkin lymphoma involvement may occur in stage IV disease.
- Non-Hodgkin lymphoma is much more common.
- **Appearances:**
  ° Large multiple nodules (the most common) (Figure 8.3)
  ° Solitary nodule
  ° Diffuse involvement (Figure 8.4)
- **On MRI and CT**
  ° *Focal Involvement:*
  ° Lesions vary in signal intensity from low to moderately high on T2-WIs.

° Low in signal intensity on T1-WIs.
° Low attenuation on precontrast CT images.
° These lesions are hypovascular. They usually show early peripheral enhancement and later progressive enhancement on postcontrast images. They may also show progressive heterogeneous enhancement on postcontrast images (Figure 8.3)
° *Diffuse Involvement:*
° Precontrast signal intensity changes are similar to focal involvement.
° Involvement of portal tracts with progressive enhancement is seen (Figure 8.4)
- **Differential Diagnosis:**
  ° Cholangiocarcinoma
  ° Inflammatory myofibroblastic tumor
  ° Metastases

Multiple myeloma

- Focal deposits of multiple myeloma rarely occur in the liver and most often in the setting of disseminated disease.
- The liver is the most commonly involved solid organ in the body.
- Focal involvement presents as nodular lesions in the liver. The lesions may vary in size and large lesions measuring more than 5 cm may also be seen.
- Diffuse involvement presents as involvement of portal tracts without formation of focal nodules.
- **On MRI and CT:**
  ° Imaging appearances of lesions are not specific.
  ° Focal nodular lesions demonstrate mild to moderately hyperintense on T2-WI and variable signal intensities on T1-WIs. High signal intensity on T1-WI may develop secondary to high protein content of lesions. These lesions

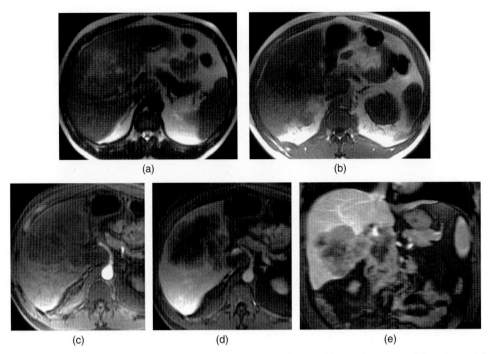

(a)   (b)   (c)   (d)   (e)

Figure 8.1 *Transverse T2-weighted SS-ETSE (a), T1-weighted 2D-GE (b), T1-weighted postgadolinium fat-suppressed hepatic arterial phase (c), hepatic venous phase (d) and interstitial phase (e) 3D-GE images show a large mass with central necrosis in the liver, which represents primary lymphoma. The lesion shows heterogeneous predominantly peripheral enhancement (d) which progresses in the later phases (e). The lesion also extends into the caudate lobe.*

show low attenuation on CT. These lesions demonstrate progressive enhancement on postcontrast images although they may occasionally be hypervascular (Figure 8.5).

° Diffuse involvement may be seen as hepatomegaly and/or infiltration of portal tracts with progressively enhancing tissue.

- **Differential Diagnosis:**
  ° Metastases
  ° Lymphoma
  ° Cholangiocarcinoma

Extramedullary hematopoiesis

- An unusual condition in which red blood cells are produced outside the bone marrow when the production of red blood cells is not sufficient to meet the demand of the body.
- This condition results from myeloproliferative disorders, hemolytic disease, and bone marrow infiltration, which lead to inadequate hematopoiesis. Focal areas of hematopoiesis may develop in various places in the body including the liver, spleen, lymph nodes, paravertebral areas, and even the kidneys or pleura.
- Hepatomegaly may be seen as a finding in patients with hematopoiesis. Focal solitary or multiple lesions may be seen in the liver with extramedullary hematopoiesis. However,

infiltrative lesions along the portal tracts (Figure 8.6) or subcapsular lesions may also be detected.

- **On CT:**
  ° Homogeneous low attenuation lesions showing mild or no enhancement on the hepatic arterial dominant phase but shows mild to moderate progressive enhancement in the later phases (Figure 8.6).

- **On MRI:**
  ° Homogeneous mild to moderate high signal intensity on T2w images.
  ° Homogeneous low signal intensity on T2w images may also be seen.
  ° No or mild enhancement in the hepatic arterial dominant phase with mild to moderate progressive enhancement in the later phases (Figure 8.6).

- **Differential Diagnosis:**
  ° Lymphoma
  ° Metastases

Epithelioid hemangioendothelioma (EHE)

- Epithelioid hemangioendothelioma (EHE) is a rare low-grade malignancy of the hepatic vasculature with an incidence of less than 0.1/100.000 per year.

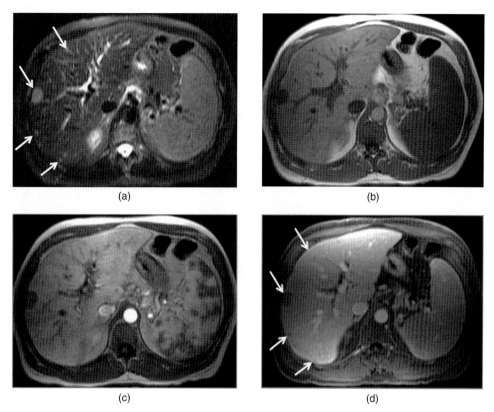

Figure 8.2 *Transverse T2-weighted SS-ETSE (a), T1-weighted 2D-GE (b), T1-weighted postgadolinium hepatic arterial dominant phase (c), hepatic venous phase (d) images show multiple foci of primary lymphoma (arrows) in the liver.* The lesions show mild enhancement on postgadolinium images.

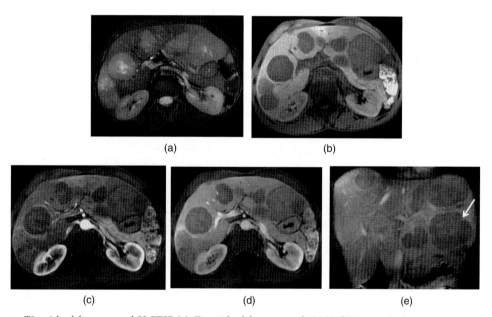

Figure 8.3 *Transverse T2-weighted fat-suppressed SS-ETSE (a), T1-weighted fat-suppressed 3D-GE (b), T1-weighted postgadolinium fat-suppressed hepatic arterial dominant phase (c), hepatic venous phase (d) and coronal interstitial phase (e) 3D-GE images show multiple foci of secondary lymphoma in the liver and spleen (arrow, e) due to Non-Hodgkin lymphoma.* The lymphoma foci show mild heterogeneous enhancement.

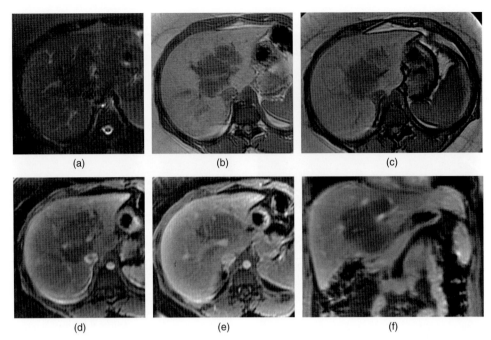

Figure 8.4 *Transverse T2-weighted fat-suppressed SS-ETSE (a), T1-weighted in-phase (b) and out-of-phase (c) 2D-GE, T1-weighted postgadolinium fat-suppressed hepatic arterial dominant phase (d), hepatic venous phase (e) and coronal interstitial phase (f) 3D-GE images show an infiltrating lymphoma in the porta hilum extending along the portal tracts.* The lymphoma shows low T2 signal due to its high cellular content and shows mild enhancement due to its hypovascularity.

- Usually occurs in middle-age (25–60) with a female predilection (F : M/3 : 2) and peak incidence occurring between 30 and 40 years of age.
- Clinically, patients are usually asymptomatic, and not uncommonly the disease may be discovered incidentally. They may present with abdominal pain, jaundice, or hepatosplenomegaly. Tumor markers are usually negative.
- Distant metastatic lesions may be seen occasionally in the lungs and other organs including lymph nodes.
- **Macroscopically:**
  - Most lesions tend to be located at the periphery of the liver and tend to occur in multiples and to coalesce over time, forming large masses. Solitary masses may also occasionally be seen.
  - The presence of fibrotic stroma may cause capsular retraction in peripherally located lesions.
- **Microscopically**:
  - There is characteristically abundant fibrotic stroma with scattered clumps of neoplastic cells invading sinusoids and vessels, which arise from endothelial cells.
- **On CT and MRI:**
  - The lesions are hypoattenuating on precontrast CT images.
  - The lesions usually show high signal on T2-WIs with a more hyperintense center. Variable heterogeneous T2 signal with low T2 signal representing its fibrous stroma may also occasionally be seen. The lesions demonstrate moderately low signal on T1-WIs (Figures 8.7 and 8.8).
  - Calcifications and capsular retraction are occasionally seen.

- On postcontrast CT and MR images, the tumor may enhance peripherally creating target appearance (Figure 8.7) with progressive enhancement in the later phases. Delayed imaging may also show the enhancing central portion, depending on the predominance of fibrosis. Aggressive tumors may show moderately intense diffuse heterogeneous enhancement on immediate postcontrast images. Peripheral hypodense/hypointense rim may also occasionally be seen on postcontrast images.
- The characteristic enhancement appearance on MR studies is initial ring enhancement, with later peripheral ring and central enhancement, with an intermediate band of minimally enhanced tissue on early and late post contrast images. This may be a characteristic appearance of this tumor, distinguishing it from metastases, which do not show an intermediate band of minimally enhanced tissue. However, this is rarely seen and the enhancement features are usually not specific (Figure 8.8)
- **Differential Diagnosis**
- Metastases. Small EHE and metastases have a similar appearance of ring enhancement. Investigation for a history of a primary extrahepatic malignancy is critical, as well as studying the images for a primary malignancy. Larger EHE exhibit the intermediate band of minimal enhancement, not observed with metastases.
- Angiosarcoma. Very rare. The enhancement pattern usually resembles hemangiomas.

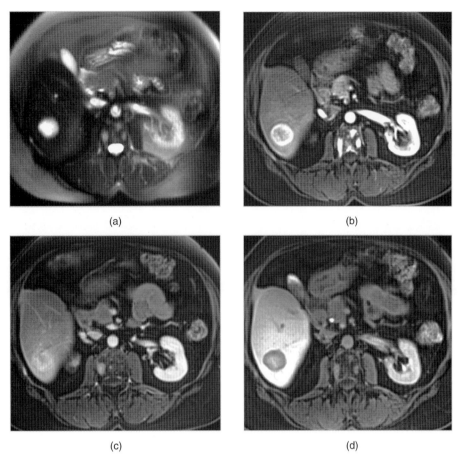

(a)

(b)

(c)

(d)

Figure 8.5 *Transverse T2-weighted fat-suppressed SS-ETSE (a), T1-weighted postgadolinium hepatic arterial dominant phase (b), hepatic venous phase (c) and hepatocyte phase (d) 3D-GE images show a multiple myeloma metastasis in the right lobe of the liver.* The metastasis shows markedly high T2 signal (a) and prominent early enhancement (b) due to its hypervascularity. The lesion appears hypointense on the hepatocyte phase acquired 20 min after the administration of gadoxetic acid, since it does not contain hepatocytes. Note the presence of nodular enhancing lesions in the vertebral body secondary to multiple myeloma.

Hepatoblastoma

- Hepatoblastoma is the most common primary malignant tumor of the liver in children.
- 70% seen in the first 2 years of life and 90% seen in patients younger than 5 years of age.
- 4% of cases are congenital.
- Nonspecific clinical presentation including abdominal enlargement and failure to thrive. Jaundice is rarely seen.
- Hepatoblastoma has been associated with several syndromes including Beckwith-Wiedemann syndrome, and Gardner syndrome.
- Markedly elevated levels of alpha fetoprotein.
- Metastatic disease most commonly involves the lungs, bones, lymph nodes, and brain.
- **On gross inspection:**
  - ° A solid, well-defined, occasionally lobulated large mass surrounded by a pseudocapsule (Figures 8.9 and 8.10).

- ° Although usually solitary, multiple lesions may be seen in less than 20% of cases.
- ° Areas of necrosis, hemorrhage (Figure 8.10) and calcifications are frequently present. Calcifications are usually coarse.
- **Imaging Features**
  - ° **On CT:** Usually appear as lobulated heterogeneously enhancing hypoattenuating masses on CT examinations. Calcifications and hyperdense areas representing hemorrhage on precontrast images may be seen. The pseudocapsule shows increased enhancement. The tumor may invade the portal and hepatic veins.
  - ° **On MRI:** Tumors demonstrate heterogeneous mild-moderate T2 signal and heterogeneous moderate low T1 signal. Focal areas of low signal on T2 and high signal on T1-weighted images represent hemorrhage. On dynamic postgadolinium T1-weighted images, they usually show progressive heterogeneous enhancement. The tumor may show wash-out and enhancement of the pseudocapsule,

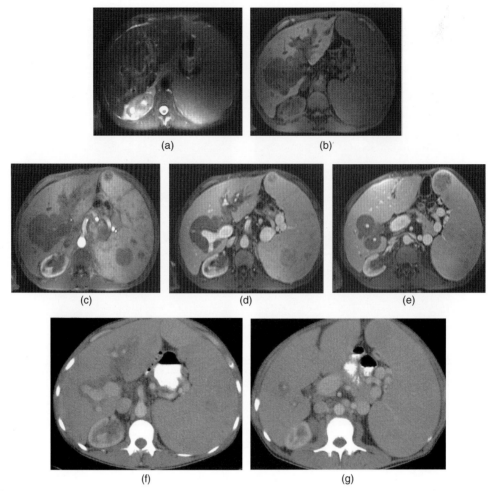

Figure 8.6 *Transverse T2-weighted fat-suppressed SS-ETSE (a), T1-weighted fat-suppressed 3D-GE (b), T1-weighted postgadolinium fat-suppressed hepatic arterial dominant phase (c), hepatic venous phase (d) and interstitial phase (e) 3D-GE images show infiltrative midly enhancing mass lesion in the porta hepatis and along the portal tracts.* This lesion shows midly high T2 signal. Additionally, multiple foci of moderately enhancing nodular foci are also noted in the enlarged spleen. These lesions develop due to extramedullary hematopoiesis. Postcontrast hepatic venous CT images (f, g) show decrease in the size of periportal infiltration during the treatment. Source: Semelka 2010. Reproduced with permission of Wiley.

which is more prominent in the later phases (Figures 8.9 and 8.10) The tumor may sometimes invade the portal and hepatic veins.

- **Differential Diagnosis**
- Infantile hemangioendothelioma
- Mesenchymal hamartoma

Infantile hemangioendothelioma

- Infantile hemangioendothelioma of the liver is the most common benign liver tumor in children.
- Vascular neoplasm, which is also known as *infantile hepatic hemangioma*.
- Commonly (90%) diagnosed in the first 6 months.

- They are usually asymptomatic but serious complications include congestive heart failure (due to hemangioma associated arteriovenous shunts), Kasabach-Merritt syndrome of coagulopathy (due to thrombocytopenia secondary intratumoral sequestration), hemoperitoneum (due to tumoral rupture), and hypothyroidism.
- AFP may be mild–elevated.
- Associated with cutaneous hemangiomas and other solid organ involvement.
- Infantile hemangioendothelioma is included in hepatic vascular malformations. Hepatic vascular malformations are categorized into three groups.
- The first group includes multifocal lesions, which are positive for erythrocyte-type glucose transporter protein 1 (GLUT-1). These lesions do not contain necrosis and may or may not be associated with cutaneous hemangiomas or arterivenous shunts. These are usually asymptomatic although heart

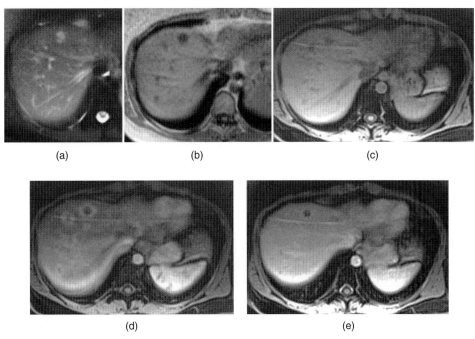

Figure 8.7 *Transverse T2-weighted fat-suppressed SS-ETSE (a), T1-weighted 2D-GE (b), T1-weighted fat-suppressed 3D-GE (c), T1-weighted postgadolinium fat-suppressed hepatic arterial dominant phase (d) and hepatic venous phase (e) 3D-GE images show multiple small foci of hemangioendothelioma with mild to moderate T2 signal and peripheral enhancement. The lesions show early prominent peripheral enhancement which fade in the later phase.*

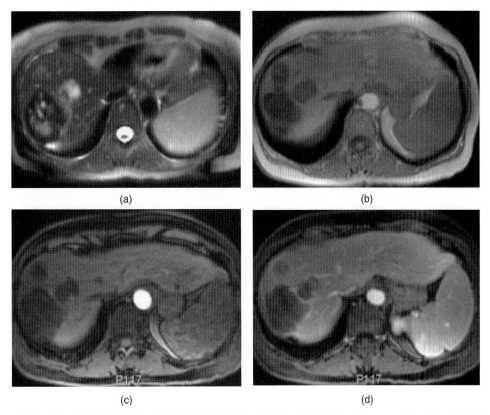

Figure 8.8 *Transverse T2-weighted SS-ETSE (a), T1-weighted 2D-GE (b), T1-weighted postgadolinium fat-suppressed hepatic arterial phase (c) and hepatic venous phase (d) 3D-GE images show multiple foci of hemangioendothelioma. The lesions show variable T2 signal. The largest lesion shows peripheral low T2 signal, whereas the other lesions show mild to moderate high T2 signal. The lesions also show mild predominantly peripheral enhancement.*

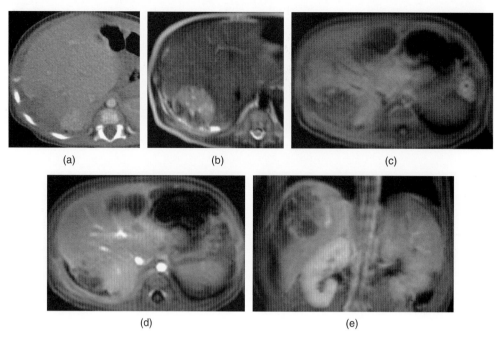

(a) (b) (c)

(d) (e)

Figure 8.9 *Transverse postcontrast CT (a), transverse T2-weighted SS-ETSE (b), T1-weighted fat-suppressed MPRAGE (c), T1-weighted postgadolinium transverse (d) and coronal MPRAGE images demonstrate a medium-sized heterogeneous mass with heterogeneous enhancement in the liver in an infant.* The lesion represents a hepatoblastoma. The images have blurring due to motion artifacts, although noncooperative patient protocol is used.

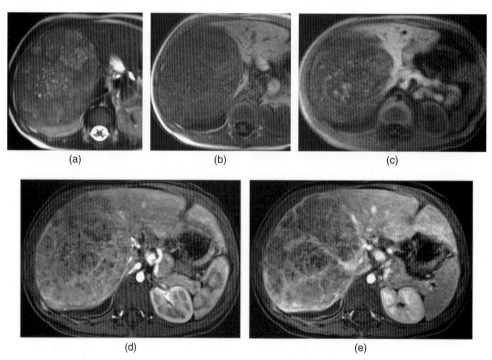

(a) (b) (c)

(d) (e)

Figure 8.10 *Transverse T2-weighted SS-ETSE (a), T1-weighted in-phase (b) 2D-GE, T1-weighted fat-suppressed 3D-GE (c), T1-weighted postgadolinium fat-suppressed hepatic arterial dominant phase (d) and hepatic venous phase (e) 3D-GE images demonstrate a large heterogeneous mass with heterogeneous enhancement in the liver.* The lesion represents a hepatoblastoma. The lesions demonstrate central mildly high signal due to mild hemorrhage. Additionally, the lesion shows mild wash-out and capsular enhancement in the later phase (e).

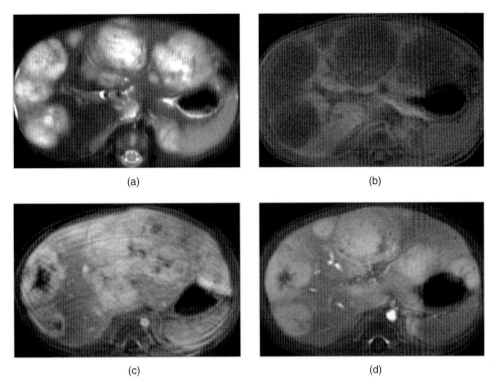

Figure 8.11 *Transverse T2-weighted fat-suppressed SS-ETSE (a), T1-weighted fat-suppressed MPRAGE (b), T1-weighted postgadolinium fat-suppressed MPRAGE (c, d) images show multiple nodular foci of infantile hemangioendothelioma in an infant.* The lesions show markedly high T2 signal and intense enhancement, which is peripheral in early phases and progresses centrally in the later phases.

failure may be seen due to shunts. They initially show proliferation followed by involution. These are termed *infantile hemangioendothelioma.*

- The second group includes focal lesions, which are negative for GLUT-1. These lesions are usually large and contain necrosis, hemorrhage, and thrombosis. These are usually symptomatic due to heart failure secondary to shunts. These are rarely associated with cutaneous hemangiomas. These lesions involute by age 12–14 months and are counterparts of cutaneous rapidly involuting hemangioma.
- The third group includes diffuse lesions largely replacing the liver and resulting in massive hepatomegaly and mass effect. Hypothyroidism is usually seen. Congestive heart failure may develop, but may be difficult to detect clinically.
- Imaging features depend on the spectrum of gross pathological appearances.
- Imaging findings include enlarged hepatic veins and hepatic arteries. Arteriovenous shunts may be detected.
- On CT: These are well-defined hypoattenuating lesions, which may present as multifocal smaller or solitary larger lesions. They may contain calcifications. They demonstrate peripheral thick rim-like and/or peripheral nodular enhancement with progressive centripedal filling, which is similar to hemangiomas. Larger lesions may have central

necrosis, which is hypoattenuated, or hemorrhage, which is hyperattenuated.

- **On MRI:** They show markedly high signal on T2-weighted images. On T1-weighted images, they demonstrate low signal, although central hemorrhage or thrombosis may be seen as central high signal intensity areas. Signal void structures representing vessels or shunts with high flow can be seen. Signal void calcifications may be detected. On dynamic postgadolinium T1-weighted images, peripheral thick rim-like enhancement/peripheral nodular enhancement with progressive centripedal filling is seen (Figure 8.11).
- **Differential Diagnosis:**
- Metastatic neuroblastoma
- Mesenchymal hamartoma
- Hepatoblastoma

Mesenchymal hamartoma

- Mesenchymal hamartoma of the liver is the second most common benign liver tumor in children.
- Commonly (95%) seen in children less than 5-years old.
- Common presentation is painless abdominal distension.
- Tumor markers are often negative.
- Calcification is not seen.

- They usually present as a large, well-marginated solitary mass. These lesions are commonly cystic (85%) although solid lesions (15%) may also be seen. The cystic lesions may appear multiloculated and contain multiple small cysts, although large cysts may also be detected in these lesions.
- Imaging features depend on the spectrum of gross pathologic appearance. Cystic components are avascular and stromal components hypervascular.
- **On CT:** The lesions appear hypoattenuated and cystic portions of the lesion show fluid attenuation on unenhanced CT images. Solid components and septa/walls of cystic components demonstrate progressive enhancement on contrast enhanced CT images.
- **On MR:** Cystic components of the lesion usually demonstrate high signal on T2-WI and low signal on T1-WI, although the signal intensity of cystic portions may occasionally vary according to protein content. Solid components and septal walls of cystic components demonstrate low signal on T2-WI and T1-WI due to the presence of fibrotic tissue, although predominantly solid lesions show mildly high signal. The solid components and septal walls show progressive enhancement.
- **Differential Diagnosis:**
- Hepatoblastoma
- Solitary form of infantile hemangioendothelioma
- Undifferentiated embryonal sarcoma

Primary sarcomas of the liver

- Various types of sarcomas including angiosarcoma, embryonal rhabdomyosarcoma, fibrosarcoma, liposarcoma, leimyosarcoma, carcinosarcoma, malignant fibrous histiocytoma, and undifferentiated embryonal sarcoma may be seen in the liver. They represent less than 1% of all malignant hepatic tumors.
- Patients are often asymptomatic until tumors attain a large size.

Angiosarcoma

- Angiosarcoma is the most common primary sarcoma arising in the liver, and accounts for 1.8% of all primary liver malignancies.
- Associated with environmental and occupational exposure to carcinogens, including thorotrast, vinyl chloride, arsenic, and radiation.
- Commonly affects older male patients in the sixth to eighth decades.
- Poor prognosis. Tumor markers are usually negative.
- Often located peripherally in the liver.
- Hemorrhage may be present.

- Metastatic lesions are usually present at the time of diagnosis. The most common metastatic sites include the lung and spleen.
- **Histopathology:**
  - Multicentric nodules throughout the liver.
  - Occasionally, tumor may present as a solitary (Figure 8.12). large mass, with or without associated micronodules.
  - Less common, diffusely infiltrative pattern with micronodules.
- **Microscopically:**
  - Ill-defined clusters of malignant endothelial cells lining and expanding the sinusoids.
  - Vascular markers are positive.
- **On CT and MRI:**
  - They appear as hypoattenuated lesions on unenhanced CT images. Intratumoral hemorrhage appears as hyperdense areas in the tumor. Spontaneous intraperitoneal hemorrhage may occur. Calcifications may be evident. Central necrosis and fibrosis may also be present.
  - Mild to moderate high signal intensity on T2-WIs.
  - Moderately low signal on T1-WIs.
  - The frequent presence of hemorrhage results in focal areas of low signal intensity on T2- and high signal on T1-WIs. The observation of hemorrhage in smaller hemangioma-like tumors is a clue to the diagnosis.
  - Demonstrate various enhancement patterns, including progressive heterogeneous enhancement, progressive enhancement with later fading, and peripheral enhancement with centripedal progression with or without nodules (Figure 8.12).
- **D.D.**
  - Hemangioma: Small hemangiomas do not show hemorrhage, whereas this is common with angiosarcoma.
  - Metastases
  - Infantile hemangioendothelioma

Undifferentiated (embryonal) sarcoma of the liver

- Undifferentiated sarcoma is a rare mesenchymal tumor occurring most frequently in pediatric patients. It most commonly affects children between 6 and 10 years of age, although it may also occur in adults. Tumor markers are usually not elevated. An abdominal mass, pain, and discomfort are usually the presenting symptoms. Undifferentiated sarcoma has a poor prognosis.
- **Histopathology:**
  - Often a solitary well-demarcated large predominantly solid mass with some cystic spaces and internal septa. A fibrous pseudocapsule commonly surrounds the tumor. Hemorrhage and necrosis may be present.
- **On CT:** Due to myxoid stroma, the lesion shows low attenuation (near water attenuation) on unenhanced CT images.

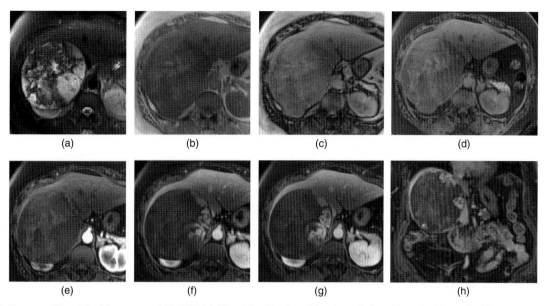

(a)   (b)   (c)   (d)

(e)   (f)   (g)   (h)

Figure 8.12 *Transverse T2-weighted fat-suppressed SS-ETSE (a), T1-weighted in-phase (b) and out-of-phase (c) 2D-GE, T1-weighted fat-suppressed 3D-GE (d), T1-weighted postgadolinium fat-suppressed late hepatic arterial phase (e), hepatic venous phase (f, g) and coronal interstitial phase (h) 3D-GE images demonstrate a large angiosarcoma in the liver.* The lesion shows very heterogeneous T2 and T1 signal and the presence of low T2 signal and high T1 signal develops due to the presence of hemorrhage. The lesion shows large peripheral nodular enhancement with centripedal progression. The enhancement pattern mimics hemangioma; however, precontrast signal characteristics and its round form are not consistent with hemangiomas. Hemangiomas almost invariably show moderate to markedly high homogeneous T2 signal and appear lobulated if > 3 cm in size.

Peripheral solid components or septa without myxoid stroma may be present. Calcifications are uncommon. Hemorrhage may be seen as hyperdense foci in the tumor. Central necrosis may be present. On postcontrast CT images, predominant peripheral enhancement, which may or may not be associated with progressive enhancement of solid components, is seen. The pseudocapsule shows prominent enhancement.

- **On MRI:** Due to myxoid stroma, the lesion shows markedly high signal on T2-weighted images and markedly low signal on T1-weighted images. Focal areas of low T2 signal and high T1 signal representing hemorrhage may be noted. Fluid levels, internal debris, or central necrosis may also be seen. Peripherally located solid tissue or septa without myxoid stroma demonstrate low T1 and T2 signal. On dynamic postgadolinium T1-weighted images, predominantly peripheral enhancement, with heterogeneous progressive enhancement of solid components, is seen.
- **Differential Diagnosis:**
- Mesenchymal hamartoma

References

1 Leite, N.P., Kased, N., Hanna, R.F. *et al.* (2007) Cross-sectional imaging of extranodal involvement in abdominopelvic lymphoproliferative malignancies. Radiographics, 27, 1613–1634.

2 Lee, S.H., Kim, H.J., Mun, J.S. *et al.* (2008) A case of primary hepatic Burkitt's lymphoma. Korean J Gastroenterol, 51, 259–264.

3 Tan, Y. and Xiao, E.H. (2013) Rare hepatic malignant tumors: dynamic CT, MRI and clinicopathologic features: with analysis of 54 cases and review of the literature. Abdom Imaging, 38, 511–526.

4 Karcaaltincaba, M., Haliloglu, M., Akpinar, E. *et al.* (2007) Multidetector CT and MR findings in periportal space pathologies. Eur J Radiol, 61, 3–10.

5 Maher, M.M., McDermott, S.R., Fenlon, H.M. *et al.* (2001) Imaging of primary non-Hodgkin's lymphoma of the liver. Clin Radiol, 56, 295–301.

6 Wong, Y., Chen, F., Tai, K.S. *et al.* (1999) Imaging features of focal intrahepatic extramedullary hematopoiesis. Br J Radiol, 72, 906–910.

7 Chung, E.M., Cube, R., Lewis, R.B., and Conran, R.M. (2010) From the archives of the AFIP: pediatric liver masses: radiologic – pathologic correlation part 1. Benign tumors. Radiographics, 30, 801–826.

8 Chung, E.M., Lattin, G.E. Jr.,, Cube, R. *et al.* (2011) From the archives of the AFIP: pediatric liver masses: radiologic – pathologic correlation part 2. Malignant tumors. Radiographics, 31, 483–507.

9 Psatha, E.A., Semelka, R.C., Fordham, L. *et al.* (2004) Undifferentiated (embryonal) sarcoma of the liver (USL): MRI findings including dynamic gadolinium enhancement. Magn Reson Imaging, 22, 897–900.

10 Leonardou, P., Semelka, R.C., Mastropasqua, M. *et al.* (2002) Epithelioid hemangioendothelioma of the liver. MR imaging findings. Magn Reson Imaging, 20, 631–633.

11 Kelekis, N.L., Semelka, R.C., Siegelman, E.S. *et al.* (1997) Focal hepatic lymphoma: magnetic resonance demonstration using current techniques including gadolinium enhancement. Magn Reson Imaging, 15, 625–636.

12 Worawattanakul, S., Semelka, R.C., Kelekis, N.L., and Wossley, J.T. (1997) Angiosarcoma of the liver: MR imaging pre- and post-chemotherapy. Magn Reson Imaging, 15, 613–617.

13 Kelekis, N.L., Semelka, R.C., Warshauer, D.M., and Sallah, S. (1997) Nodular liver involvement in light chain multiple myeloma: appearance on US and MRI. Clin Imaging, 21, 207–209.

14 Miller, W.J., Dodd, G.D. 3rd,, Federle, M.P., and Baron, R.L. (1992) Epitheloid hemangioendothelioma of the liver: imaging findings with pathologic correlation. AJR Am J Roentgenol, 159, 53–57.

CHAPTER 9
Cholangiocarcinoma

Ersan Altun[1], Mohamed El-Azzazi[1,2,3,4], Richard C. Semelka[1], and Miguel Ramalho[1,5]

[1] The University of North Carolina at Chapel Hill, Department of Radiology, Chapel Hill, NC, USA
[2] University of Dammam, Department of Radiology, Dammam, Saudi Arabia
[3] King Fahd Hospital of the University, Department of Radiology, Khobar, Saudi Arabia
[4] University of Al Azhar, Department of Radiology, Cairo, Egypt
[5] Hospital Garcia de Orta, Department of Radiology, Almada, Portugal

- Cholangiocarcinoma is the second most common primary liver malignancy and accounts for 10–20% of primary tumors.
- More common in areas with endemic fluke infestation (O. Viverini and C. Sinensis). Hepatolithiasis developing secondary to recurrent pyogenic cholangitis is another risk factor.
- Other risk factors include congenital biliopancreatic anomalies, cirrhosis, primary sclerosing cholangitis, hepatitis B or C virus infection, and heavy alcohol consumption.
- Classified into three types:
  - Mass-forming cholangiocarcinoma
  - Periductal infiltrative cholangiocarcinoma
  - Intraductal cholangiocarcinoma
- **Mass-forming intrahepatic cholangiocarcinoma**
- Usually presents as a solitary intrahepatic heterogeneous mass with irregular well-defined margins. They are usually hypovascular (Figures 9.1–9.3) although hypervascular cholangiocarcinomas (Figure 9.4) may also be seen occasionally.
- May show biliary dilatation at the periphery of the lesion (Figures 9.2 and 9.5), when the tumor is more central in location.
- Vascular compression (especially portal vein) is common (Figure 14.8). Development of intravascular thrombosis is rare and is a distinguishing feature from HCC.
- Capsular retraction (Figures 9.1 and 9.3), central necrosis, and satellite nodules may be seen. Capsular retraction overlying the tumor is considered a hallmark of this tumor, but is seen only occasionally.
- Atrophy of the involved segment may be detected (Figure 9.1).
- **Microscopy:**
  - Tumors with glandular configurations surrounded by abundant, dense fibrous stroma.

- **On CT:**
  - Hypoattenuating mass with irregular and undulating but moderately defined margins (Figure 9.6).
  - Mild to moderate irregular peripheral enhancement with gradual centripedal enhancement and pooling of contrast material on delayed images due to its abundant fibrotic stroma.
- **On MRI:**
  - Usually demonstrate mild to moderate high signal intensity on T2-WIs. Higher T2 signal compared to HCCs. They usually have irregular and undulating contours (Figures 9.2 and 9.3).
  - Moderately low signal intensity on T1-WIs.
  - Mild to moderate early irregular peripheral contrast enhancement with progressive enhancement on delayed images (Figures 9.2, 9.3, and 9.5). Note that in hypovascular tumors, the peripheral tumor border zone enhancement may simulate ring enhancement of metastases, but subtle diffuse heterogeneous enhancement may be seen on arterial phase images. Note that tumors show progressive enhancement and do not show wash-out and late capsule enhancement as seen with HCC.
  - Although they are generally hypovascular, hypervascular tumors showing homogeneous or heterogeneous prominent enhancement, usually without central necrosis, on the hepatic arterial dominant phase may be seen.
- **Differential Diagnosis**
- Hepatocellular carcinoma (HCC) with sclerosis and HCC-cholangiocarcinoma may demonstrate similar imaging features to cholangiocarcinoma.
- Metastases
- Gallbladder carcinoma (Figure 9.7).

Liver Imaging: MRI with CT Correlation, First Edition. Edited by Ersan Altun, Mohamed El-Azzazi and Richard C. Semelka.
© 2015 John Wiley & Sons, Inc. Published 2015 by John Wiley & Sons, Inc.

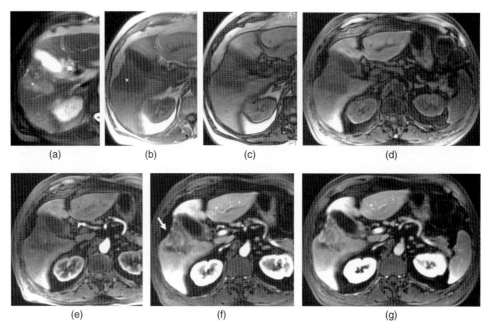

Figure 9.1 *Transverse T2-weighted fat-suppressed SS-ETSE (a), T1-weighted in-phase (b) and out-of-phase (c) 2D-GE, T1-weighted fat-suppressed 3D-GE (d), T1-weighted postgadolinium fat-suppressed late hepatic arterial phase (e), hepatic venous phase (f) and interstitial phase (g) 3D-GE images show a mass forming hypovascular cholangiocarcinoma (asteriks; a, b) in the right lobe of the liver.* The lesion shows mildly high T2 signal. It is associated with capsular retraction (arrow, f) and prominent delayed enhancement in the later phases (f, g), due to its significant fibrosis component.

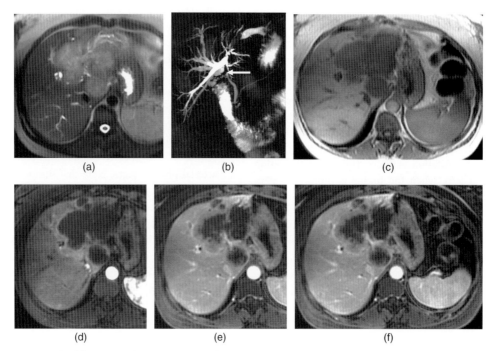

Figure 9.2 *Transverse T2-weighted fat-suppressed SS-ETSE (a), coronal 3D reconstructed MRCP images (b), T1-weighted in-phase 2D-GE (c), T1-weighted postgadolinium fat-suppressed late hepatic arterial phase (d), hepatic venous phase (e) and interstitial phase (f) 3D-GE images show a large mass-forming cholangiocarcinoma associated with portal hilum invasion and intrahepatic biliary dilatation.* The lesion is located predominantly in the left lobe of the liver and has lobulated contours. The lesion causes compresses/invades the proximal common hepatic duct which is seen as a cut-off sign (arrow, c) on MRCP image. The intrahepatic bile ducts appear dilated while the common bile duct is in normal calibration. The lesion shows predominantly peripheral early enhancement (d), which progresses in the later phases (e, f).

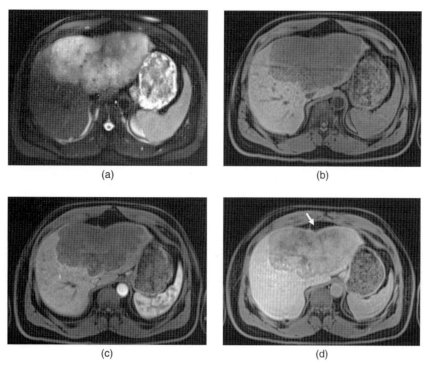

Figure 9.3 *Transverse T2-weighted fat-suppressed SS-ETSE (a), T1-weighted fat-suppressed 3D-GE (b), T1-weighted postgadolinium fat-suppressed hepatic arterial dominant phase (c) and interstitial phase (d) 3D-GE images demonstrate a large mass-forming cholangiocarcinoma.* The lesion shows moderately high T2 signal. Prominent capsular retraction (arrow, d) and delayed interstitial phase enhancement (d) are seen due to its prominent fibrous content. The lesion is hypovascular and does not depict enhancement on the hepatic arterial dominant phase (c).

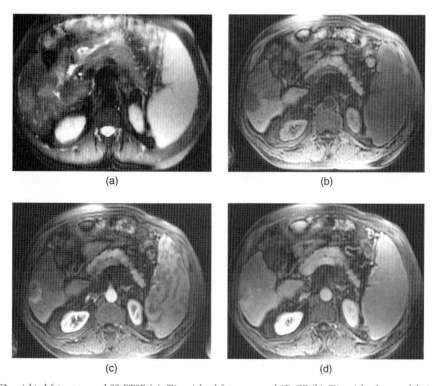

Figure 9.4 *Transverse T2-weighted fat-suppressed SS-ETSE (a), T1-weighted fat-suppressed 3D-GE (b), T1-weighted postgadolinium fat-suppressed hepatic arterial dominant phase (c) and interstitial phase (d) 3D-GE images show a mass-forming cholangiocarcinoma in the right lobe of the liver.* The liver is cirrhotic and the spleen is enlarged due to portal hypertension. The lesion is relatively hypervascular and demonstrates predominantly peripheral early increased enhancement (c) which progresses in the later phase (d).

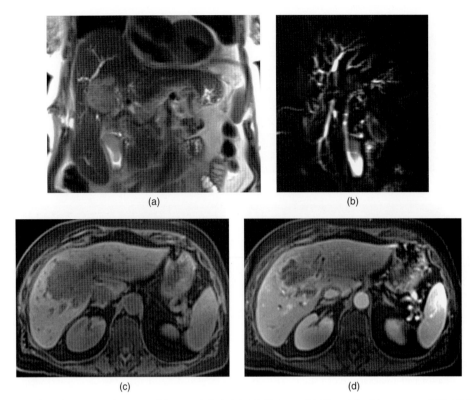

Figure 9.5 *Coronal T2-weighted fat-suppressed SS-ETSE (a), coronal thick slab MRCP image (b), T1-weighted fat-suppressed 3D-GE (c), T1-weighted post-gadolinium fat-suppressed hepatic venous phase (d) 3D-GE images show a large perihilar mass-forming cholangiocarcinoma.* The tumor causes intrahepatic biliary dilatation associated with cut-off sign on MRCP image and demonstrates heterogeneous enhancement (d).

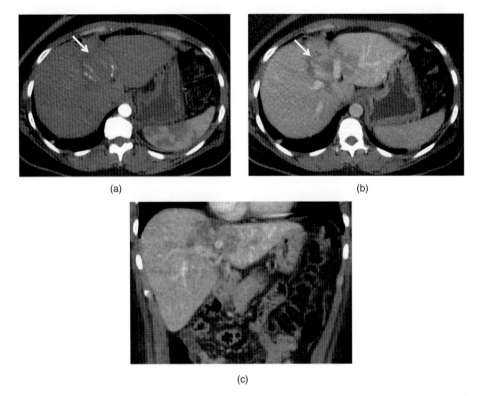

Figure 9.6 *Postcontrast transverse hepatic arterial dominant (a), transverse (b) and coronal (c) hepatic venous phase CT images demonstrate a perihilar ill-defined enhancing mass representing a mass forming cholangiocarcinoma (arrows).*

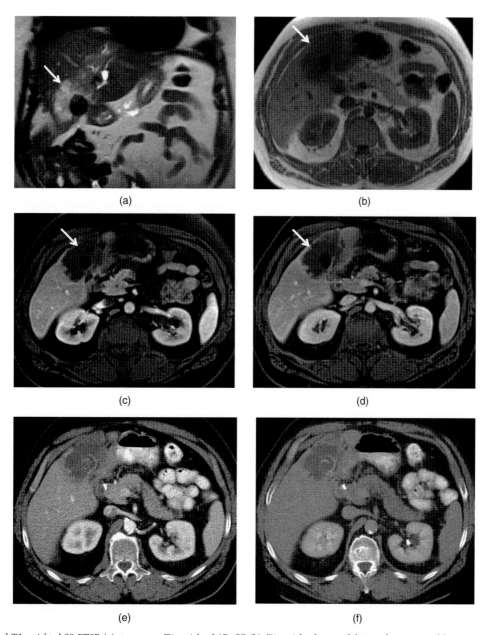

Figure 9.7 *Coronal T2-weighted SS-ETSE (a), transverse T1-weighted 2D-GE (b), T1-weighted postgadolinium fat-suppressed hepatic venous phase (c) and interstitial phase (d) MR images and transverse postcontrast CT images (e, f) demonstrate a gallbladder cancer invading the adjacent liver parenchyma. The tumor is hypovascular and does not show significant enhancement. Note the presence of gallstones in the gallbladder lumen.*

- Abscesses, hepatic tuberculosis, and inflammatory myofibroblastic tumor may mimic cholangiocarcinomas.
- **Periductal infiltrating cholangiocarcinoma**
- Infiltrative tumoral growth is seen along the irregularly narrowed thick walled biliary ducts without mass formation. Note that a critical imaging feature is high grade intrahepatic biliary obstruction, despite relatively small tumor thickness (3 mm at presentation) involving the bile duct, in contrast to inflammatory conditions such as primary sclerosing cholangitis that will show only mild to moderate intrahepatic ductal dilation for the same thickness of disease. For this reason, it is important to try to image patients prior to placement of a biliary stent, as the biliary stent results in decreased intrahepatic dilation, the presence of which is a cardinal finding in cholangiocarcinoma.

- Characterized by diffuse ductal thickening and increased enhancement due to tumor infiltration (Figure 9.8), which is associated with irregularly narrowed duct and significantly dilated proximal peripheral biliary ducts.

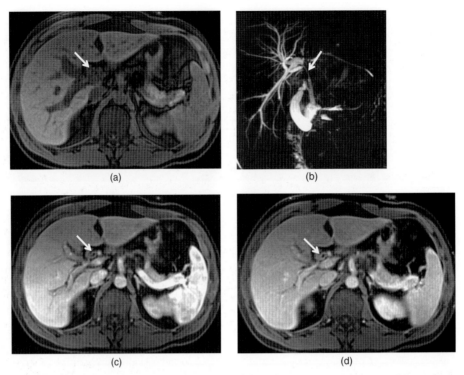

Figure 9.8 *Transverse T1-weighted fat-suppressed 3D-GE (a), coronal 3D reconstructed MRCP (b), T1-weighted postgadolinium hepatic arterial dominant (c) and hepatic venous phase (d) images show an infiltrative perihilar (Klatskin tumor) cholangiocarcinoma which is characterized by enhancing wall-thickening of the common hepatic duct (arrows; a, c, d).* MRCP image shows intrahepatic biliary dilatation, which is associated with cut-off sign (arrow, b). Note the presence of stent in the common hepatic duct (arrow, b).

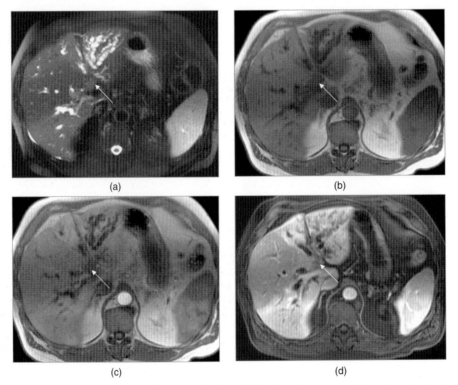

Figure 9.9 *Transverse T2-weighted fat-suppressed SS-ETSE (a), T1-weighted 2D-GE (b), T1-weighted postgadolinium hepatic arterial dominant phase 2D-GE (c) and fat-suppressed hepatic venous phase (d) 3D-GE images show a small perihilar (Klatskin tumor) mass forming cholangiocarcinoma (arrows; a–d).* The lesion shows mild enhancement on the later phase (d) and cause prominent intrahepatic biliary ductal dilatation, which is also associated with differential increased enhancement. Source: Semelka 2010. Reproduced with permission of Wiley.

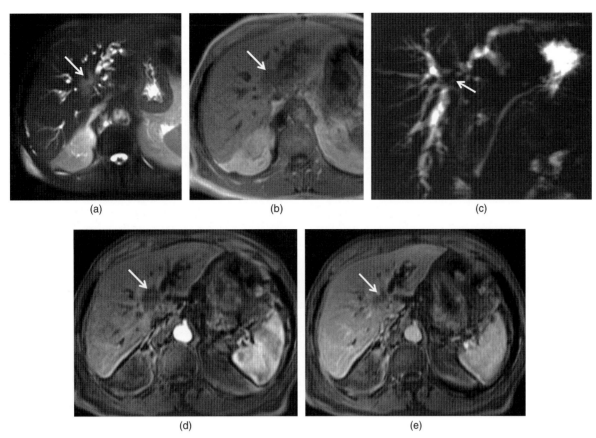

Figure 9.10 *Transverse T2-weighted fat-suppressed SS-ETSE (a), T1-weighted in-phase 2D-GE (b), coronal thick slab MRCP image (c), T1-weighted post-gadolinium fat-suppressed late hepatic arterial phase (d) and hepatic venous phase (e) 3D-GE images show a small perihilar (Klatskin tumor) mass-forming cholangiocarcinoma (arrows; a–e).* The tumor demonstrates mild enhancement on the hepatic venous phase (e) and is associated with intrahepatic biliary dilatation and cut-off sign on MRCP image (arrow, c).

- This type of cholangiocarcinoma is common in the hilar region, where it is termed Klatskin tumor, and is uncommon more distally in the CBD or isolated within the liver parenchyma.
- These tumors may be associated with small enhancing mass-like soft tissues at the porta hepatis or adjacent to the common hepatic bifurcation (Figures 9.9 and 9.10).
- *Differential Diagnosis*
- Periportal lymphangitic metastases which are usually not associated with a comparable level of ductal dilatation.
- Benign inflammatory and fibrotic strictures are usually not associated with irregular margins, asymmetric narrowing, prominent ductal wall thickening and enhancement, lymph node enlargement, and periductal soft tissue. A critical difference is that benign disease does not result in severe intrahepatic ductal dilation.
- **Intraductal polypoid cholangiocarcinoma**
- Presents as a polypoid mass, which is usually associated with focal biliary ductal wall thickening and ductal dilatation.
- Polypoid masses show enhancement with proximal biliary ductal dilatation.

- Ductal dilatation without obvious mass formation and wall thickening may also be seen due to mucin production.
- *Differential Diagnosis*
- Metastases
- Benign inflammatory and fibrotic strictures.
- Impacted stones, which do not show enhancement.

References

1 Ruys, A.T., van Beem, B.E., Engelbrecht, M.R. *et al.* (2012) Radiological staging in patients with hilar cholangiocarcinoma: systematic review and meta-analysis. Br J Radiol, 85, 1255–1262.
2 Chung, Y.E., Kim, M.J., Park, Y.N. *et al.* (2009) Varying appearances of cholangiocarcinoma: radiologic – pathologic correlation. Radiographics, 29, 683–700.
3 Gakhal, M.S., Gheyi, V.K., Brock, R.E., and Andrews, G.S. (2009) Multimodality imaging of biliary malignancies. Surg Oncol Clin N Am, 18, 225–239.
4 Van Beers, B.E. (2008) Diagnosis of cholangiocarcinoma. HPB (Oxford), 10, 87–93.

5 Vilgrain, V. (2008) Staging cholangiocarcinoma by imaging studies. HPB (Oxford), 10, 106–109.

6 Sainani, N.I., Catalona, O.A., Holalkere, N.S. *et al.* (2008) Cholangiocarcinoma: current and novel imaging techniques. Radiographics, 28, 1263–1287.

7 Menias, C.O., Surabhi, V.R., Prasad, S.R. *et al.* (2008) Mimics of cholangiocarcinoma: spectrum of disease. Radiographics, 28, 1115–1129.

8 Al Ansari, N., Kim, B.S., Sriattanapong, S. *et al.* (2014) Mass-forming cholangiocarcinoma and adenocarcinoma of unknown primary: can they be distinguished on liver MRI? Abdom Imaging, 39, 1228–1240.

9 Fowler, K.J., Sheybani, A., Parker, R.A. 3rd, *et al.* (2013) Combined hepatocellular and cholangiocarcinoma (biphenotypic) tumors: imaging features and diagnostic accuracy of contrast enhanced CT and MRI. AJR Am J Roentgenol, 201, 332–339.

10 De Campos, R.O., Semelka, R.C., Azevedo, R.M. *et al.* (2012) Combined hepatocellular carcinoma – cholangiocarcinoma: report of MR appearance in eleven patients. J Magn Reson Imaging, 36, 1139–1147.

11 Worawattanakul, S., Semelka, R.C., Noone, T.C. *et al.* (1998) Cholangiocarcinoma: spectrum of appearances on MR images using current techniques. Magn Reson Imaging, 16, 993–1003.

CHAPTER 10

Infectious diseases of the liver

Ersan Altun[1], Mohamed El-Azzazi[1,2,3,4], and Richard C. Semelka[1]

[1] The University of North Carolina at Chapel Hill, Department of Radiology, Chapel Hill, NC, USA
[2] University of Dammam, Department of Radiology, Dammam, Saudi Arabia
[3] King Fahd Hospital of the University, Department of Radiology, Khobar, Saudi Arabia
[4] University of Al Azhar, Department of Radiology, Cairo, Egypt

Abscess

- Hepatic abscesses can be classified as pyogenic, amebic, and fungal.
- They may occur as single or multiple lesions.
- Infectious agents reach the liver through the hepatic artery, portal vein, biliary tract, and direct extension from contiguous organs.
- Pathology:
  ○ **Early stages:** Liver abscesses are ill-defined with intense acute inflammation.
  ○ **Later stages:** Liver abscesses become well-circumscribed and surrounded by a shell of granulation tissue.
  ○ **End stages:** Liver abscesses show complete fibrous encapsulation.
- Pyogenic Abscesses
  ○ Commonly occur as complications of ascending cholangitis and portal phlebitis.
  ○ Common causative organisms include *Escherichia coli*, Clostridia species, *Staphylococcus aureus,* and Bacteriodes species.
  ○ Presents with fever, right upper quadrant pain, tender hepatomegaly, and high white blood cell counts.
  ○ Portal vein thrombosis may be associated with abscess.
  ○ Pyogenic abscesses may be composed of small abscesses coalescing into and forming a multiloculated larger abscess cavity. This characteristic finding is known as the *cluster of grapes sign* (Figure 10.1).
  ○ Localized edema may surround the abscess cavity. When peripheral edema is present surrounding the enhancing pseudocapsule of abscess cavity, the appearance is called *double target appearance* on CT and MRI, which is described as the presence of the following from internal to external: hypodense/hypointense central area (abscess cavity); hyperdense/hyperintense enhancing pseudocapsule; and external hypodense/hypointense surrounding localized edema (Figures 10.2 and 10.3).
  ○ Gas may be present in pyogenic abscesses.
  ○ **On CT:**
  ○ Pyogenic abscesses are seen as round or irregularly shaped hypoattenuating lesions on pre- and postcontrast examinations. Surrounding transient peripheral parenchymal enhancement on the hepatic arterial dominant phase is usually present, indicating the presence of hyperemia and inflammatory response in the surrounding liver parenchyma. Progressively intense rim enhancement of the pseudocapsule and enhancement of internal septations are seen on hepatic venous and interstitial phases of postcontrast examinations (Figure 10.3).
  ○ **On MRI:**
  ○ Pyogenic abscesses usually have high signal intensity on T2-WI, but mixed signal is a common feature among a population of lesions (Figure 10.4).
  ○ Pyogenic abscesses usually have low signal intensity on T1-WI (Figure 10.4).
  ○ Depending on their protein content, abscesses may have variable signal intensities on T2-WI and T1-WI. If an abscess has high protein content, it usually shows low signal on T2-WI and high signal on T1-WI. The feature of mixed T2 signal is helpful, if present, to distinguish from cysts/biliary hamartomas which generally do not contain protein/blood in the liver.
  ○ Pyogenic abscesses are usually associated with moderate perilesional parenchymal transient enhancement with indistinct outer margins on the hepatic arterial dominant phase, which rapidly fade to isointensity with the remaining liver parenchyma on later phases on postgadolinium sequences (Figures 10.1, 10.2, 10.4–10.6). Moderate

Liver Imaging: MRI with CT Correlation, First Edition. Edited by Ersan Altun, Mohamed El-Azzazi and Richard C. Semelka.
© 2015 John Wiley & Sons, Inc. Published 2015 by John Wiley & Sons, Inc.

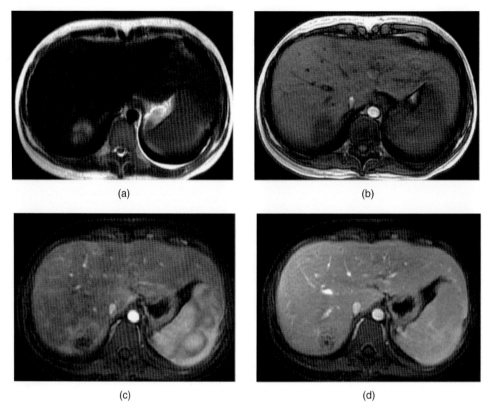

(a)

(b)

(c)

(d)

Figure 10.1 *Transverse T2-weighted SS-ETSE (a), transverse T1-weighted 2D-GE (b), transverse T1-weighted hepatic arterial dominant phase (c), and hepatic venous phase (d) 3D-GE images demonstrate pyogenic abscess in the immunocompromised patient.* The lesions show high signal on T2-weighted images (a), peripheral parenchymal transient enhancement on the hepatic arterial dominant phase images (c) and progressive enhancement on postgadolinium images (c, d). The lesion displays the "cluster of grapes" sign. Progressive rim enhancement and enhancement of internal septations are seen on postgadolinium images (c, d). The lesions are composed of small abscesses coalescing into and forming multiloculated larger abscess cavities.

perilesional parenchymal transient enhancement reflects hyperemic inflammatory response in the adjacent liver parenchyma.

° Progressive moderate to intense enhancement of the wall and internal septations of abscesses are seen on all phases of postgadolinium sequences (Figures 10.1, 10.2, 10.4–10.6).

° Double target or cluster of grapes signs may be present (Figure 10.1).

° Layering of gas (signal void on both T2- and T1-WIs) (Figure 10.6) and debris (variable signal on T1-WI or T2-WI, most often low signal on T2- and high signal on T1-WI) due to high protein within the abscess cavity may be seen.

° Small abscesses may also show moderate enhancement due to enhancement of internal septations and prominent inflammatory response (Figure 10.7).

° Some pyogenic abscesses may also have very thick walls (Figure 10.5).

° Peripheral subcapsular abscesses especially develop secondary to operations and interventions (Figure 10.8)

° If the portal vein or its branches is thrombosed, the most important imaging finding is the absence of contrast

enhancement of the portal vein on examination of all postgadolinium series. The infected bland thrombus may show high signal intensity on T2-WI and low to intermediate signal on T1-WI. Additionally, the portal vein wall may also show a moderate to intense enhancement, best seen on hepatic venous and interstitial phases of enhancement, which is the clue to its infected nature.

• **Amebic Abscesses**

° Caused by *Entameba histolytica*.

° Presents with right upper quadrant pain, tender hepatomegaly, and diarrhea.

° Associated with a history of travel to an endemic area and positive serology.

° Lesions are usually solitary and affect the right lobe more often than the left lobe.

° Due to right lobe involvement and large size of the abscess, the diaphragm may be involved and pulmonary consolidation and empyema may be present.

° The radiologic features of amebic abscesses usually overlap with pyogenic abscesses. Lesions are encapsulated, thick-walled (5 to 10-mm), and demonstrate progressive substantial enhancement of the capsule on postcontrast

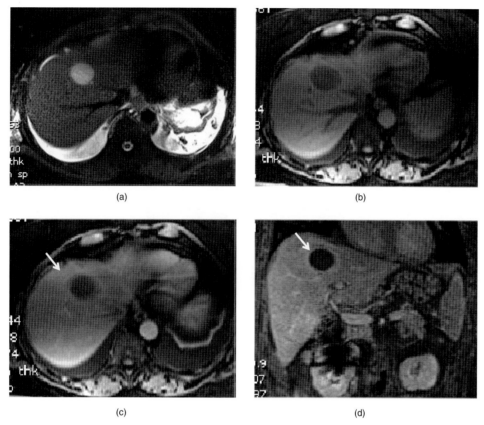

(a)　　　　　　　　　　　　　(b)

(c)　　　　　　　　　　　　　(d)

Figure 10.2 *Transverse T2-weighted fat-suppressed SS-ETSE (a), T1-weighted fat-suppressed 3D-GE (b), T1-weighted fat-suppressed postgadolinium hepatic arterial dominant phase (d) and coronal hepatic venous phase (e) 3D-GE images demonstrate a solitary bacterial abscess.* The abscess shows high signal intensity due to its high fluid content on T2-weighted image (a). Mild peripheral parenchymal transient enhancement (arrow, c) surrounding the abscess is noted on the hepatic arterial dominant phase (c). The enhancement of the wall of abscess (arrow, d) is noted on the hepatic venous phase image. Mild edema is also seen surrounding the abscess.

images on MRI and CT. Amebic walls have thicker walls compared to the majority of pyogenic abscesses.
° Gas is usually not present within amebic abscesses.
° The differentiation of amebic abscesses from pyogenic abscesses is based on the clinical, radiologic, and serologic data, and is critical to determine as the treatment strategies are different for pyogenic abscesses compared to amebic abscesses. Amebic abscesses generally do not require drainage, whereas pyogenic abscesses may require intervention.

- **Fungal Abscesses**
  ° Are generally caused by Candida species, especially Candida Albicans, and seen in immune-compromised patients including AIDS patients, patients on chemotherapy especially for leukemia, patients undergoing bone marrow transplantation, and prolonged duration of neutropenia (Figure 10.9).
  ° Spleen is usually involved in combination with the liver (Figure 10.10).
  ° The kidneys may also be occasionally involved (Figure 10.10).
  ° Histoplasmosis, cryptococcus, mucormycosis, or aspergillus may also sometimes involve the liver.

° Imaging features of various fungal organism infections are similar.
° Candidiasis or other fungal infections may produce either little or no inflammatory/suppurative response, or occasionally granulomas in the liver. It is critical to be aware of this in immunocompromised patients, as, unlike pyogenic abscesses, little indication of the infective nature of the lesions is apparent, reflecting the inability of the host to mount an immune response.
° Hepatic candidiasis is typically characterized by the presence of microabscesses which contain the fungi in the center of the lesion, surrounded by necrosis and polymorphonuclear infiltrate.
° In the healing stage, microabscesses decrease in size and the amount of surrounding peripheral fibrous tissue increases (Figures 10.10 and 10.11)
° **On CT:**
° Abscesses are frequently smaller than 1-cm and are generally between 2 and 20 mm in size.
° Multiple small hypoattenuating lesions involving the liver and spleen are usually seen on contrast-enhanced CT examinations (Figure 10.10).

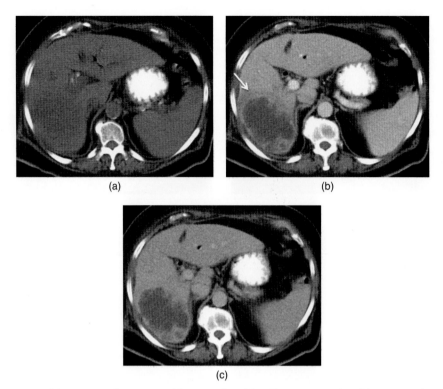

(a)

(b)

(c)

Figure 10.3 *Transverse precontrast (a), postcontrast hepatic arterial dominant phase (b) and hepatic venous phase (c) CT images show a large abscess in the right lobe of the liver.* The abscess has thick irregular walls. Peripheral surrounding parenchymal edema and early transient increased enhancement are detected in the early phase of enhancement (arrow, b). The walls of the abscess demonstrate thick irregular enhancement in the early and late phase of enhancement. Note that no stromal enhancement is seen in the abscess, which is a feature distinguishing abscess from metastasis.

° They may not be detected on non-contrast enhanced CT examinations.

° Lesions may show no enhancement reflecting neutropenic state of patients, although in normal immune status patients, they usually display peripheral enhancement on contrast enhanced CT examinations. Additionally, lesions may occasionally show central enhancement on contrast enhanced CT examinations reflecting abundant inflammatory response or granuloma formation.

° **On MR:**

° **Untreated Lesions – Acute Phase:**

° Abscesses are frequently smaller than 1-cm and are generally between 2 and 20 mm in size.

° Multiple small foci of lesions with moderate to marked high signal on T2-WI, mild to moderate low signal on T1-WI. Peripheral rim enhancement on postgadolinium images (Figure 10.9) is apparent in normal immune status patients. Central enhancement is occasionally seen, which reflects that the lesions are in a phlegmonous or fibrinous state.

° Lesions may show no rim or perilesional enhancement in patients in a neutropenic state, although at least faint rim enhancement may be observed on later postgadolinium hepatic venous and interstitial phase images.

° **Partially Treated Lesions – Subacute Phase (After the start of treatment)**

° Lesions show mild to moderate high signal on T2-WI

° Lesions show variable signal ranging from mildly low signal to mild to moderately high signal on T1-WI.

° Dark perilesional rings may be observed on T1-WI or T2-WI, representing collections of iron-laden macrophages throughout granulation tissue surrounding and within the periphery of lesions (Figure 10.10).

° Lesions usually demonstrate peripheral enhancement on postgadolinium hepatic venous and interstitial phase images. Additionally, lesions may display central enhancement on postgadolinium hepatic venous and interstitial phase images, reflecting the reconstitution of immune response and granuloma formation.

° **Completely Treated Lesions – Chronic Healed Lesions**

° Lesions show mildly low signal on T1-WI and variable and mildly to moderately low-high signal on T2-WI (Figure 10.11).

° Lesions show negligible enhancement on postgadolinium images.

° Capsular retraction may be observed adjacent to the lesions due to their fibrotic nature.

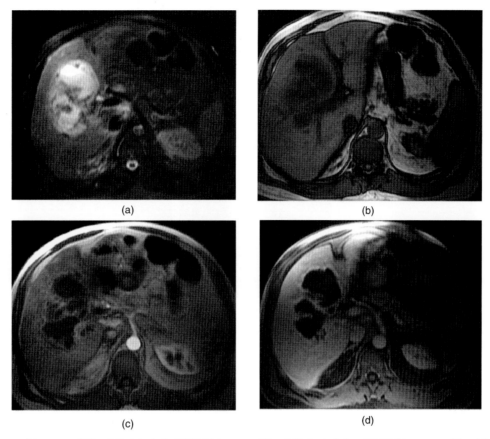

(a)　　　　(b)

(c)　　　　(d)

Figure 10.4 *Transverse fat-suppressed T2-weighted single shot ETSE (a), transverse T1-weighted out-of-phase 2D-GE (b), transverse T1-weighted hepatic arterial dominant phase (c) and hepatic venous phase (d) 3D-GE images demonstrate an abscess, which is a complex multiloculated cystic mass with thick wall and internal septations showing progressive enhancement on postgadolinium images (c, d).* Note the presence of peripheral transient enhancement around the cystic lesion on the hepatic arterial dominant phase image (c).

- **Differential Diagnosis and Pearls for Abscesses**
  - ° Clinical history and laboratory findings are critical.
  - ° Metastases may mimic abscesses as both show peripheral rim type of enhancement. Metastases can be distinguished from abscesses by observing progressive centripetal enhancement in late phases of contrast enhancement, which is a typical feature of metastases. Generally, any stroma related to abscesses exhibits enhancement on arterial phase images, with no progressive enhancement of previously unenhanced tissue; abscesses show progressively intense enhancement of already enhanced stroma (which can be marked) rather than progressive enhancement of previously unenhanced stroma. Progressively intense enhancement of internal septations of abscesses should not be confused with centripetal enhancement of solid metastatic tissue.
  - ° Metastases with large necrotic components may mimic the appearance of hepatic abscesses, and the differentiation of these type of metastases from abscesses is difficult. This reflects that progressive centripetal enhancement, which is a distinguishing marker for metastases, is not present (due to necrosis) and therefore cannot be used

as the distinctive feature. Clinical history therefore is of paramount importance. Although pyogenic abscesses always should have perilesional enhancement on optimally timed hepatic arterial dominant phase images, metastases exhibit this only for mucinous type tumors such as colon cancer. Attention therefore to this opposing phenomenon is also essential, as metastases may also show perilesional enhancement.
  - ° Metastases may also mimic abscesses clinically if they become secondarily infected. This may sometimes be observed, particularly with colon cancer metastases.

Hydatid disease

- Hydatid disease is a zoonosis with worldwide distribution, produced by the larval stage of Echinococcus tapeworm. The two main types of hydatid disease are caused by the larval form of two different tapeworms: *Echinococcus granulosus* and *Echinococcus multilocularis*. *E. granulosus* is more common than *E. multilocularis*, but the latter is the more aggressive form.

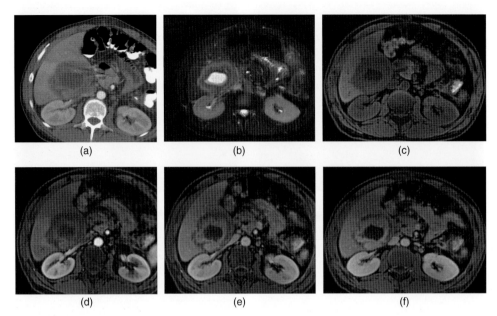

(a) (b) (c)

(d) (e) (f)

Figure 10.5 *Transverse postcontrast hepatic arterial dominant phase CT image (a), T2-weighted SS-ETSE (b), T1-weighted fat-suppressed 3D-GE (c), T1-weighted fat-suppressed postgadolinium hepatic arterial dominant phase (d), hepatic venous phase (e) and interstitial phase (e) 3D-GE MR images illustrate a large abscess with thick enhancing walls. The abscess cavity shows low attenuation on CT image (a) and high fluid content on T2-weighted MR image (b). Note the presence of early increased enhancement in the liver parenchyma adjacent to the abscess (a, d). The wall of the abscess is very thick and shows progressive enhancement (d–f).*

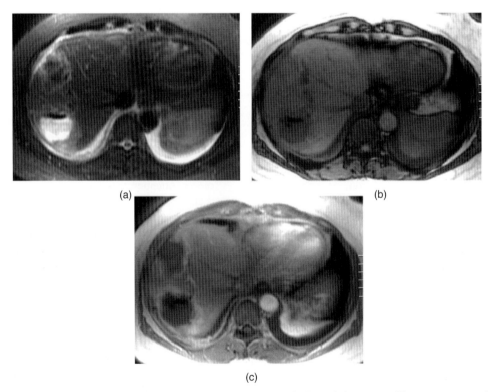

(a) (b)

(c)

Figure 10.6 *Transverse T2-weighted fat-suppressed single shot ETSE (a), transverse T1-weighted out-of-phase 2D-GE (b), transverse T1-weighted hepatic arterial dominant phase 2D-GE (c) images acquired at 1.5 T demonstrate two abscess cavities showing prominent peripheral enhancement in the hepatic arterial dominant phase (c). One of the abscesses, which is located more posteriorly, contains an air–fluid level.*

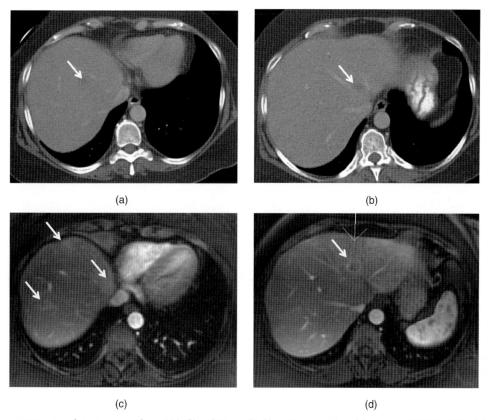

(a)

(b)

(c)

(d)

Figure 10.7 *Transverse postcontrast hepatic venous phase CT (a, b) and T1-weighted hepatic venous phase fat-suppressed 3D-GE MR (c, d) images demonstrate multifocal pyogenic abscesses in the liver.* The lesions appear ill-defined and mildly hypodense on CT. They show moderate enhancement due to a combination of factors including their small size, enhancement of internal septations, and prominent inflammatory response.

- **Hydatid Cyst**
- Hydatid cyst is caused by *E. granulosus.*
- Hydatid cyst is endemic primarily in the Mediterranean region, Middle East, and temperate grazing regions of the world, including New Zealand, South America, and Africa.
- The life cycle of *E. granulosus* involves two hosts. The definitive host is usually a dog or another carnivore. The adult worm of the parasite inhabits the proximal small bowel of the definitive host, releases eggs with larvae (oncospheres) into the feces. Sheep are the most common intermediate hosts. They ingest oncospheres while grazing on contaminated ground. The larvae hatch in the intestines of the intermediate host, penetrate the intestinal mucosa, and migrate to the visceral organs where they form cysts. When the definitive host eats the viscera of the intermediate host, the life cycle of *E. granulosus* is completed. Humans may become incidental intermediate hosts by ingesting *E. granulosus* eggs.
- After the ingestion of eggs of *E. granulosus* or *E. multilocularis* with contaminated food, the larvae invade the intestinal wall, migrate to the liver via the portal vein, and form hepatic hydatid cysts.
- Each hydatid cyst consists of three layers: (i) the outer pericyst which is composed of dense fibrotic host tissue; (ii) the middle

laminated membrane which is acellular and allows the passage of nutrients; and (iii) the inner germinal layer where the scolices, namely the larval stage of the parasite, and the laminated membrane, are produced.
- Daughter cysts, or vesicles, develop on the periphery as a result of germinal layer invagination in the mother cyst.
- Cyst fluid is clear or pale yellow and antigenic as it contains scolices or hooklets. When vesicles rupture within the mother cyst, scolices pass into the cyst fluid and form a white sediment known as *hydatid sand.*
- Hydatid disease involves the liver in 75% of patients, the lung in 15%, and other organs in the remaining 10%.
- The patients are usually asymptomatic, although the cysts may cause pain or jaundice.
- Biochemical analysis usually demonstrates eosinophilia, but a serologic test is positive only in 25% of patients.
- One of the intrahepatic complications of hydatid cyst is cyst rupture. Contained cyst ruptures occur when the endocyst ruptures but the pericyst remains intact. Endocyst detachment, which is a sign of endocyst rupture, is seen as floating membranes within the cyst and known as *water lily sign.* Hydatid cyst may rupture into the biliary tree or may directly rupture into the peritoneal cavity, pleural cavity, abdominal

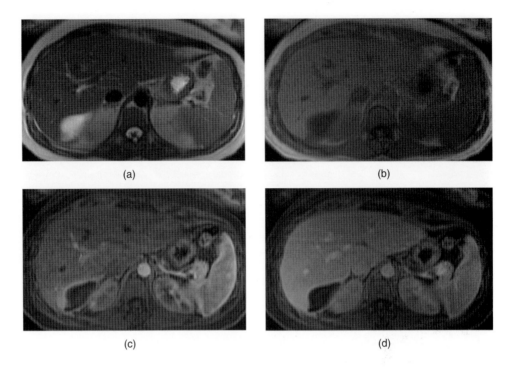

Figure 10.8 *Transverse T2-weighted SS-ETSE (a), T1-weighted 2D-GE (b), T1-weighted fat-suppressed postgadolinium hepatic arterial dominant phase (c) and hepatic venous phase (d) 3D-GE images show a subcapsular abscess in the posterior segment of the right lobe of the liver. The abscess shows typical features including high fluid content (a), early transient peripheral parenchymal enhancement (c), and late wall enhancement (d).*

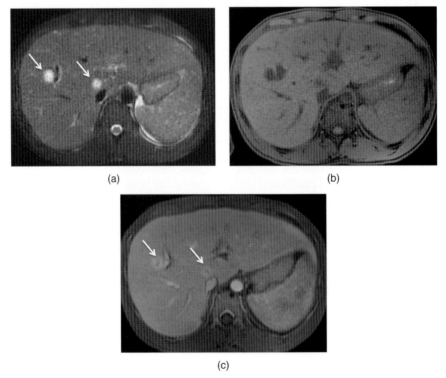

Figure 10.9 *Transverse T2-weighted fat-suppressed single shot ETSE (a), T1-weighted fat-suppressed 3D-GE (b), T1-weighted fat-suppressed postgadolinium hepatic venous phase 3D-GE (c) images demonstrate fungal abscesses (arrows) in an immunocompromised patient.* MRI (a–c) shows two hepatic lesions with thick walls at the same imaging plane. The lesions show high signal on T2-weighted image, and prominent wall enhancement on postgadolinium image (c). The thick walls of fungal abscesses may show prominent enhancement due to their abundant inflammatory component.

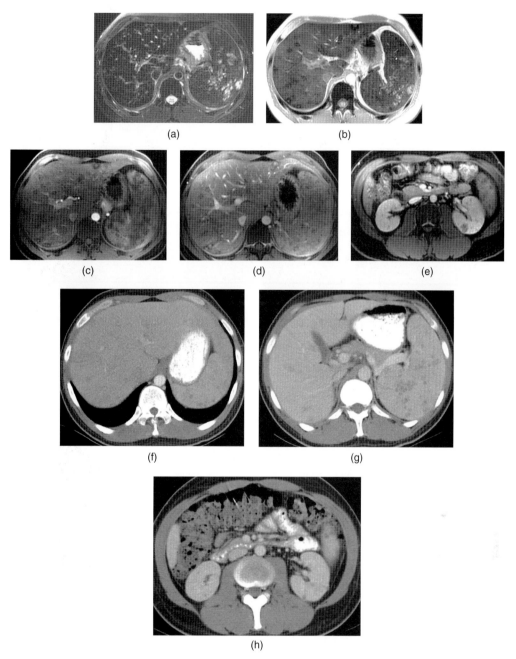

Figure 10.10 *Transverse T2-weighted fat-suppressed SS-ETSE (a), T1-weighted 2D-GE (b), T1-weighted fat-suppressed postgadolinium hepatic arterial dominant phase (c) and hepatic venous phase (d, e) 3D-GE images demonstrate multiple, partially-treated fungal abscesses in the liver, spleen, and kidneys. The lesions show mildly high signal or isointense signal on T2-weighted image (a). They show dark perilesional rings on T1-weighted image (b). They also show mild peripheral and central enhancement on postgadolinium images (c–e). Hemorrhagic changes are also detected in the splenic lesions. Transverse post-contrast hepatic venous phase images (f–h) show further response to the treatment in the same patient. The lesions are smaller and demonstrate negligible enhancement.*

wall, or hollow viscera. The rupture of hydatid cyst into the biliary tree, circulation, or other adjacent abdominal structures may elicit anaphylaxis due to the antigenic nature of the cyst fluid.

• Another intrahepatic complication is infection, which results from the rupture of cysts into the biliary tree or other adjacent abdominal structures. Secondarily infected hydatid cysts may form pyogenic abscesses and cholangitis may coexist. Fat-fluid level may be present due to the communication between biliary tree and hydatid cyst.

• Hydatid cysts may show exophytic growth through the bare area of the liver and gastrohepatic ligament. They may involve

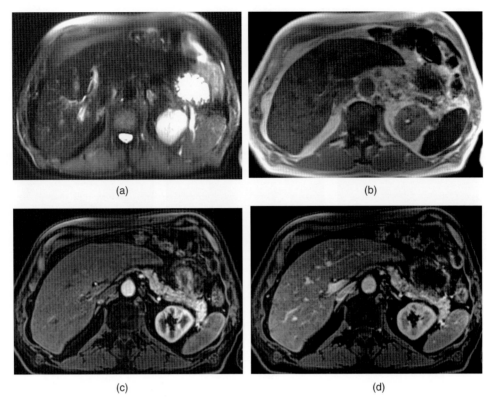

(a)

(b)

(c)

(d)

Figure 10.11 *Transverse T2-weighted fat-suppressed SS-ETSE (a), T1-weighted 2D-GE (b), T1-weighted fat-suppressed postgadolinium hepatic arterial dominant phase (c) and hepatic venous phase (d) 3D-GE images demonstrate treated fungal abscesses in the liver.* Multiple liver lesions with isointense T2 signal (a) and low T1 signal (b) show subtle enhancement.

the diaphragm and may extend or rupture into the pleural cavity via the transdiaphragmatic route, especially from the bare area of the liver in the right lobe. This is a distinctive feature for a hydatid cyst. Hydatid cysts may also invade the abdominal wall. Disseminated peritoneal hydatid cysts may result from the rupture of hydatid cysts. Air--fluid may be present due to the rupture of hydatid cyst into the hollow viscera.

- **On CT:**
  - Hydatid cysts are seen as intermediate or large-sized unilocular or multilocular hypoattenuating liver cysts. Hydatid cysts may appear as a unilocular cyst with a thick or thin wall. They may also appear as multilocular–multivesicular cysts with multiple daughter cysts or septations. Daughter cysts may be seen as round peripheral structures that may have lower attenuation compared to the fluid within the mother cyst. Cysts may contain hydatid sand (matrix) which is seen as hyperdense material. Hydatid sand may be located in the central part or may show layering along the dependent aspect of the cyst. A cyst with a detached membrane, known as the *water lily sign*, is a specific finding for hydatid cysts. Coarse calcifications may be present in the wall of the cysts and within the cysts. Hydatid cysts do not show contrast enhancement on postcontrast examinations.

- Unilocular cysts (WHO classification CL and CE1) and multilocular cysts (WHO classification CE2) (Figure 10.12) are active viable hydatid cysts.
  - A cyst with detached membrane (WHO classification CE3) (Figure 10.13) is in the transition period (active or inactive). It may degenerate or may produce daughter cysts.
  - A non-enhancing hypoattenuating lesion with heterogeneous content with or without any coarse calcification (WHO classification CE4), and prominent large coarse calcifications (WHO classification CE5) is inactive.

- **On MRI:**
  - Pericyst appears as a hypointense rim on both T1-WI and T2-WI. The signal intensity of internal fluid content of the cyst, including the hydatid sand or matrix, is variable on T2-WI and T1-WI. Therefore, the mother cysts may be seen as hyperintense or hypointense on both T1-WI and T2-WI, depending on the protein content. Daughter cysts usually show individually high or low signal on T2-WI and T1-WI (Figure 10.12); respectively, and they may show lower signal compared to the internal matrix of mother cysts on T2-WI and T1-WI. Detached germinal membrane may also appear as high signal on T2-WI and low signal on T1-WI (Figure 10.13). The pericyst may show subtle enhancement, but the internal contents of hydatid cysts do not show contrast enhancement on postgadolinium images.

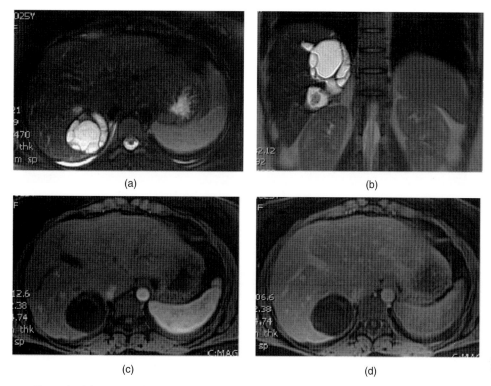

(a)

(b)

(c)

(d)

Figure 10.12 *Transverse T2-weighted fat-suppressed SS-ETSE (a), coronal T2-weighted SS-ETSE (b), transverse T1-weighted fat-suppressed postgadolinium hepatic arterial dominant phase (c) and hepatic venous phase (d) 3D-GE images illustrate a hepatic hydatid cyst containing daughter cysts.* At this stage, the hydatid cyst is a multilocular cyst and this suggests the presence of active disease. The cyst does not show any enhancement.

- **Differential Diagnosis and Pearls:**
  - Unilocular cysts with thin or thick wall may be confused with simple cysts, cystic metastases, or pyogenic abscesses. Cystic metastases usually demonstrate more intense wall enhancement in comparison to hydatid cysts on postcontrast examinations. Pyogenic abscesses usually demonstrate progressive central stromal enhancement on postcontrast examinations and are usually associated with the presence of early perilesional parenchymal enhancement on the hepatic arterial dominant phase.
  - Clinical and serologic data help to differentiate these entities from each other.
- ***E. multilocularis* Cyst**
- *E. multilocularis* is rarer and endemic to the upper Midwest of the United States, Alaska, Canada, Japan, Central Europe, and parts of Russia.
- Definitive hosts are foxes and, less commonly, cats and dogs. Humans are infected either by direct contact with a definitive host or indirectly by ingestion of contaminated water or contaminated plants.
- *E. multilocularis* produces multilocular cysts that resemble alveoli. The liver is the most commonly involved organ and is affected in 90% of patients.
- CT and MR demonstrate multiple irregular lesions composed of multiple small-sized cysts. The lesions are hypoattenuating

on CT examinations and show high signal on T2-weighted images. They may contain calcifications and central necrosis. The lesions do not show enhancement on postcontrast examination on CT and MRI.

- Hilar infiltration may be present and may result in intrahepatic bile duct dilatation and invasion of vascular structures.

Tuberculosis

- Tuberculosis is a very common granulomatous infection caused by *Mycobacterium tuberculosis* and may involve the liver hematogeneously in two different patterns: miliary or local.
- Miliary tuberculosis of the liver is the most common form and seen in 50–80% of patients with advanced tuberculosis or miliary tuberculosis.
- Local hepatic tuberculosis is seen as nodular (focal) tuberculosis and/or tubular (hepatobiliary) tuberculosis. Nodular tuberculosis forms tuberculous abscesses and tuberculomas while tubular tuberculosis affects the intrahepatic bile ducts.
- Imaging findings of miliary and nodular forms are similar to fungal abscesses/infections.

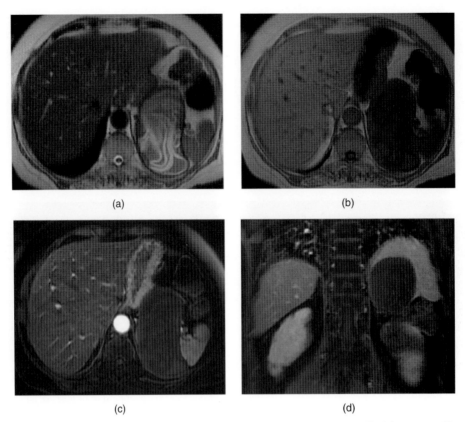

(a)   (b)

(c)   (d)

Figure 10.13 *Transverse T2-weighted SS-ETSE (a), transverse T1-weighted 2D-GE (b), postgadolinium T1-weighted fat-suppressed hepatic arterial dominant (c) and coronal hepatic venous phase (d) 3D-GE images demonstrate a hydatid cyst with detached germinal membrane.* Hydatid cysts may be seen in any part of the body. The hydatid cyst is located between the spleen and stomach in this patient. The water-lily sign is noted in the cyst due to detached membrane. The cyst does not show any enhancement.

- Tubular tuberculosis involves the intrahepatic bile ducts and portal triads/hilus. Imaging findings include periportal high signal intensity on T2-WI and moderate/intense enhancement on late-phase postgadolinium images.
- Associated porta hepatis nodes are also common.

Acute viral hepatitis

- Acute viral hepatitis is a systemic infection affecting the liver and caused by viral agents. The most common viral agents are hepatotropic viruses, including hepatitis A, B, C, D, and E. However, other viruses including, but not limited to, herpes virus, rubella virus, yellow fever, and Coxsackie virus may also cause hepatitis.
- These viruses usually produce clinically similar disease patterns ranging from asymptomatic unapparent infections to fulminant fatal acute infections. They may also cause subclinical persistent infections progressing to chronic liver disease with cirrhosis (commonly blood borne agents including hepatitis B, C, and D), which will be the subject of Chapter 11.

- The major histopathologic findings of acute hepatitis are necrosis of hepatocytes with diffuse cell injury and portal tract inflammatory infiltrate. Hepatocyte regeneration occurs in the recovery phase and confluent necrosis leading to bridging necrosis may be seen with more severe forms.
- Imaging findings on CT and MRI include hepatomegaly, periportal edema, and periportal enlarged lymph nodes. Periportal edema is seen as low attenuation density changes along the portal tracts,veins, on CT and is characterized by high signal intensity on T2-weighted images and low signal intensity on T1-weighted images on MRI. Focal edema may be seen as an increased parenchymal signal on T2-weighted and low signal on T1-weighted MR images. Diffuse or segmental/focal heterogeneously increased enhancement may be seen on contrast enhanced CT, especially on the hepatic arterial dominant phase. Diffuse or segmental/focal heterogeneously increased enhancement is seen on the hepatic arterial dominant phase, which usually fades to isointensity on the hepatic venous phase on MRI. Enhancement of periportal tracking tissue on late postcontrast images is an important feature to examine for in the setting of possible viral disease, as this is consistent

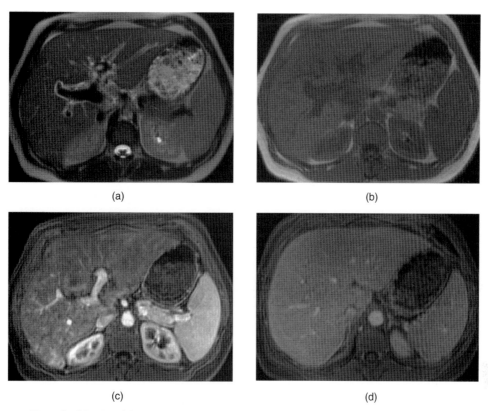

(a)

(b)

(c)

(d)

Figure 10.14 *Transverse T2-weighted SS-ETSE (a), transverse T1-weighted 2D-GE (b), postgadolinium T1-weighted fat-suppressed hepatic arterial dominant (c) and hepatic venous phase (d) 3D-GE images illustrate acute viral hepatitis.* Mild edema of the liver parenchyma in combination with moderate periportal edema is detected on T2-weighted image (a). The liver shows diffuse heterogeneous enhancement on the hepatic arterial dominant phase (c), which becomes isointense in the later phase (d).

with true inflammatory tissue rather than simple periportal edema, a finding more in keeping with infection.

- Gallbladder wall thickening due to edema is a frequent finding. However, ascites is not commonly seen.
- Figures 10.14 and 10.15.

Bacterial acute cholangitis

- The development of bacterial acute cholangitis occurs in the setting of stagnant bile, high intra-biliary pressure, and contamination of the biliary tree with bacteria. Therefore, it is usually observed in the presence of biliary obstruction (Figure 10.16).
- The clinical picture of the Charcot triad refers to the presence of fever, right upper quadrant pain, and jaundice.
- Biliary obstruction facilitates and leads to bacterial colonization of the biliary tree by interfering with and impairing the protective mechanisms of the biliary system, which under normal circumstances enable the production and transport of sterile bile into the duodenum. Elevated intrabiliary pressure resulting from the obstruction increases permeability of biliary ductules, allowing bacteria and their toxins entry into the bloodstream and liver parenchyma. Additionally,

impaired IgA secretion due to elevated intrabiliary pressure decreases the antibacterial properties of bile.

- Bile duct stones are the most common cause of bacterial cholangitis and are present in 70–80% of patients with acute cholangitis (Figure 10.16), although the incidence of bacterial cholangitis developing secondary to malignant obstruction, instrumentation of biliary tree, surgery, or sclerosing cholangitis has increased in recent years. Bacterial acute cholangitis is present in 6–9% of patients with gallstones.
- Biliary cultures are usually polymicrobial and gram negative rods are seen in 80–90% of patients.
- Hepatic abscesses (Figure 10.17) and portal vein thrombosis (Figure 10.18) may be associated with acute bacterial cholangitis.
- Intrahepatic and extrahepatic bile duct dilatation, including the common bile duct, and symmetrical thickening and enhancement of bile duct walls are typical imaging findings. Bile duct dilatation and wall thickening are observed on T2W and T1W precontrast images. Bile duct wall enhancement is best seen in the interstitial phase of enhancement on postgadolinium images. Associated parenchymal changes include peribiliary, peribiliary- patchy, wedge-shaped high signal intensity changes on T2W images. Corresponding peribiliary, peribiliary-patchy and wedge-shaped enhancements are seen

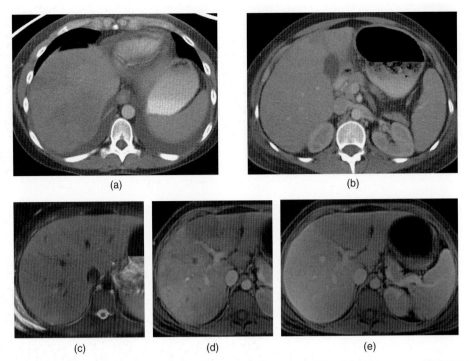

(a) (b)

(c) (d) (e)

Figure 10.15 *Transverse postcontrast hepatic arterial dominant phase CT images (a, b), transverse T2-weighted fat-suppressed SS-ETSE (c), T1-weighted post-gadolinium fat-suppressed hepatic arterial dominant (d) and hepatic venous phase (e) 3D-GE MR images demonstrate acute hepatitis, which is characterized by enlarged edematous liver with heterogeneous enhancement.* The liver shows mildly increased T2 signal due to edema (c). Heterogeneous enhancement is seen as patchy, segmental, and wedge-shaped areas of decreased and increased enhancement in the hepatic arterial dominant phase (a, b, d). The liver tends to show more homogeneous enhancement in the hepatic venous phase (e).

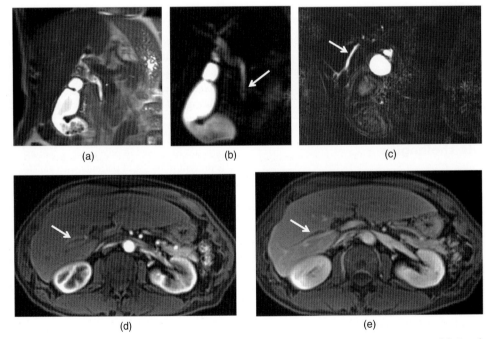

(a) (b) (c)

(d) (e)

Figure 10.16 *Coronal T2-weighted SS-ETSE (a), coronal thick slab MRCP (b), coronal thin slab MRCP (c), transverse postgadolinium fat-suppressed hepatic arterial dominant phase (d) and hepatic venous phase (e) images illustrate ascending cholangitis.* The gallbladder is hydropic and contains multiple stones (a, b). Additionally, a common bile duct stone is seen (arrow, b). A focally dilated bile duct (arrow, c) is seen in the right lobe with adjacent early transient increased enhancement in the hepatic arterial dominant phase (arrow, d) and bile duct wall enhancement on the hepatic venous phase (e). These findings are consistent with ascending cholangitis and develop secondary to the obstruction of the common bile duct due to stone disease.

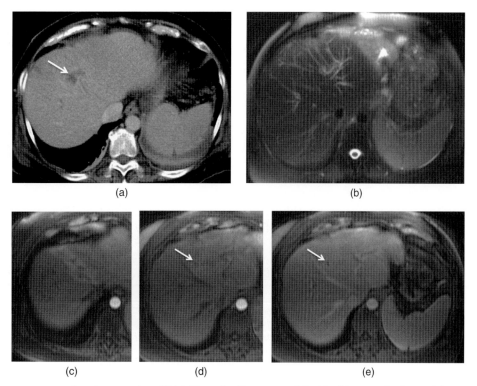

Figure 10.17 *Transverse postcontrast hepatic venous phase CT (a), T2-weighted fat-suppressed SS-ETSE (b), T1-weighted postgadolinium fat-suppressed hepatic arterial dominant phase (c, d), and hepatic venous phase (e) 3D-GE images illustrate ascending cholangitis.* Mild focal hypodense area (arrow, a) associated with intrahepatic biliary dilatation is seen on CT image, which represents focal abscess associated with ascending cholangitis. Focal segmental increased transient enhancement is detected on the hepatic arterial dominant phase with enhancing focal abscess (d, e). The transient segmental enhancement fades in the later phase (e).

in the hepatic arterial dominant phase and tend to fade to isointensity with the remaining liver parenchyma on later phases of postgadolinium T1W images (Figures 10.16 and 10.17). Enhancing and enlarged papilla may be seen on postgadolinium T1W images.

- Although CT findings are similar to the findings detected on postgadolinium T1W images, MRI is superior to CT in the diagnosis of bacterial acute cholangitis. This primarily reflects the greater sensitivity to contrast enhancement, and therefore the better appreciation of the transient arterial phase periduct hepatic parenchymal enhancement.
- Antibiotic therapy associated with emergent or elective endoscopic or percutaneous drainage is the therapeutic approach, which is necessary to decompress the biliary tree and to stop the spread of infection.

Recurrent pyogenic cholangitis

- Recurrent episodes of bacterial cholangitis lead to the formation of ectasia, focal strictures, and intrahepatic stones. Chronic intrahepatic ductal dilatation or associated portal vein thrombosis causes lobar or segmental atrophy.

- *Ascaris lumbrocoides* and *Clonorchis sinensis* infestations are associated with recurrent pyogenic cholangitis. It has been proposed that chronic infestation of the biliary tree causes the formation of subsequent bile duct fibrosis, strictures, stagnant biliary flow, and stones, which together allow the development of recurrent bacterial infections.
- More commonly seen in Asian population, hence the clinical moniker oriental cholangiohepatitis, although the incidence has been rising in Western countries.
- Hepatic abscesses and portal vein thrombosis may be associated.
- Focal dilatation and stenosis or strictures of peripheral intrahepatic bile ducts, disproportionate dilatation of central and extrahepatic bile ducts, intrahepatic biliary stone formation, and thickened periportal space due to periductal inflammation and fibrosis are the common findings of recurrent pyogenic cholangitis.
- Stenoses rarely affect the extrahepatic biliary tree. Intraductal stones are found in the majority of patients. Pnemobilia resulting from the reflux of gas from the gastrointestinal tract or gas forming organism may frequently be seen. Atrophy of the parenchyma is seen in chronic infections.

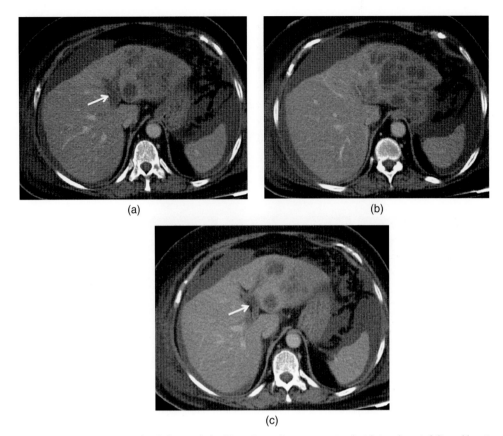

Figure 10.18 *Transverse postcontrast CT images (a–c) show multifocal hypodense abscesses associated with intrahepatic biliary dilatation in the left hepatic lobe.* The left portal vein is thrombosed due to associated ascending cholangitis. Note the ascites and nodular contour of the liver.

- Recurrent pyogenic cholangitis is associated with increased risk of developing cholangiocarcinomas centrally or peripherally. In order to detect cholangiocarcinomas early, patients with RPC should be tested with MRI.
- Treatment is directed to control the acute episodes of cholangitis and to remove the predisposing causes. Percutaneous or endoscopic drainage, stone removal or stenting with antibiotic treatment, and supportive measures with good follow-up are usually successful in the majority of cases. Surgery is reserved for patients with recurrent and persistent disease and the resection of involved segments is usually performed.

HIV-related cholangitis

- Human immunodeficiency virus (HIV) infection may also involve the liver and biliary tree, especially in patients with markedly depressed immune system. The biliary tree may be affected when the CD4 count is <100/mm.
- Liver function test abnormalities and right upper quadrant pain are usually the initial nonspecific findings. Liver function test abnormalities may be commonly encountered in HIV (+) patients due to various conditions ranging from drug reactions to hepatitis. Right upper quadrant pain in combination with fever may also be seen due to ascending cholangitis in this patient group.
- Transaminases and cholestasis enzymes are usually elevated, although bilirubin level is normal or mildly elevated. Therefore, jaundice is only observed if there is liver failure or common bile duct obstruction.
- Because the clinical findings and symptoms are not specific, CT and MRI may be helpful to determine the etiology and to differentiate the biliary infection or involvement from parenchymal infection or inflammation.
- Acquired immunodeficiency syndrome (AIDS) cholangiopathy causes secondary sclerosing cholangitis. AIDS cholangiopathy results from inflammation, ischemia, autonomic nerve damage of bile ducts due to opportunistic biliary infections involving bile ducts, or direct invasion of biliary epithelium by HIV virus.
- *Mycobacterium avium* complex, *Cryptosporidium parvum*, cytomegalovirus, and herpes simplex virus are the usual causative agents in AIDS cholangiopathy, although no pathogens are identified in 50% of patients.
- Typical imaging findings include intrahepatic and extrahepatic bile duct strictures, irregular wall thickening, beading, and pruning of bile ducts (Figure 10.19). Papillary stenosis

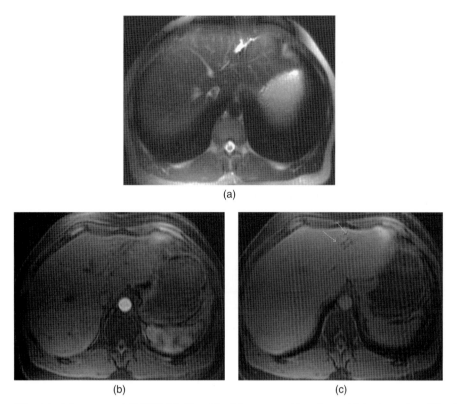

Figure 10.19 *Transverse T2-weighted fat-suppressed SS-ETSE (a), T1-weighted fat-suppressed hepatic arterial dominant phase (b) and hepatic venous phase 3D-GE images demonstrate focally dilated bile duct in the left lobe with associated ductal wall enhancement in a HIV (+) patient, illustrating HIV related cholangitis.*

and acalculous cholecystitis are the other common imaging findings.

- Endoscopic retrograde pancreatiography may be used for the demonstration of biliary inflammation and pathogens. Biliary sphincterotomy stent placement and antibiotherapy are used in the treatment.

References

1 Mortele, K.J., Segatto, E., and Ros, P.R. (2004) The infected liver: radiologic–pathologic correlation. Radiographics, 24, 937–955.

2 Kawamoto, S., Soyer, P.A., Fishman, E.K., and Bluemke, D.A. (1998) Nonneoplastic liver disease: evaluation with CT and MR imaging. Radiographics, 18, 827–848.

3 Catalona, O.A., Sahani, D.V., Forcione, D.G. et al. (2009) Biliary infections: spectrum of imaging findings and management. Radiographics, 29, 2059–2080.

4 Marrone, G., Crino, F., Caruso, S. et al. (2012) Multidisciplinary imaging of liver hydatidosis. World J Gastroenterol, 18, 1438–1447.

5 Balci, N.C., Semelka, R.C., Noone, T.C. et al. (1999) Pyogenic hepatic abscesses: MRI findings on T1- and T2-weighted and serial gadolinium-enhanced gradient-echo images. J Magn Reson Imaging, 9, 285–290.

6 Sallah, S., Semelka, R.C., Sallah, W. et al. (1999) Amphotericin B lipid complex for the treatment of patients with acute leukemia and hepatosplenic candidiasis. Leuk Res, 23, 995–999.

7 Sallah, S., Semelka, R., Kelekis, N. et al. (1998) Diagnosis and monitoring response to treatment of hepatosplenic candidiasis in patients with acute leukemia using magnetic resonance imaging. Acta Hematol, 100, 77–81.

8 Balci, N.C., Tunaci, A., Semelka, R.C. et al. (2000) Hepatic alveolar echinococcosis: MRI findings. Magn Reson Imaging, 18, 537–541.

9 Semelka, R.C., Kelekis, N.L., Sallah, S. et al. (1997) Hepatosplenic fungal disease: diagnostic accuracy and spectrum of appearances on MR imaging. AJR Am J Roentgenol, 169, 1311–1316.

10 Bilgin, M., Balci, N.C., Erdogan, A. et al. (2008) Hepatobiliary and pancreatic MRI and MRCP findings in patients with HIV infection. AJR Am J Roentgenol, 191, 228–232.

CHAPTER 11

Chronic hepatitis and liver cirrhosis

Ersan Altun[1], Mohamed El-Azzazi[1,2,3,4], Richard C. Semelka[1], and Mamdoh AlObaidy[1,5]
[1] The University of North Carolina at Chapel Hill, Department of Radiology, Chapel Hill, NC, USA
[2] University of Dammam, Department of Radiology, Dammam, Saudi Arabia
[3] King Fahd Hospital of the University, Department of Radiology, Khobar, Saudi Arabia
[4] University of Al Azhar, Department of Radiology, Cairo, Egypt
[5] King Faisal Specialist Hospital & Research Center, Department of Radiology, Riyadh, Saudi Arabia

- Chronic liver diseases progress to the formation of liver fibrosis and cirrhosis. The most common chronic liver diseases are non-alcoholic fatty liver disease, chronic hepatitis C infection, chronic hepatitis B infection, and alcoholic hepatitis. Other, less prevalent chronic liver diseases include autoimmune hepatitis, primary biliary cirrhosis, primary sclerosing cholangitis, Wilson's disease, hereditary hemochromatosis, congenital hepatic fibrosis, alpha-1-antitrypsin deficiency, and cystic fibrosis.
- Repetitive hepatocyte injury from various causes leads to the development of liver fibrosis, which is characterized by deposition of an abundant volume of collagen and proteoglycans in the extracellular matrix. Collagen is produced in excess amounts by hepatic stellate cells induced by fibrogenic cytokines.
- Development of liver fibrosis is a component of wound-healing mechanism. Therefore, liver fibrosis on its own is reversible and may regress initially. However, progressive liver fibrosis due to repetitive and chronic injury may lead to cirrhosis, which is an irreversible condition.
- The pattern of fibrosis pathologically differs for chronic viral hepatitis, and fatty liver disease/alcoholic hepatitis.
- In chronic viral hepatitis, fibrosis starts in the portal triads characterized by focal fibrotic expansion of portal triads (stage F1). The extension of thin fibrous septa, arising from the expanded portal triads, into the adjacent liver parenchyma occurs in the next stage (stage F2). Further thickening and elongation of fibrous septa lead to the formation of fibrous bridges connecting adjacent portal triads and central veins (stage F3). Further enlargement and merging of fibrous bridges divide the liver parenchyma and lead to the formation of regenerative nodules surrounded by fibrous tissue (stage F4).

- In alcoholic hepatitis and nonalcoholic fatty liver disease, fibrosis starts adjacent to the central veins in a perisinusoidal manner (zone 3 perisinusoidal fibrosis) (stage F1). Further involvement of portal tracts with fibrosis (zone 1 periportal fibrosis) occurs in the next stage (stage F2). Further thickening and elongation of fibrous septa lead to the formation of fibrous bridges connecting adjacent portal triads and central veins (stage F3). Further enlargement and merging of fibrous bridges divide the liver parenchyma and lead to the formation of regenerative nodules surrounded by fibrous tissue (stage F4).
- Advanced stages of liver fibrosis and cirrhosis may present similar pathological findings and may be indistinguishable from each other because histopathological features of fatty liver disease is lost with advanced fibrosis and cirrhosis.
- Cirrhosis is not a static phenomenon but a dynamic process, including the histopathological findings of inflammation, cell injury and death, fibrosis and regeneration.
- The presence of regenerative nodules surrounded by fibrosis is the hallmark of cirrhosis. Regenerative nodules may also be occasionally seen without the development of fibrosis, as in nodular regenerative hyperplasia, Budd-Chiari syndrome, portal vein thrombosis, or massive hepatic injury. Extensive fibrosis without formation of regenerative nodules may also be seen occasionally as in congenital hepatic fibrosis.
- **Classification of Cirrhosis based on Nodule Size:**
- *Micronodular:* Often observed with diffuse liver injury due to alcohol or metabolic disorders such as nonalcoholic steatohepatitis. Primary biliary cirrhosis, primary sclerosing cholangitis, hereditary hemochromatosis, and Wilson's disease may cause micronodular cirrhosis.
  ° Small regenerative nodules (<3-mm in diameter).
  ° Figure 11.1.

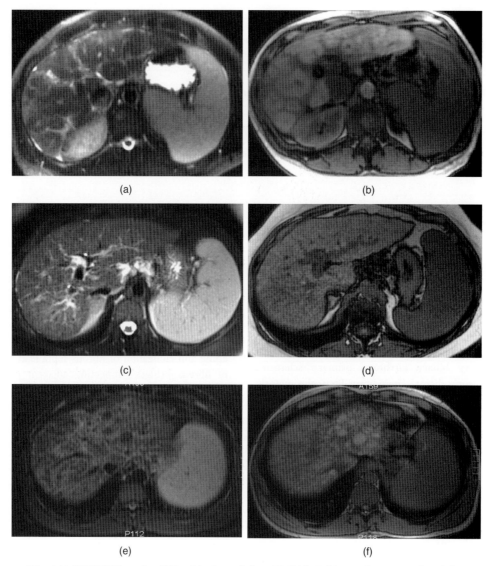

(a)

(b)

(c)

(d)

(e)

(f)

Figure 11.1 *Transverse T2-weighted SS-ETSE (a, c, e) and T1-weighted out-of-phase 2D-GE (b, d, f) images demonstrate three different patients with macronodular, micronodular, and mixed macronodular-micronodular cirrhosis.* The first patient with macronodular cirrhosis shows multiple large regenerative nodules (a, b). The second patient with micronodular cirrhosis shows multiple diffuse small regenerative nodules (c, d). The third patient with mixed macronodular–micronodular type cirrhosis shows the presence of combination of small and large regenerative nodules. Note that regenerative nodules show similar signal or low signal compared to the background liver on T2-weighted images and similar signal or high signal (due to protein content) on out-of-phase T1-weighted images.

- *Macronodular:* Liver injury predominantly resulting in hepatocellular regeneration is more commonly associated with this pattern. Viral hepatitis and toxic hepatitis are the most common cause. Primary sclerosing cholangitis, Wilson's disease and alpha-1-antitrypsin deficiency can also cause macronodular cirrhosis.
  ° Large regenerative nodules (>3-mm in diameter)
  ° Figure 11.1.
- *Mixed:* Macronodular pattern develops with advancing cirrhosis, and therefore micronodular and macronodular patterns are both seen in most disease processes (Figure 11.1).

The differentiation between micronodular and macronodular pattern has very limited clinical value.
- **General Morphologic features of Chronic Hepatitis and Cirrhosis of the liver on MRI and CT:**
  ° *Features of Chronic Hepatitis*
  ° The liver appears normal in the early stages of chronic hepatitis.
  ° Chronic hepatitis may progress to cirrhosis, showing the development of fibrosis.
  ° Enlarged portahepatis, gastrohepatic, reptroperitoneal lymph nodes may be present.

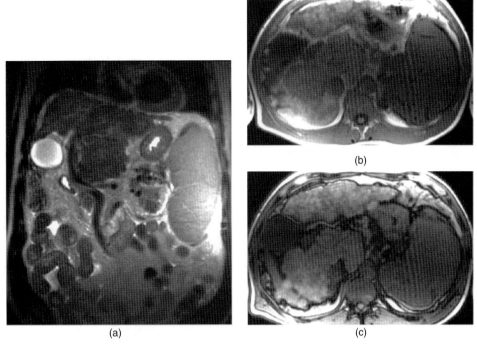

(a) (b) (c)

Figure 11.2 *Coronal T2-weighted SS-ETSE (a), T1-weighted 2D-GE in-phase (b) and out-of-phase (c) images demonstrate a cirrhotic liver with severely nodular contours, caudate lobe hypertrophy, right lobe atrophy and left lobe hypertrophy.* Note the enlarged spleen containing Gamna–Gandy bodies which are seen as hypointense nodules on in-phase T1-weighted image (b) and less distinct on out-of-phase image (c) due to their iron deposition.

° *Features of Cirrhosis*
° Atrophy of the right lobe and the medial segment of the left lobe (Figure 11.2).
° Relative sparing and/or hypertrophy of the caudate lobe and lateral segment of the left lobe (Figure 11.2).
° Irregular hepatic contour due to the presence of regenerative nodules and fibrosis.
° Enlargement of the hilar periportal space.
° Expansion of the major interlobar fissure causing extrahepatic fat to fill the space between the left medial and lateral segments.
° Expanded gallbladder fossa, which is filled with fat.
° Enlarged porta hepatis, gastrohepatic, celiac, paracaval or retroperitonel lymph nodes.
° Associated with mesenteric, omental, retroperitoneal edema and omental hypertrophy.
• **Morphologic features of Fibrosis of the liver on MRI and CT:**
° Liver fibrosis may be classified into two types, reticular and confluent.
° ***Reticular type:*** A network of linear fibrotic stroma of varying thickness. Reticular type of fibrosis can be classified morphologically into three major types according to the thickness of reticular fibers (Figure 11.3).
° *Mild:* <2 mm. The contours of the liver appear normal (Figure 11.4).

° *Moderate:* >2 mm. The contours of the liver appear mildly undulating (Figures 11.5 and 11.6).
° *Severe:* >2 mm. The contours of the liver appear nodular and undulating (Figure 11.7).
° ***Confluent type:*** Commonly appears as a peripheral triangular area with its apex directed to the porta hepatis. It is commonly seen in segment VIII.
° **On CT:** The sensitivity of CT is low and therefore mild to moderate reticular fibrosis is not seen. Severe reticular fibrotic network appears as hypoattenuating fibrotic bands associated with contour undulation. Postcontrast CT examination on the interstitial phase is more sensitive compared to noncontrast CT examination. Confluent fibrosis appears as a focal hypoattenuating lesion, which shows progressive enhancement.
° **On MRI:**
° On T1-weighted images: Out-of-phase SGE is the most sensitive precontrast sequence for the demonstration of reticular fibrosis, including mild and moderate fibrosis. Confluent fibrosis appears as a hypointense lesion, which may be associated with volume loss and capsular retraction.
° On T2-weighted images: Acute fibrous tissue displays high signal due to higher fluid content, whereas chronic fibrous tissue displays low signal on T2-weighted images. Mild to moderate reticular fibrotic network is not usually seen. Severe fibrosis may be detected as low and/or high intensity

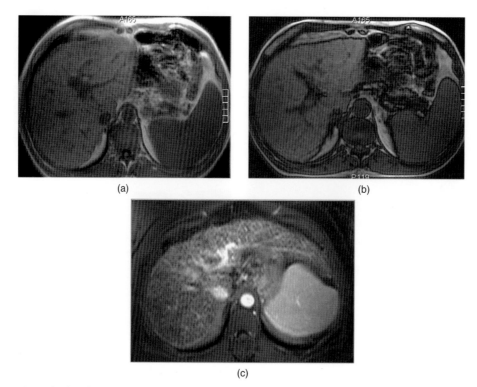

Figure 11.3 *Transverse T1-weighted in-phase 2D-GE (a), out-of-phase 2D-GE (b) and postgadolinium interstitial phase 3D-GE (c) images show cirrhotic liver in three different patients with cirrhosis.* The first two patients demonstrate moderate fibrosis (a, b) and the third patient shows severe fibrosis (c). The contours of the liver appear mildly nodular in the first two patients and reticular fibers are appreciated particularly on the periphery. The contours of the liver appear again mildly nodular in the third patient; however, the reticular fibers are very prominent and thick. Note that the out-of-phase image (b) shows the nodular contours better compared to the in-phase image (a).

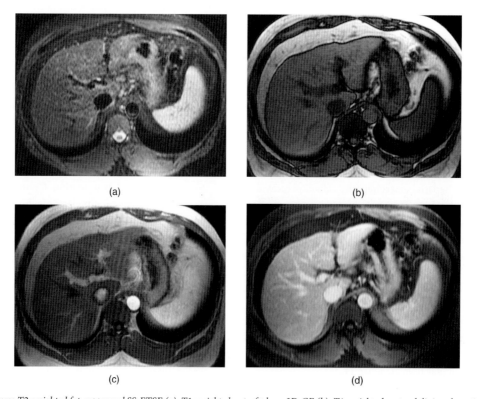

Figure 11.4 *Transverse T2-weighted fat-suppressed SS-ETSE (a), T1-weighted out-of-phase 2D-GE (b), T1-weighted postgadolinium hepatic arterial dominant phase 2D-GE (c) and T1-weighted fat-suppressed interstitial phase 3D-GE images show mild reticular fibrosis.* Note that the contours of the liver appear normal. Mild reticular network is seen on T2-weighted (a), T1-weighted out-of-phase (b) and postgadolinium interstitial phase (d) images.

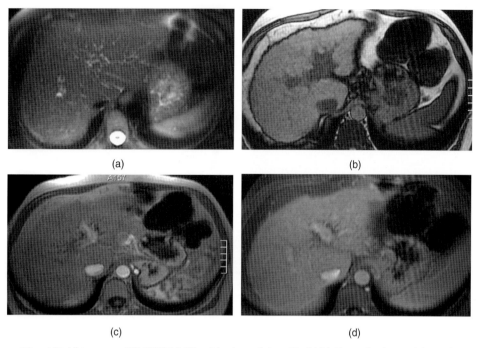

(a)   (b)

(c)   (d)

Figure 11.5 *Transverse T2-weighted fat-suppressed SS-ETSE (a), T1-weighted out-of-phase 2D-GE (b), T1-weighted postgadolinium hepatic arterial dominant phase 2D-GE (c) and T1-weighted fat-suppressed interstitial phase 3D-GE images show moderate reticular fibrosis.* Note that the contours of the liver appear mildly nodular and moderate reticular network is well seen on out-of-phase image (b) and postgadolinium interstitial phase image (d).

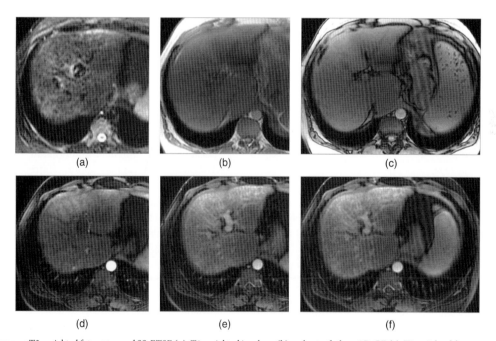

(a)   (b)   (c)

(d)   (e)   (f)

Figure 11.6 *Transverse T2-weighted fat-suppressed SS-ETSE (a), T1-weighted in-phase (b) and out-of-phase 2D-GE (c), T1-weighted fat-suppressed postgadolinium hepatic arterial dominant phase (d), hepatic venous (e) and interstitial phase (f) 3D-GE images show moderate reticular fibrosis.* The contours of the liver appear normal to mildly nodular. Moderate reticular network is best seen on the interstitial phase postgadolinium image (f). The fibrotic network is not well seen on the out-of-phase image due to low contrast resolution of T1-weighted images, which are acquired at 3.0 T. Note that the caudate lobe is hypertrophic and right lobe is atrophic.

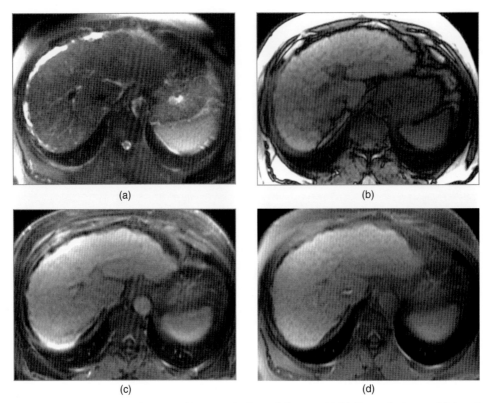

Figure 11.7 *Transverse T2-weighted fat-suppressed SS-ETSE (a), T1-weighted out-of-phase 2D-GE (b), T1-weighted postgadolinium fat-suppressed hepatic venous phase (c) and interstitial phase (d) 3D-GE images show severely nodular liver contour and severe reticular fibrotic network, which are best seen on out-of-phase image (b) and interstitial phase image (d).*

bands. Confluent fibrosis usually shows high signal on T2-weighted images.

  ° Postgadolinium T1-weighted images: Reticular and confluent fibrotic changes demonstrate negligible enhancement in the hepatic arterial dominant phase and progressive enhancement in later phases, which is more prominent in the interstitial phase.

  ° Figures 11.8 and 11.9.

- **Distinctive Morphological Features of Cirrhosis Depending on the Etiology**
  ° Morphological pattern of cirrhosis is usually not helpful and distinctive for the identification of etiology except primary sclerosing cholangitis and sarcoidosis.
  ° Advanced form of primary sclerosing cholangitis and sarcoidosis cause central regeneration with peripheral atrophy resulting in the most severe distortion of liver morphology (Figure 11.10) Early form of primary sclerosing cholangitis may show left lobe hypertrophy associated with bile duct changes, including multifocal stenosis, beading, and dilatation with or without pruned tree appearance (Figure 11.11).
  ° Other causes of cirrhosis may either cause prominent fibrosis associated with normal liver morphology (more common with primary biliary cirrhosis or autoimmune hepatitis) (Figures 11.12 and 11.13) or classic morphology of cirrhosis, including caudate lobe hypertrophy and

lateral segment of hypertrophy (alcohol, Hepatitis B and C, NASH) (Figures 11.14 and 11.15).

- **Ancillary Features of Chronic Hepatitis and Cirrhosis**
  ° Omental hypertrophy (Figure 11.16).
  ° Enlarged gallbladder fossa (Figure 11.16).
  ° Gallbladder wall edema (Figure 11.17).
  ° Focal or diffuse iron deposition (Figure 11.18).
  ° Transient perfusional abnormalities/vascular shunting (Figures 11.19 and 11.20).

- **Acute on Chronic Hepatitis**
  ° Acute inflammation may be seen in the presence of chronic hepatitis. Acute inflammation is usually seen as patchy and wedge-shaped areas.
  ° **On MRI:** Acute inflammation is usually characterized by the presence of edema as demonstrated by high T2 signal and increased early transient enhancement in the hepatic arterial dominant phase. Acute inflammation may show isointense or mildly low signal on precontrast T1-weighted image. The enhancement fades in the later phases, including the hepatic venous phase and interstitial phase (Figure 11.21).
  ° **On CT:** Acute inflammation is usually characterized by the presence of early increased enhancement on the hepatic arterial dominant phase (Figure 11.21), which fades in the later phases. However, mild acute inflammation may

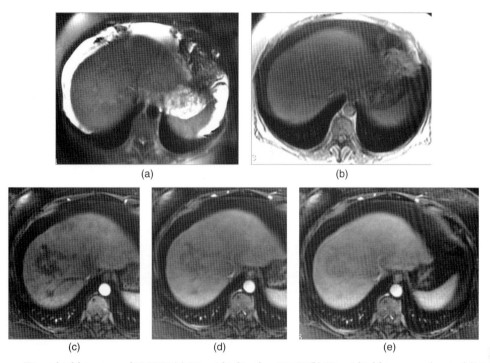

Figure 11.8 *Transverse T2-weighted fat-suppressed SS-ETSE (a), T1-weighted in-phase 2D-GE (b), T1-weighted fat-suppressed postgadolinium hepatic arterial dominant phase (c), hepatic venous (d) and interstitial phase (e) 3D-GE images show confluent fibrosis at segment VIII.* The confluent fibrosis shows mild T2 signal on T2-weighted image (a) and isointense signal on T1-weighted image (b). On postgadolinium images, the confluent fibrosis does not show enhancement in the hepatic arterial dominant phase (c) but demonstrates progressive enhancement in the later phases, which is more prominent in the interstitial phase. The fibrosis shows subtle high T2 signal representing its chronic nature.

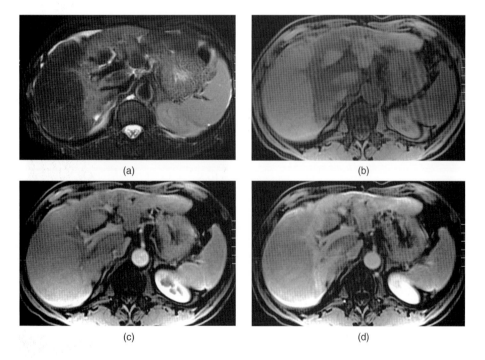

Figure 11.9 *Transverse T2-weighted fat-suppressed SS-ETSE (a), T1-weighted fat-suppressed 3D-GE (b), T1-weighted fat-suppressed postgadolinium hepatic arterial dominant phase (c), hepatic venous (d) and interstitial phase (e) 3D-GE images show prominent wedge-shaped and patchy confluent fibrosis in this patient with cirrhosis.* The fibrosis shows moderately high T2 signal due to its relatively acute nature. The fibrosis shows mild enhancement in the hepatic arterial dominant phase and prominent enhancement in the interstitial phase.

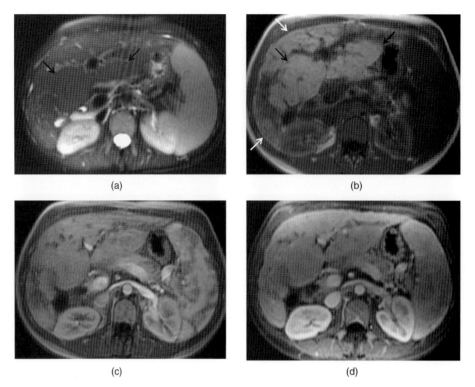

Figure 11.10 *Transverse T2-weighted fat-suppressed SS-ETSE (a), T1-weighted in-phase 2D-GE (b), T1-weighted postgadolinium hepatic arterial dominant phase (c) and fat-suppressed hepatic venous phase (d) 3D-GE images demonstrate advanced cirrhosis due to primary sclerosing cholangitis.* The right lobe is prominently atrophic. Prominent central regeneration of the left lobe and caudate lobe (black arrows; a, b) and peripheral atrophy of the left and right lobes (white arrows; b) are seen.

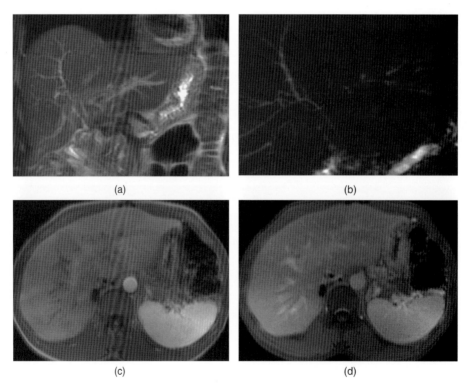

Figure 11.11 *Coronal T2-weighted SS-ETSE (a), coronal MIP MRCP (b), transverse T1-weighted hepatic arterial dominant phase 2D-GE (c) and fat-suppressed interstitial phase 3D-GE (d) images demonstrate findings of early cirrhosis secondary to primary sclerosing cholangitis in a patient with liver transplant.* Intrahepatic bile ducts demonstrate pruned tree appearance associated with focal mild dilatation and strictures, which are more prominent on the left sided intrahepatic ducts (a, b). The lateral segment of the left lobe appears enlarged and shows central regeneration. Diffuse wedge-shaped and patchy early increased enhancement in the liver on the hepatic arterial dominant phase (c), which fade on the later phases (d). Early increased enhancement likely results from early transient perfusional abnormality.

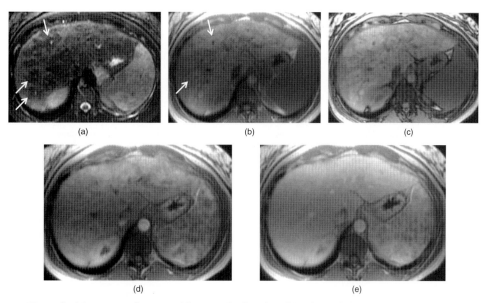

(a)　　　　　　　　　　(b)　　　　　　　　　　(c)

(d)　　　　　　　　　　(e)

Figure 11.12 *Transverse T2-weighted fat-suppressed SS-ETSE (a), T1-weighted in-phase (b) and out-of-phase 2D-GE (c), T1-weighted postgadolinium hepatic arterial dominant phase (d), hepatic venous phase (e) 2D-GE images demonstrate a patient with primary biliary cirrhosis.* The contours of the liver appear mildly nodular. Multiple T2 hypointense and T1 isointense nodular areas surrounding T2 hyperintense and T1 hypointense portal tracts are seen in the liver representing halo sign (arrows; a, b). These nodules represent regenerative nodules. The nodules demonstrate similar enhancement to the background liver. Moderate fibrotic network is also noted on pre- and postgadolinium images.

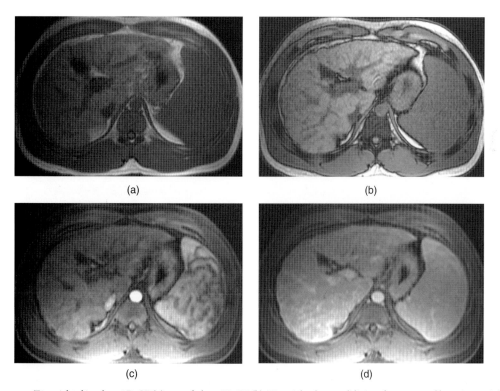

(a)　　　　　　　　　　(b)

(c)　　　　　　　　　　(d)

Figure 11.13 *Transverse T1-weighted in-phase 2D-GE (a), out-of-phase 2D-GE (b), T1-weighted postgadolinium fat-suppressed hepatic arterial dominant phase (c) and interstitial phase 3D-GE (d) images demonstrate the cirrhotic liver developing secondary to autoimmune hepatitis.* The lateral segment of the left lobe is hypertrophic. Note the nodular contours and severe fibrotic network of the liver on out-of-phase image (b) and interstitial phase postgadolinium image (d).

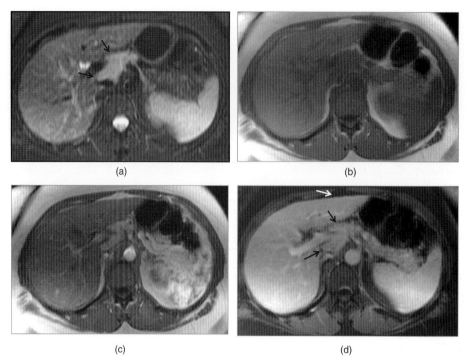

Figure 11.14 *Transverse T2-weighted fat-suppressed SS-ETSE (a), T1-weighted in-phase 2D-GE (b), T1-weighted postgadolinium hepatic arterial dominant phase (c) and fat-suppressed hepatic venous phase (d) 3D-GE images demonstrate mildly cirrhotic liver developing secondary to chronic hepatitis C infection.* The contour of the liver is mildly undulating and nodular (white arrow, d). Note the presence of multiple enlarged porta hepatis, celiac and portacaval lymph nodes (black arrows; a, d). The lymph nodes show high signal on T2-weighted image (a) and show homogeneous enhancement on postgadolinium images (d).

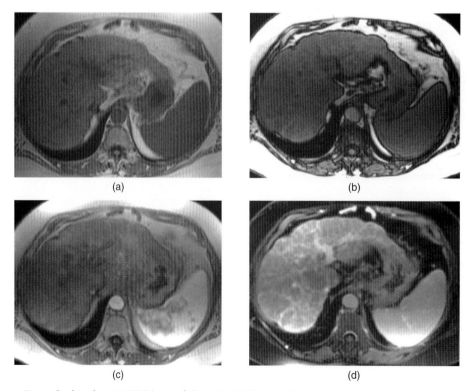

Figure 11.15 *Transverse T1-weighted in-phase 2D-GE (a), out-of-phase 2D-GE (b), T1-weighted postgadolinium hepatic arterial dominant phase 2D-GE (c) and interstitial phase fat-suppressed 3D-GE (d) images demonstrate cirrhosis due to NASH.* The liver has nodular contours and shows severe fibrosis. Fibrotic network is visualized on out-of-phase image (b) and prominently enhances on the interstitial phase image (d). Heterogeneous fat deposition which is characterized by signal drop on out-of-phase image (b) is seen. Note the presence of heterogeneous early enhancement on the hepatic arterial dominant phase, which results from the inflammation.

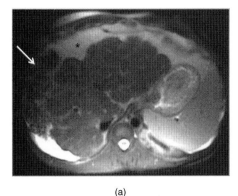
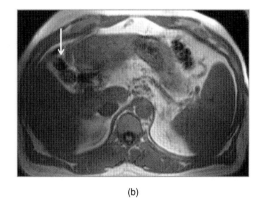

(a)   (b)

Figure 11.16 *Transverse T2-weighted fat-suppressed SS-ETSE (a) show the presence of a large amount of ascites (asterisk, a), omental hypertrophy (arrow, a) and mild splenomegaly in a patient with advanced cirrhosis and portal hypertension.* T1-weighted 2D-GE (b) images demonstrate the mild enlargement of gallbladder fossa (arrow, b).

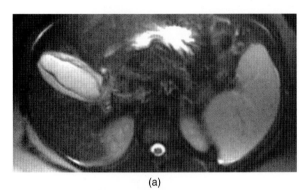

(a)

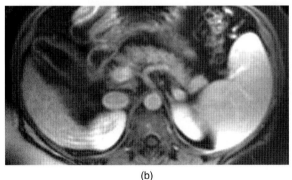

(b)

Figure 11.17 *Transverse T2-weighted fat-suppressed SS-ETSE (a), T1-weighted fat-suppressed postgadolinium interstitial phase 3D-GE (b) images show the development of gallbladder edema secondary to the chronic hepatitis/liver disease.* The mucosa and submucosa of the gallbladder wall show enhancement but the gallbladder wall does not show increased enhancement.

not be detected on CT due to its lower contrast resolution compared to MRI.

° The differential diagnosis includes transient perfusional abnormality/vascular shunting, which shows the same enhancement features as acute or chronic hepatitis. However, edema is not associated with perfusional abnormality/vascular shunting, which is a distinguishing feature.

- **Features of Portal Hypertension**
  ° Dilated portal vein and the presence of varices.
  ° Ascites.
  ° Splenomegaly with or without Gamna Gandy bodies.
  ° Major sites of portosystemic collateralization/varices include gastroesophageal, paraumbilical, retroperitoneal, perigastric, splenorenal, omental, peritoneal, and hemorrhoidal varices. The paraumbilical vein becomes patent.
  ° **On CT:** Varices appear as tortuous tubular vascular structures that enhance after administration of intravenous contrast medium.
  ° **On MRI:** Varices demonstrate variable signal intensities due to their flow pattern. They may appear as signal void vascular structures (in high flow states) on T1- and T2-weighted images, or demonstrate high or low signal on T2- and T1-weighted images, respectively. On postgadolinium T1-weighted images, varices enhance on the hepatic venous and interstitial phase images.
  ° Figures 11.22, 11.23, and 11.24.
- **Morphologic Features of Cirrhotic Nodules**
- *Regenerative Nodules (RNs)*
  ° Representing a benign proliferation of hepatocytes surrounded by fibrous septal tissue.
  ° **On CT:**
  ° RNs appear as isodense or mildly hyperdense nodular lesions on unenhanced or enhanced CT images.
  ° **On MRI:**
  ° The majority are isointense on both T2- and T1-weighted images (Figure 11.25).
  ° Occasionally, RNs may appear:
  ° Low in signal intensity on T2-weighted images due to high protein or iron content (Figure 11.25).
  ° Hyperintense on T1-weighted images due to high protein content (Figure 11.25).

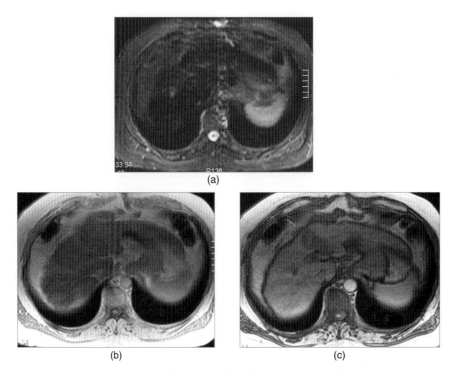

Figure 11.18 *Transverse T2-weighted STIR (a), T1-weighted in-phase 2D-GE (b) and out-of-phase 2D-GE (c) images show iron deposition in the liver.* The liver shows prominently decreased signal on T2-weighted image due to iron deposition. The liver shows decreased signal on T1-weighted in-phase image and the liver signal is mildly higher on out-of-phase image compared to in-phase image secondary to iron deposition. The liver is cirrhotic with nodular contours. The spleen or bones do not demonstrate iron deposition and the pancreas (not shown) does not show iron deposition. Therefore, the iron deposition is not due to hemosiderosis or hemochromatosis but the cirrhosis itself.

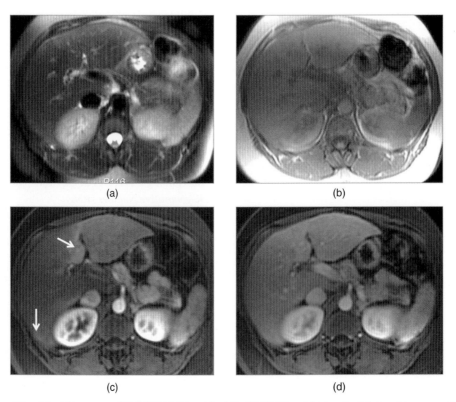

Figure 11.19 *Transverse T2-weighted fat-suppressed SS-ETSE (a), T1-weighted 2D-GE (b), T1-weighted postgadolinium fat-suppressed hepatic arterial dominant phase (c) and hepatic venous phase (d) 3D-GE images demonstrate transient perfusional abnormality in a patient with cirrhosis.* Patchy and wedge shaped areas of peripheral early transient increased enhancement (arrows, c), which fade on the later phase (d), are detected in the right lobe posterior segment and left lobe medial segment.

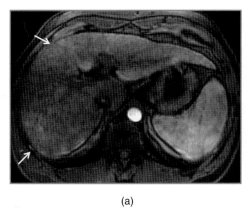
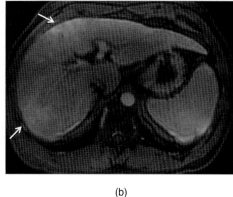

(a)   (b)

Figure 11.20 *Transverse T1-weighted fat-suppressed hepatic arterial phase (a) and hepatic venous phase (b) 3D-GE images show early transient patchy and wedge-shaped areas of early increased enhancement.* These transient areas of early increased enhancement tend to become isointense in the later phases and are due to transient perfusional abnormalities secondary to cirrhosis.

◦ Hypointense on T1-weighted images due to iron content. They show relatively increased signal on out-of-phase images compared to in-phase images (Figure 11.26).

◦ Hypointense on T1-weighted out-of-phase images compared to in-phase images due to fat content (Figure 11.26).

◦ Enhance minimally on postgadolinium images and therefore they usually maintain their precontrast signal intensities on postgadolinium images (Figures 11.26 and 11.27).

◦ However, isovascular or hypovascular HCCs, which do not show wash-out or capsule on the later phases, may mimic regenerative nodules. Therefore, large regenerative nodules or any nodules appearing distinctively different from the background liver should be followed up to exclude HCC (Figure 11.28).

• *Dysplastic nodules (DNs)*

   ◦ Dysplasia is characterized by cellular atypia and represents progressive change from regenerative nodules. HCCs may develop in dysplastic nodules and therefore dysplastic nodules are premalignant nodules.

   ◦ Dysplastic nodules are considered an intermediate step in the pathogenesis of HCC in stepwise progression.

   ◦ **On CT:** Dysplastic nodules appear isoattenuating or mildly hyperattenuating nodules on unenhanced images. High grade dysplastic nodules demonstrate early increased enhancement in the hepatic arterial dominant phase, which fade to isodensity with the background liver parenchyma in the later phases. Low grade dysplastic nodules cannot be recognized on CT.

   ◦ **On MRI:**

   ◦ Dysplastic nodules commonly show isointense or hypointense signal on T2-weighted images and isointense or hyperintense signal on T1- weighted images. They may rarely show high T2 signal and low T1 signal.

   ◦ Figures 11.29 and 11.30.

   ◦ Correlations exist between the extent of enhancement on the hepatic arterial dominant phase images and the grade of DNs. Increase in arterial blood supply and decrease of portal blood supply of hepatic nodules is closely related to the process of development of high grade dysplastic nodules and malignant transformation of high grade dysplastic nodules to HCC.

   ◦ On postgadolinium T1-weighted images:

   ◦ There are three types of DNs:

   ◦ *Low grade DNs:*

      • Show negligible or similar enhancement to the background parenchyma (i.e., isointense) in the hepatic arterial dominant phase and in the later phases. They are difficult to differentiate from regenerative nodules, and generally we employ size of lesions. Lesions that are mildly high signal on T1 and >3 cm in size are called low grade DNs.

   ◦ *High grade DNs:*

      • Demonstrate mild to marked increased enhancement in the hepatic arterial dominant phase images.

      • Show fading towards background signal of the liver in the later phases without evidence of wash-out or late capsule enhancement.

      • Usually <1.5 cm.

      • Figures 11.29–11.31.

      • The differential diagnosis includes small HCC and focal perfusional abnormalities/vascular shunts. Small HCCs demonstrate increased enhancement in the hepatic arterial dominant phase and wash-out with capsular enhancement in the later phases. Perfusional abnormalities/vascular shunts are usually wedge-shaped and linear but not nodular (Figure 11.32).

      • High grade dysplastic nodules are usually followed by imaging, particularly in high risk patients, to detect the progression to HCC (Figures 11.33 and 11.34).

   ◦ *High grade DN with "a nodule within a nodule" appearance*

      • Appears as foci of small HCC that develop in a high-grade DN.

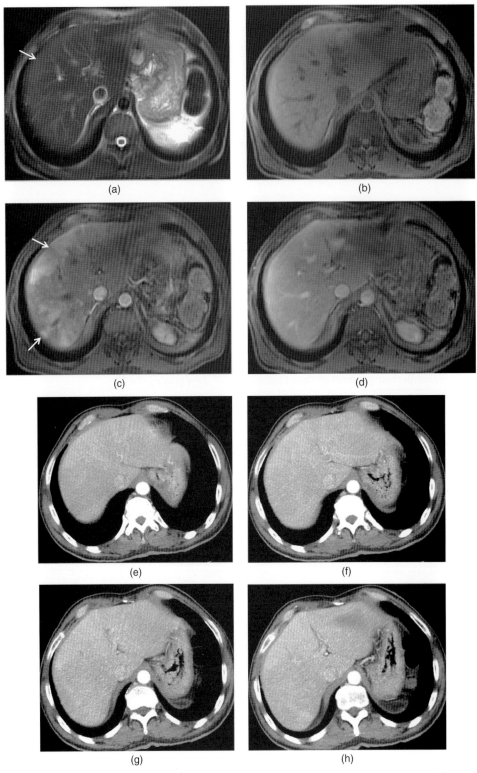

Figure 11.21 *Transverse T2-weighted fat-suppressed SS-ETSE (a), T1-weighted fat-suppressed 3D-GE (b), T1-weighted postgadolinium fat-suppressed hepatic arterial dominant phase (c) and hepatic venous phase (d) 3D-GE images demonstrate wedge-shaped, patchy, mildly increased T2 signal (arrow, a) and early transient increased enhancement (arrows, c), which are suggestive of acute on chronic hepatitis.* This area shows isointense signal on T1-weighted image (b) and early increased enhancement (arrows, c) in the hepatic arterial dominant phase (c) fades on the hepatic venous phase (d). Note that the liver has normal morphology despite chronic hepatitis. Transverse postcontrast hepatic arterial dominant phase CT images show patchy and wedge-shaped areas of increased enhancement on CT in the same patient. The CT examination was performed a few months earlier compared to MRI. Note that MRI shows enhancement better compared to CT, due to higher soft tissue contrast resolution.

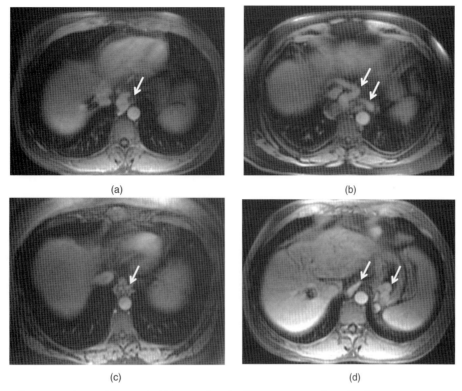

Figure 11.22 *Transverse fat-suppressed postgadolinium 3D-GE images show distal gastric, gastroesophageal, and gastric wall varices in four different patients.* Large caliber distal esophageal and gastroesophageal varices are seen in the first two patients (a, b). Small caliber distal esophageal varices are seen in the third patient (c). Medium caliber distal esophageal and large caliber gastric wall varices are seen in the fourth patient (d).

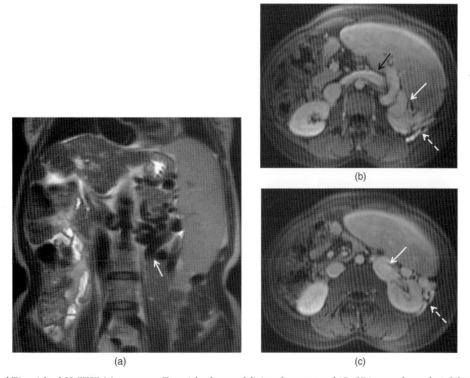

Figure 11.23 *Coronal T2-weighted SS-ETSE (a), transverse T1-weighted postgadolinium fat-suppressed 3D-GE images show splenic hilum varices, perisplenic varices, and splenorenal shunt in a patient with advanced cirrhosis and portal hypertension.* Note the huge splenomegaly. Splenic hilar varices show high flow state and therefore appear as signal void tubular structures (arrow, a). Large caliber perisplenic varices are noted (white arrows; b, c). Small caliber retroperitoneal varices are seen (posterior white arrows; b, c). The left renal vein appears enlarged due to splenorenal shunt (black arrow, b).

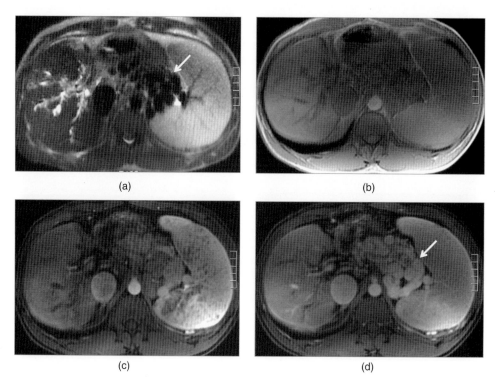

(a) (b)

(c) (d)

Figure 11.24 *Transverse T2-weighted SS-ETSE (a), T1-weighted in-phase 2D-GE (b), T1-weighted postgadolinium fat-suppressed hepatic arterial dominant phase (c) and hepatic venous phase (d) 3D-GE images show cirrhosis and portal hypertension secondary to primary sclerosing cholangitis.* Intrahepatic bile ducts are mildly dilated and show focal dilatations and strictures, which are seen on T2-weighted image (a) and postgadolinium hepatic venous image (d). The liver is small and the spleen is enlarged. The portal vein is chronically thrombosed and not visualized. Note the presence of extensive high flow state perisplenic and perigastric varices (arrows; a, d) and very large IVC.

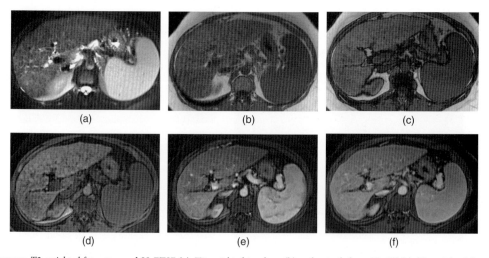

(a) (b) (c)

(d) (e) (f)

Figure 11.25 *Transverse T2-weighted fat-suppressed SS-ETSE (a), T1-weighted in-phase (b) and out-of-phase 2D-GE (c), T1-weighted fat-suppressed 3D-GE, T1-weighted fat-suppressed postgadolinium hepatic arterial dominant phase (e) and hepatic venous (f) 3D-GE images show multiple regenerative nodules in a patient with cirrhosis.* The regenerative nodules show isointense to hypointense signal on T2-weighted images and isointense to hyperintense signal on T1-weighted images. The nodules showing low T2 signal and high T1 signal have high protein content. The nodules show homogeneous enhancement and similar enhancement compared to the background liver. Severe fibrotic network is also noted. Note the presence of splenomegaly and enlarged splenic vein.

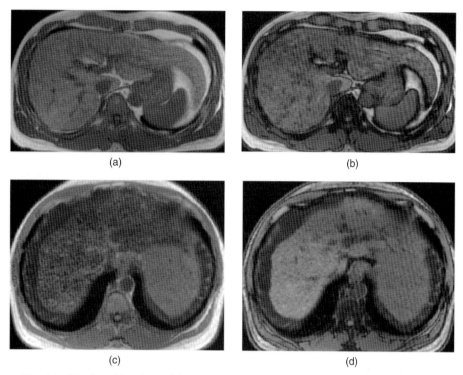

(a)　　　　　　　　　　　(b)

(c)　　　　　　　　　　　(d)

Figure 11.26 *Transverse T1-weighted in-phase (a) and out-of-phase (b) 2D-GE images demonstrate multiple regenerative nodules having fat content in a patient with cirrhotic liver.* Some of the regenerative nodules show decreased signal on out-of-phase image (b) compared to in-phase image (a) due to their fat content. T1-weighted in-phase (c) and out-of-phase (d) 2D-GE images demonstrate multiple regenerative nodules having iron content in another patient with cirrhotic liver. Some of these regenerative nodules show prominently decreased signal on in-phase image (c) compared to out-of-phase (d) image due to their iron content.

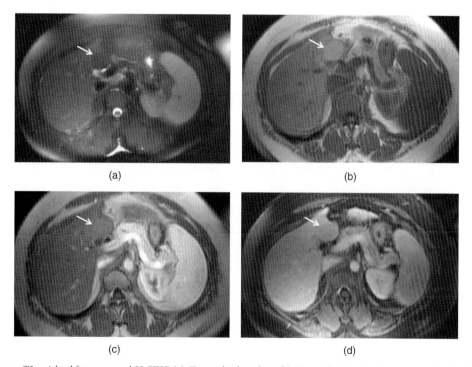

(a)　　　　　　　　　　　(b)

(c)　　　　　　　　　　　(d)

Figure 11.27 *Transverse T2-weighted fat-suppressed SS-ETSE (a), T1-weighted in-phase (b), T1-weighted postgadolinium hepatic arterial dominant phase (c) and interstitial phase (d) images show an exophytic large regenerative nodule (arrows) located in the gallbladder fossa. The regenerative nodule demonstrates low T2 signal, high T1 signal, and similar enhancement compared to the background liver on postgadolinium images.*

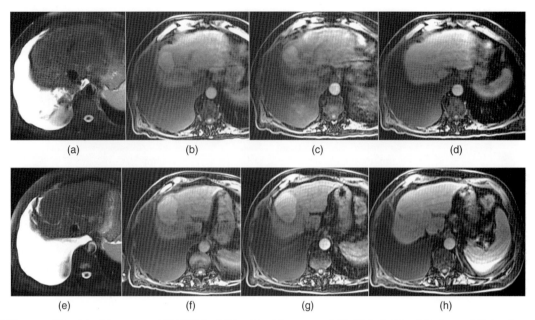

(a) (b) (c) (d)

(e) (f) (g) (h)

Figure 11.28 *Transverse T2-weighted fat-suppressed SS-ETSE (a, e), T1-weighted fat-suppressed 3D-GE (b, f), T1-weighted postgadolinium fat-suppressed hepatic arterial phase (c, g), hepatic venous phase (d, h) 3D-GE images demonstrate interval enlargement of a large nodular isovascular HCC in 6 months.* The first set of images (a–d) demonstrate a nodular lesion with isointense T2 signal and high T1 signal. The lesion shows mild arterial phase enhancement (c) and becomes isointense on the hepatic venous phase (d). The second set of images (e–h) show the interval enlargement of the lesion in 6 months. The lesion shows similar morphologic features and enhancement features compared to prior examination. This lesion represents an isovascular HCC with mild arterial enhancement and shows no wash-out. This case illustrates that HCC may be isovascular and may not show wash-out and emphasizes the importance of follow-up. Note the large right pleural effusion and cirrhotic liver.

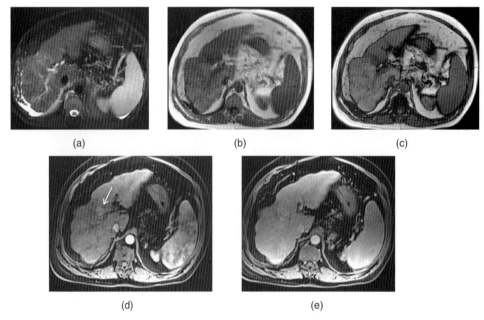

(a) (b) (c)

(d) (e)

Figure 11.29 *Transverse T2-weighted fat-suppressed SS-ETSE (a), T1-weighted in-phase (b) and out-of-phase 2D-GE (c), T1-weighted fat-suppressed postgadolinium hepatic arterial dominant phase (d) and hepatic venous (e) 3D-GE images show a high grade dysplastic nodule in a cirrhotic liver.* The high grade dysplastic nodule shows a 1 cm nodule with early enhancement in the hepatic arterial dominant phase, which fades in the hepatic venous phase. The dysplastic nodule demonstrates mildly low signal on T2-weighted image (a) and low signal on T1-weighted images (b, c).

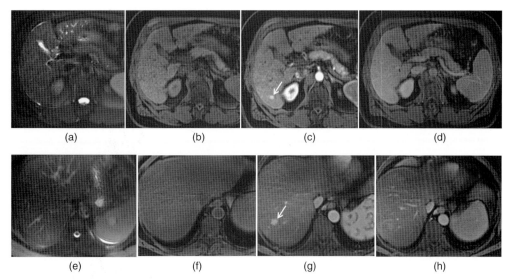

(a) (b) (c) (d)

(e) (f) (g) (h)

Figure 11.30 *Transverse T2-weighted fat-suppressed SS-ETSE (a), T1-weighted fat-suppressed 3D-GE (b), T1-weighted postgadolinium fat-suppressed hepatic arterial phase (c) and hepatic venous phase (d) images show a small subcentimeter high grade dysplastic nodule (arrow, c) in a patient with chronic liver disease.* The nodule demonstrates early increased enhancement (c) and later fading (d) and is isointense on precontrast images (a, b). Transverse T2-weighted fat-suppressed SS-ETSE (e), T1-weighted fat-suppressed 3D-GE (f), T1-weighted postgadolinium fat-suppressed hepatic arterial phase (g) and hepatic venous phase (h) images show a 1 cm high grade dysplastic nodule (arrow, g) in another patient with chronic liver disease. The nodule shows isointense T2 signal and high T1 signal on precontrast images and early increased enhancement (g) with later fading (h).

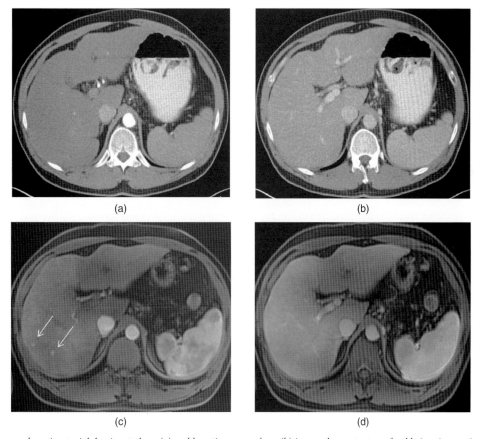

(a) (b)

(c) (d)

Figure 11.31 *Transverse hepatic arterial dominant phase (a) and hepatic venous phase (b) images demonstrate no focal lesions in a patient with chronic liver disease.* Transverse T1-weighted postgadolinium fat-suppressed hepatic arterial dominant phase (c) and hepatic venous phase (d) images show two nodular foci of early increased enhancement, which fade in the hepatic venous phase (d). These lesions represent dysplastic nodules and are well visualized on MRI compared to CT, due to higher soft tissue contrast resolution.

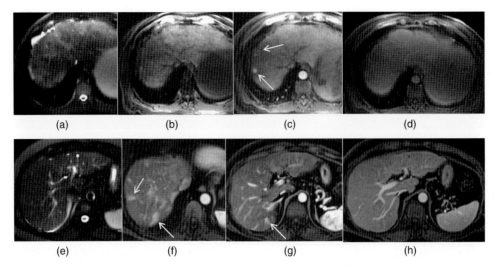

Figure 11.32 *Transverse T2-weighted fat-suppressed SS-ETSE (a), T1-weighted fat-suppressed 3D-GE (b), T1-weighted postgadolinium fat-suppressed hepatic arterial phase (c), hepatic venous phase (d) 3D-GE images show two small high grade dysplastic nodules (arrows, c), which show early increased enhancement (c) and later fading without wash-out (d).* The larger nodule shows also low T2 and high T1 signal on precontrast images. The other smaller lesion is isointense on precontrast images. Transverse T2-weighted fat-suppressed SS-ETSE (e), T1-weighted postgadolinium hepatic arterial dominant phase (f, g) and hepatic venous phase (h) images show linear wedge- shaped areas of early increased enhancement (arrows; f, g) on the hepatic arterial dominant phase, which become isointense on the hepatic venous phase. These areas do not have precontrast correlation and appear isointense on precontrast images and they represent perfusional abnormalities and vascular shunts.

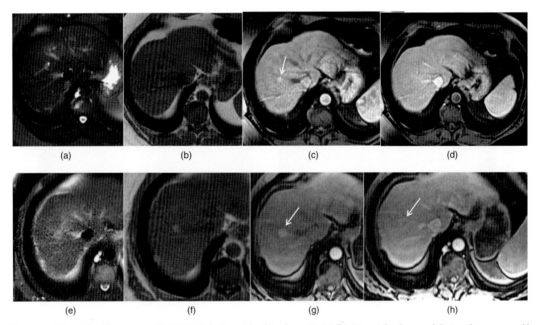

Figure 11.33 *Transverse T2-weighted fat-suppressed SS-ETSE (a), T1-weighted in-phase 2D-GE (b), T1-weighted postgadolinium fat-suppressed hepatic arterial dominant phase (c) and hepatic venous phase (d) 3D-GE images show a small high grade dysplastic nodule (arrow, c) with isointense signal on T2 (a) and T1-weighted (b) images.* The dysplastic nodule shows early enhancement on the hepatic arterial dominant phase (c) with fading on the hepatic venous phase (d). Transverse T2-weighted fat-suppressed SS-ETSE (e), T1-weighted in-phase 2D-GE (f), T1-weighted postgadolinium fat-suppressed hepatic arterial dominant phase (g) and hepatic venous phase (h) images demonstrate the interval enlargement of the lesion (arrows; g, h) in 6 months. The lesion shows high T2 (e) and T1 (f) signal on precontrast images. The lesion (arrows; g, h) showing interval-increased size demonstrates early increased enhancement on the hepatic arterial dominant phase (g) and later washout on the hepatic venous phase (h). This case illustrates the conversion of a high grade dysplastic nodule into HCC.

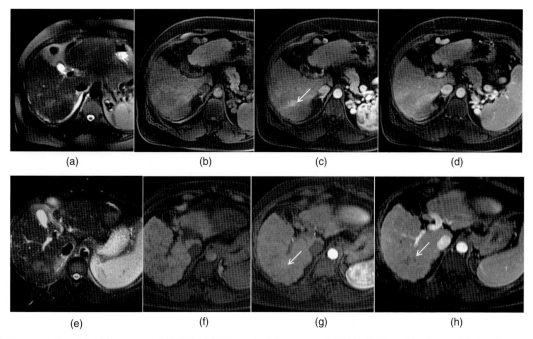

Figure 11.34 *Transverse T2-weighted fat-suppressed SS-ETSE (a), T1-weighted fat-suppressed 3D-GE (b), T1-weighted postgadolinium fat-suppressed hepatic arterial dominant phase (c) and hepatic venous phase (d) 3D-GE images show a high grade dysplastic nodule (arrow, c) with high T2 (a) and low T1 (b) signal.* The nodule shows early increased enhancement in the hepatic arterial dominant phase (c) and fading in the hepatic venous phase (d). Transverse T2-weighted fat-suppressed SS-ETSE (e), T1-weighted fat-suppressed 3D-GE (f), T1-weighted postgadolinium fat-suppressed hepatic arterial dominant phase (g) and hepatic venous phase (h) 3D-GE images show the interval enlargement of the lesion (arrows; g, h) and progression to HCC in 6 months. The lesion shows similar signal characteristics on precontrast images (e, f). The lesion shows early enhancement in the hepatic arterial dominant phase (g) and wash-out in the hepatic venous phase (h).

- On T2-weighted images: Appears as moderately high signal intensity focus within a low signal intensity nodule.
- On T1-weighted images: Appears as low signal intensity focus within high signal intensity nodule.
- On postgadolinium T1-weighted image: Small HCC focus shows increased or similar enhancement compared to the dysplastic nodule on the hepatic arterial dominant phase with relative wash-out compared to the dysplastic nodule in the later phases.

- **Risk of Developing HCC**
  ° *Low risk:* Hepatitis or cirrhosis due to autoimmune hepatitis, primary sclerosing cholangitis, or primary biliary cirrhosis. One-year follow-up is usually done to screen for HCC.
  ° *Medium risk:* Hepatitis or cirrhosis due to NAFLD and NASH, primary hemochromatosis. Six-month follow-up is usually done to screen for HCC.
  ° *High risk:* Hepatitis or cirrhosis due to alcoholic hepatitis–cirrhosis, Hepatitis B, Hepatitis C. Three to six-month follow-up is usually done to screen for HCC, depending on the clinical and imaging findings.
  ° *Highest risk:* Hepatitis or cirrhosis due to combination of alcohol with Hepatitis B or Hepatitis C. Three to six-month

follow-up is usually done to screen for HCC, depending on the clinical and imaging findings.

References

1 Hussain, S.M., Reinhold, C., and Mitchell, D.G. (2009) Cirrhosis and lesion characterization at MR imaging. Radiographics, 29, 1637–1652.

2 Faria, S.C., Ganesan, K., Mwangi, I. *et al.* (2009) MR imaging of liver fibrosis: current state of the art. Radiographics, 29, 1615–1635.

3 Hyslop, W.B., Kierans, A.S., Leonardou, P. *et al.* (2010) Overlap syndrome of autoimmune chronic liver diseases: MRI findings. J Magn Reson Imaging, 31, 383–389.

4 Elias, J. Jr.,, Altun, E., Zacks, S. *et al.* (2009) MRI findings in nonalcoholic steatohepatitis: correlation with histopathology and clinical staging. Magn Reson Imaging, 27, 976–987.

5 Zapparoli, M., Semelka, R.C., Altun, E. *et al.* (2008) 3.0-T MRI evaluation of patients with chronic liver diseases: initial observations. Magn Reson Imaging, 26, 650–660.

6 Heredia, V., Altun, E., Ramalho, M., and Semelka, R.C. (2007) Magnetic resonance imaging of the liver: a review. Expert Opin Med Diagn, 1, 213–223.

7 Ramalho, M., Altun, E., Heredia, V. *et al.* (2007) Liver MR imaging: 1.5 T versus 3.0 T. Magn Reson Imaging Clin N Am., 15, 321–347.

CHAPTER 12

Hepatic fat and iron deposition

Ersan Altun[1], Mohamed El-Azzazi[1,2,3,4] and Richard C. Semelka[1]

[1] The University of North Carolina at Chapel Hill, Department of Radiology, Chapel Hill, NC, USA
[2] University of Dammam, Department of Radiology, Dammam, Saudi Arabia
[3] King Fahd Hospital of the University, Department of Radiology, Khobar, Saudi Arabia
[4] University of Al Azhar, Department of Radiology, Cairo, Egypt

Fatty liver disease

- Fatty liver disease is the most common chronic liver disease in North America and its prevalence is about 15% in the general population.
- It results from the accumulation of triglycerides within the cytoplasm of hepatocytes.
- The two most common conditions associated with fatty liver are alcoholic liver disease and nonalcoholic fatty liver disease.
- Alcoholic liver disease is caused by excess alcohol consumption.
- Nonalcoholic fatty liver disease is associated with insulin resistance and metabolic syndrome. Therefore, diabetes mellitus and obesity are risk factors for nonalcoholic fatty liver disease. Additionally, viral hepatitis, some toxins, drugs including steroids, rapid weight loss, malnutrition, and some congenital disorders including glycogen storage disorders also cause fatty liver.
- Clinical presentation:
  ° Usually asymptomatic
  ° May be associated with hepatomegaly, right upper quadrant abdominal pain, or elevated liver function tests
- Forms:
  1 Diffuse fatty deposition
  2 Focal deposition with focal sparing
  3 Multifocal deposition
  4 Subcapsular deposition
- On CT:
  ° Fatty deposition in the liver causes lower attenuation in the liver, which is lower than that of the spleen. Quantitatively, absolute liver density measuring less than 40 HU or more than 10 HU relative density decrease of the liver compared to the spleen suggests fat deposition in the liver on precontrast images. Additionally, more than 25

HU density decrease of the liver compared to the spleen suggests fat deposition in the liver on postcontrast images on the hepatic venous phase.
- **On MRI:**
- Three different techniques are used for fat detection and quantification.
  ° Chemical shift imaging
  ° Fat suppression
  ° MR spectroscopy
- Chemical shift imaging including in-phase and out-of-phase gradient echo imaging is the most commonly used fat detection method in the liver. Chemical shift imaging is based on the detection of signal loss on out-of-phase T1-gradient echo sequence compared to in-phase T1-gradient echo sequence due to the presence of microscopic fat. This arises from the different precessional frequencies of fat and water protons; the opposite phase of fat and water protons located in the same voxel leads to signal loss of fat-and-water containing structures, compared to in-phase T1-gradient echo sequence, in which fat and water protons are in-phase with one another. The relative signal loss on out-of-phase image, which is approximately 16%, suggests the presence of fat with high accuracy. The presence of macroscopic/abundant fat does not cause signal loss on out-of-phase images, but creates a signal void (also termed as India ink) artifact at water-fat interfaces. To minimize T2* signal decay effects, chemical shift imaging should be performed with the shortest possible TE times and at 1.5 T. The out-of-phase gradient echo sequence should be acquired with a shorter TE than the in-phase sequence.
- Fat suppression techniques include either fat saturation or water excitation. With the use of these techniques, tissues containing macroscopic fat show maximal fat signal loss when fat represents near 100% of the tissue on T1- and T2-weighted sequences. This is in contrast to chemical shift

Liver Imaging: MRI with CT Correlation, First Edition. Edited by Ersan Altun, Mohamed El-Azzazi and Richard C. Semelka.
© 2015 John Wiley & Sons, Inc. Published 2015 by John Wiley & Sons, Inc.

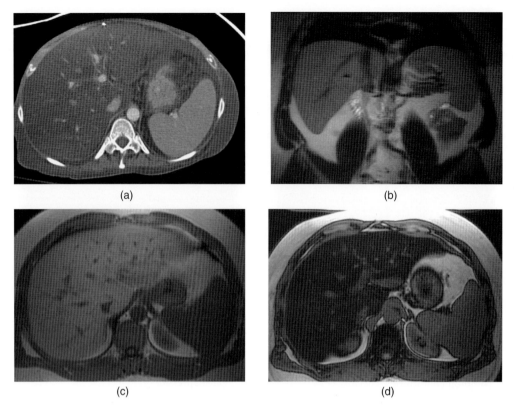

Figure 12.1 *Transverse postcontrast CT (a), coronal T2-weighted SS-ETSE (b), transverse T1-weighted in-phase (c) and out-of-phase (d) 2D-GE images demonstrate diffuse fatty liver.* The liver shows prominently decreased density compared to the spleen. The liver shows prominently high T2 signal compared to the psoas muscle suggestive of edema or fat (b). The liver shows diffusely and homogeneously prominent signal drop on out-of-phase image (d) compared to in-phase image (c).

imaging where signal loss is maximal when fat and water are approximately 50% each in the volume of tissue.

- These three methods are also used for fat quantification. Chemical shift imaging is a successful method for fat quantification. The accuracy of chemical shift imaging for fat quantification is increased with the use of techniques minimizing T1-weighting and correcting T2* signal decay. MR spectroscopy is the most specific technique for fat quantification, although it is not practical due to its small volume sampling (single voxel technique) and long acquisition times (multivoxel technique). The accuracy of fat quantification with MR spectroscopy can be improved by obtaining spectra at multiple echo times and correcting for the T2* decay.
- Fat quantification is performed with the calculation of fat signal fraction with the following formula: Fat Signal Fraction = Fat Signal/Water Signal + Fat Signal.
- Chemical shift imaging may quantify fat content in the liver with the calculation of fat signal fraction based on the following formulae:
  ° Signal (In-phase) = Water signal + Fat signal
  ° Signal (Out-of-phase) = Water signal − Fat signal
  ° Fat Signal Fraction = Signal (In-phase) − Signal (Out-of-phase)/2 Signal (In-phase)

- **Diffuse Fat Deposition**
- Diffuse fat deposition may be uniform or heterogeneous.
- The liver shows prominent decreased density on CT and the portal/hepatic vessels appear hyperdense compared to steatotic liver parenchyma (Figure 12.1).
- The liver shows decreased signal on out-of-phase images compared to in-phase images (Figures 12.1–12.5).
- FNH and metastases are the most common focal lesions associated with diffuse fatty liver.
- Nonfat-suppressed T1-WIs and fat-suppressed T2-WIs maximize the contrast between the background liver and focal lesions.
- On nonfat-suppressed T1-WIs, the fatty liver may be higher in signal intensity than normal liver, maximizing the contrast with low signal intensity masses.
- On fat-suppressed T2-WIs, fatty liver is lower in signal intensity than normal liver, maximizing the contrast with moderately high signal intensity masses.
- On postgadolinum fat-suppressed T1-weighted images, simple fat deposition shows comparable enhancement to background liver, which is a critical observation. Many fatty lesions (e.g., hepatic adenomas, HCC) show greater

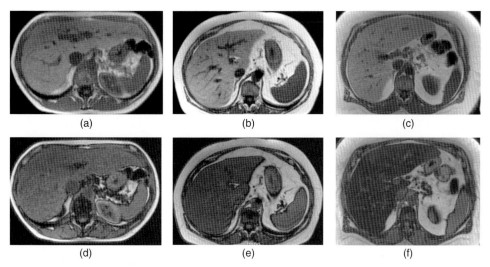

Figure 12.2 *Transverse in-phase (a–c) and out-of-phase (d–f) 2D-GE images show diffuse mild (a, d), moderate (b, e) and severe (c, f) fat deposition in the liver according to the mild, moderate and severe signal drop on out-of-phase images (d–f) compared to in-phase images (a–c).*

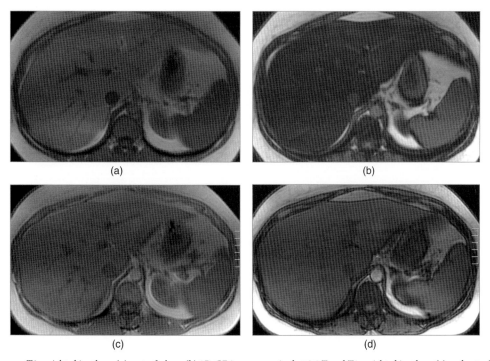

Figure 12.3 *Transverse T1-weighted in-phase (a), out-of-phase (b) 2D-GE images acquired at 3.0 T and T1-weighted in-phase (c) and out-of-phase (d) 2D-GE images acquired at 3.0 T demonstrate diffuse homogeneously fatty liver in the same patient. The acquisitions were performed within one week of each other. The liver shows diffuse signal drop on out-of-phase images (b, d) compared to in-phase image (a, c). Note that 1.5 T imaging illustrates the signal drop better compared to 3.0 T due to its higher T1 spatial resolution.*

enhancement than background liver on the hepatic arterial dominant phase images.

- **Focal Fat Deposition**
- Commonly occurs adjacent to the falciform ligament, central tip of segment IV, gallbladder, and portal/hepatic veins (Figures 12.6 and 12.7).

- Characterized by:
  - ° Lack of mass effect; as shown by no displacement of adjacent or internal vessels and no focal bulging of the liver contour.
  - ° The presence of traversing internal vessels.

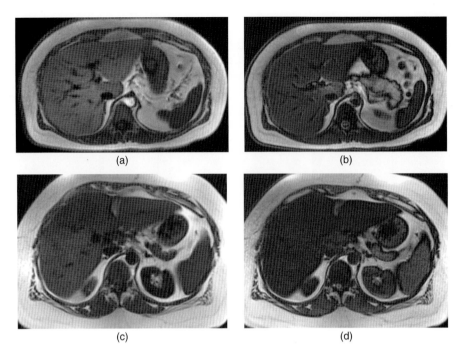

Figure 12.4 *Transverse T1-weighted in-phase (a, c) and out-of-phase (b, d) MPRAGE images acquired at 3.0 T demonstrate mild (a, b) and moderate (c, d) diffuse fat deposition in the liver.* Note that MPRAGE provides good T1 contrast resolution and provides better visualization of fat content compared to 2D-GE images at 3.0 T.

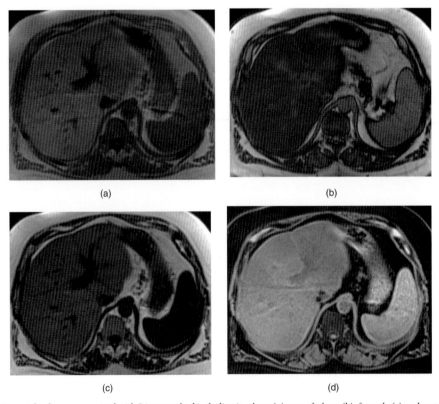

Figure 12.5 *Transverse T1-weighted images acquired with Dixon method including in-phase (a), out-of-phase (b), fat-only (c) and water only (d) 3D-GE images acquired at 3.0 T demonstrate diffuse fatty infiltration.* Out-of-phase image shows prominently decreased signal due to fat deposition. The fat only image shows increased liver signal due to increased fat content. Note that the spleen demonstrates prominently low signal due to the lack of fat. Therefore, as the fat content increases in the liver, the signal of the liver also increases on the fat-only image.

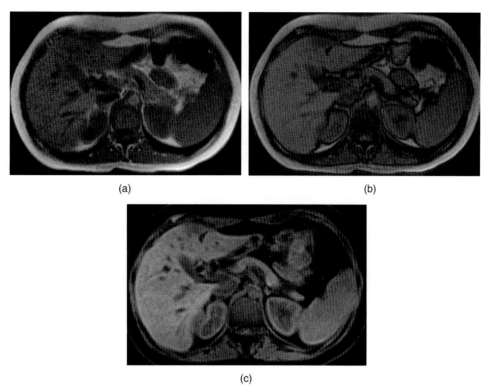

(a)   (b)

(c)

Figure 12.6 *Transverse T1-weighted in-phase (a), out-of-phase (b) 2D-GE and fat-suppressed 3D-GE (c) images show a focal area of decreased signal on out-of-phase (b) and fat-suppressed (c) images compared to in-phase image (a) adjacent to the falciform ligament, which is suggestive of focal fat deposition.*

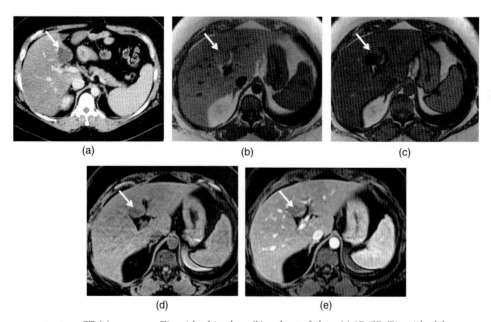

(a)   (b)   (c)

(d)   (e)

Figure 12.7 *Transverse postcontrast CT (a), transverse T1-weighted in-phase (b) and out-of-phase (c) 2D-GE, T1-weighted fat-suppressed 3D-GE (d) and T1-weighted postgadolinium hepatic venous phase 3D-GE (e) MR images show focal fat deposition (arrows) adjacent to the falciform ligament and portal vein. A focal hypodense area is seen in the liver showing diffuse fat deposition on CT (a). Note that the liver demonstrates moderately low density compared to the spleen. A similar hypointense area is noted on out-of-phase image due to prominent focal fat deposition and the liver also shows diffuse fat deposition. This area appears as a hypointense area due to fat-suppression effect on fat-suppressed precontrast (d) and postcontrast (e) images. No increased enhancement is seen in this area.*

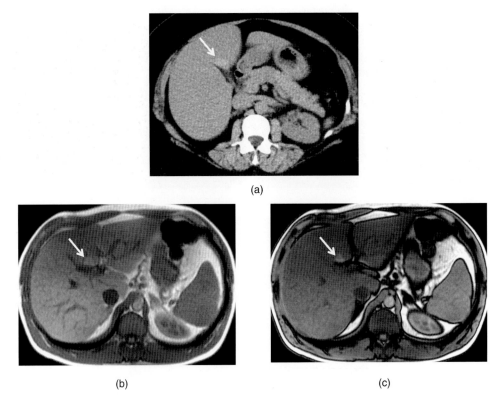

(a)

(b)   (c)

Figure 12.8 *Transverse precontrast CT (a), T1-weighted in-phase (b) and out-of-phase (c) 2D-GE MR images show mild diffuse fat deposition in the liver.* Note the presence of small focal fatty sparing (arrows) adjacent to the portal vein. This area appears as a small focal hyperdense area on CT (a). Additionally, this area is seen as a hyperintense area on out-of-phase image (c) compared to in-phase image (b).

- ° The morphology of focal fat usually has angular, wedge-shaped margins, and the region may or may not be well demarcated.
- ° Variations in blood supply and anomalous vessels may often account for focal fat or sparing. The common occurrence of anomalous vessels in the tip of segment IV and along the *ligamentum teres* explains the frequent observation of differing fat content in these regions.
- On in-phase: Isointense or hyperintense to surrounding background parenchyma.
- On out-of-phase: Shows loss of signal.
- On postgadolinium images:
  - ° Shows similar enhancement compared to background liver.
  - ° Minimally lesser enhancement most often reflects a fat suppression effect rather than a contrast wash-out, but careful distinction between these two is warranted.
- **Focal Fat Sparing**
- An area of normal liver in the setting of diffuse fatty infiltration.
- Commonly occurs adjacent to the falciform ligament, central tip of segment IV, gallbladder and portal/hepatic veins (Figure 12.8).
- Appears as an area of high signal intensity on out-of-phase images compared to the darker diffusely fatty background liver.

- Focal fat sparing may be due to arterioportal shunting, decreased portal perfusion, focal inflammation/biliary ductal dilatation (Figure 12.9), and compression of liver parenchyma by focal liver lesions (Figure 12.10).
- Focal fat sparing may mimic an enhancing lesion; however, the identification of high signal on precontrast out-of-phase T1-weighted images and the absence of increased enhancement relative to background liver, which may be determined with the help of region of interest measurements or subtraction images, are helpful for the differentiation.
- **Multifocal Fat Deposition**
- An uncommon pattern, which is characterized by multiple foci of fat scattered throughout the liver (Figures 12.11 – 12.14).
- Heterogeneous and multifocal deposition may be seen in patients with NAFLD and NASH, and may be associated with inflammatory and fibrotic changes (Figures 12.11 – 12.13).
- The foci may be round or oval and may mimic nodules (Figure 12.14).
- These foci show signal loss on out-of-phase images compared to in-phase images.
- On postgadolinium images, these lesions demonstrate similar enhancement compared to background liver parenchyma.
- Differential diagnosis of multifocal fat deposition:
  - ° Multifocal hepatic adenomatosis
  - ° Fat containing regenerative nodules

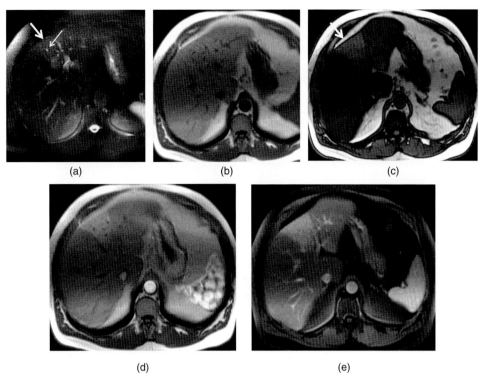

(a)   (b)   (c)

(d)   (e)

Figure 12.9 *Transverse T2-weighted fat-suppressed SS-ETSE (a), transverse T1-weighted in-phase (b) and out-of-phase (c) 2D-GE, postgadolinium T1-weighted hepatic arterial dominant 2D-GE (d) and fat-suppressed hepatic venous phase (e) 3D-GE images demonstrate a focal segmental fatty sparing at segment IVA (thick arrows).* This triangularwedge-shaped area shows mild edema (thick arrow, a) on T2-weighted image (a) which is associated with slight intrahepatic biliary ductal dilatation (thin arrow, a). The liver shows diffuse prominent fat deposition, which is characterized by decreased signal on out-of-phase image (c) compared to in-phase image (b) except the fatty sparing area. This area also shows increased enhancement on postgadolinium images due to focal cholangitis. Focal intrahepatic biliary dilatation and cholangitis may cause fatty sparing.

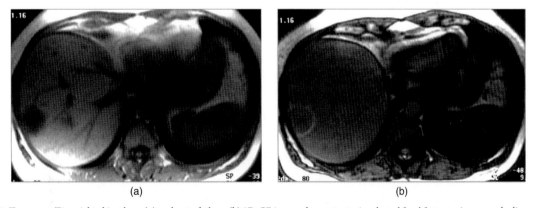

(a)   (b)

Figure 12.10 *Transverse T1-weighted in-phase (a) and out-of-phase (b) 2D-GE images demonstrate rim-shaped focal fatty sparing around a liver metastases in a patient with diffuse fatty liver.*

- **Subcapsular Deposition**
- Observed in patients with renal failure and insulin-dependent diabetes.
- The insulin added to the peritoneal dialysate in these patients results in peripheral and subcapsular deposition in the liver.

Hepatic iron overload

- Hepatic iron deposition may be classified into two forms, primary and secondary.
- *Primary Hemochromatosis*
- Primary form is hereditary hemochromatosis (HH), which is an autosomal recessive genetic disorder. HH is a common

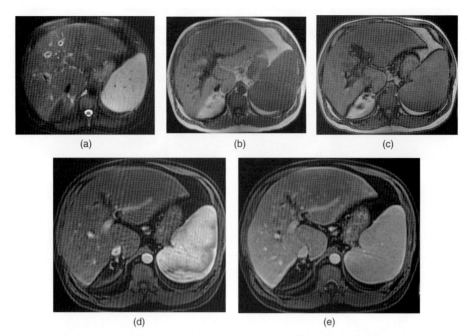

Figure 12.11 *Transverse T2-weighted fat-suppressed SS-ETSE (a), T1-weighted in-phase (b) and out-of-phase (c) 2D-GE, T1-weighted postgadolinium fat-suppressed hepatic arterial dominant phase (d) and hepatic venous phase (e) 3D-GE images illustrate enlarged fatty edemotous liver secondary to hepatitis.* The liver has enlarged caudate and left lobes. The liver shows mildly high T2 signal and periportal edema on T2-weighted image (a). Mild heterogeneous multifocal fat deposition is seen on out-of-phase image (c) as heterogeneous decreased signal compared to in-phase image (b).

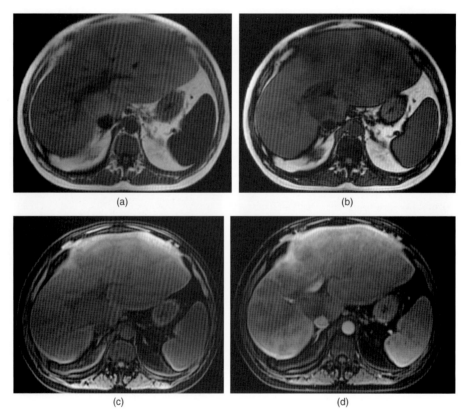

Figure 12.12 *Transverse T1-weighted in-phase (a) and out-of-phase (b) 2D-GE, T1-weighted fat-suppressed 3D-GE (c) and T1-weighted postgadolinium fat-suppressed hepatic arterial dominant phase 3D-GE (d) images show enlarged liver secondary to NASH.* The left lobe is especially enlarged. Multifocal patchy fat deposition is seen in the liver. Heterogeneous enhancement of the liver is suggestive of associated inflammation.

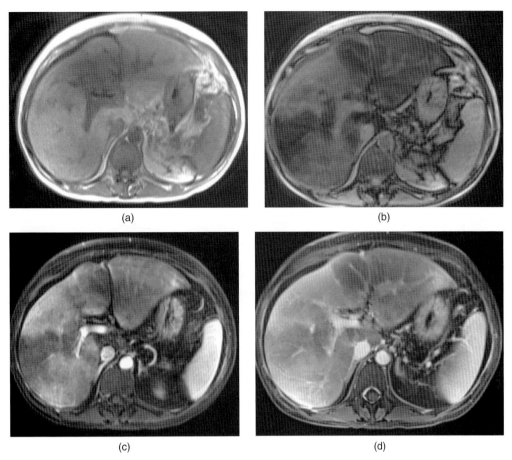

Figure 12.13 *Transverse T1-weighted in-phase (a) and out-of-phase (b) 2D-GE, T1-weighted fat-suppressed 3D-GE (c) and T1-weighted postgadolinium fat-suppressed hepatic arterial dominant phase 3D-GE (d) images demonstrate multifocal fat deposition in the liver secondary to NAFLD.* The liver shows heterogeneous enhancement due to the presence of prominent multifocal fat deposition.

genetic disease in the Caucasian population. In HH, a protein involved in the regulation of iron absorption is altered, which has the result of increased intestinal iron absorption and consequent increased iron deposition (two or three times more) in tissues, compared to the unaffected population.

- The deposition of iron in tissues commonly starts in the liver; and over time, iron deposition progresses to involve other organs, such as the heart, pancreas, anterior pituitary, thyroid, synovium and skin.
- Iron is a direct hepatotoxin and its deposition causes fibrosis and progresses to cirrhosis.
- Serologic abnormalities and mild symptoms may occur earlier in life, but the clinical signs and symptoms generally do not appear until the fifth or sixth decade of life.
- HH increases the risk of hepatocellular carcinoma.
- Iron deposition may be homogeneous or heterogeneous.
- **On CT:**
- Iron deposition may cause increased attenuation on nonenhanced CT examination. Increased hepatic attenuation over 70 HU has high specificity for iron deposition. In contrast to MRI, the detection of this condition is difficult via CT. Other

causes of increased attenuation are Wilson's disease, long-term use of amiodarone, or gold treatment.

- **On MRI:**
- Iron deposition results in decreased signal on longer TE sequences, and as it is generally performed at 1.5 T this will show lower signal on the longer TE in-phase T1-weighted gradient echo sequence compared to the shorter TE out-of-phase T1-weighted gradient sequence. Iron deposition is most visually apparent as decreased signal on T2-weighted images because of the increased T2* effect.
- Iron deposition in the liver, pancreas, myocardium, pituitary gland, and synovium causes signal decrease on T2-weighted sequences, and decreased signal on in-phase T1-weighted gradient echo sequence compared to out-of-phase T1-weighted gradient echo sequence (Figures 12.15 and 12.16).
- A diagnostic feature of HH is that signal intensity of the spleen is not substantially decreased on T2-weighted or T1-weighted images. This finding is due to accumulation of iron within the parenchyma of the liver and pancreas, and lack of selective

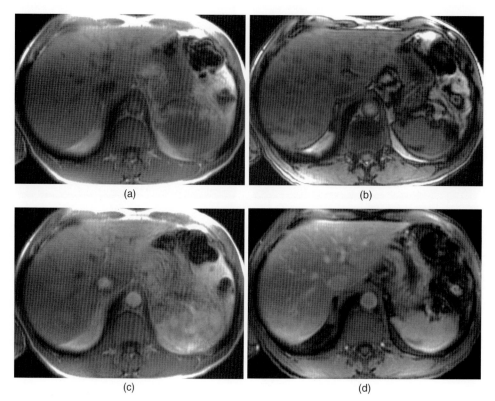

(a)

(b)

(c)

(d)

Figure 12.14 *Transverse T1-weighted in-phase (a), out-of-phase (b) 2D-GE, T1-weighted postgadolinium hepatic arterial dominant phase 2D-GE (c) and hepatic venous phase 3D-GE (d) images demonstrate multifocal nodular fat deposition in the liver.* Multifocal nodular hypointense areas are seen on out-of-phase image (b) compared to in-phase image (a) suggestive of fat deposition. These areas of fat deposition show similar enhancement to the background liver on postgadolinium images (c, d) and therefore are not visualized.

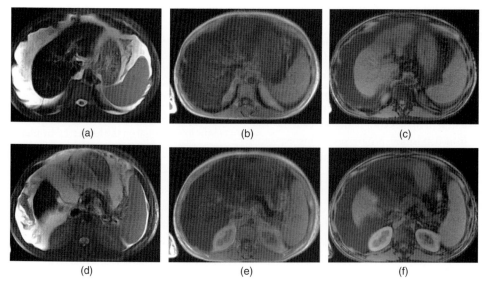

(a)

(b)

(c)

(d)

(e)

(f)

Figure 12.15 *Transverse T2-weighted fat-suppressed SS-ETSE (a, d), T1-weighted in-phase (b, e) and out-of-phase (c, f) 2D-GE images demonstrate diffuse iron deposition in the liver and pancreas secondary to primary hemochromatosis.* The liver is cirrhotic due to primary hemochromatosis. Note the presence of ascites and splenomegaly due to portal hypertension. The liver and pancreas show diffusely low signal on T1-weighted in-phase images (b, e) compared to out-of-phase images (c, d) and diffusely low signal T2-weighted images (a, d) secondary to iron deposition. The spleen does not show any iron deposition in primary hemochromatosis, which is a distinguishing feature of primary hemochromatosis from secondary hemochromatosis. The bone marrow also does not show iron deposition.

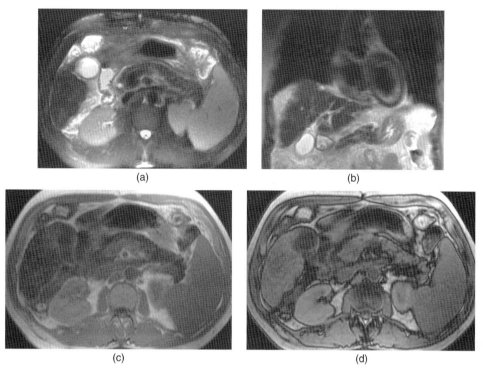

Figure 12.16 *Transverse T2-weighted fat-suppressed SS-ETSE (a), coronal T2-weighted SS-ETSE, transverse T1-weighted in-phase (c) and out-of-phase (d) 2D-GE images show iron deposition in the liver and pancreas due to primary hemochromatosis.* The liver and pancreas demonstrate diffusely low signal on T1-weighted in-phase image (c) compared to out-of-phase image (d) and diffusely low signal on T2-weighted images (a, b). The spleen does not show any iron deposition in primary hemochromatosis, which is a distinguishing feature of primary hemochromatosis from secondary hemochromatosis. The bone marrow also does not show iron deposition.

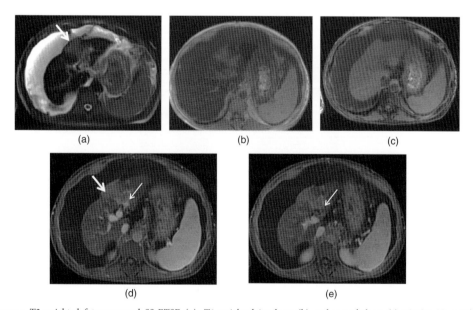

Figure 12.17 *Transverse T2-weighted fat-suppressed SS-ETSE (a), T1-weighted in-phase (b) and out-of-phase (c) 2D-GE, T1-weighted postgadolinium fat-suppressed hepatic venous phase (d, e) 3D-GE images illustrate a diffuse HCC (thick arrows; a, d) developing in a background cirrhotic liver with iron deposition due to primary hemochromatosis.* The liver shows diffusely low T2 signal and T1 in-phase signal due to iron deposition. A wedge-shaped segmental T2 mildly hyperintense (a), T1 hyperintense lesion (b) showing enhancement is detected at segment IV. The lesion also extends into the left portal vein causing tumor thrombosis (thin arrows; d, e). Note the ascites and enlarged spleen due to portal hypertension. The spleen does not show iron deposition. The bone marrow also does not show iron deposition.

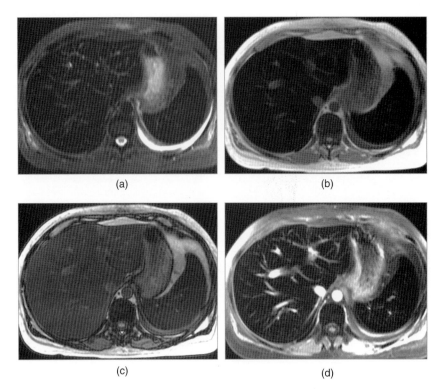

Figure 12.18 *Transverse T2-weighted fat-suppressed SS-ETSE (a), T1-weighted in-phase (b) and out-of-phase (c) 2D-GE, T1-weighted postgadolinium fat-suppressed hepatic venous phase (d) 2D-GE images illustrate iron deposition in the liver, spleen, and bone marrow due to secondary hemochromatosis, which develops following intense blood transfusions.* The liver, spleen, and bone marrow demonstrate prominent signal decrease on T2 and T1-weighted images. The signal decrease is less prominent on out-of-phase image (c) compared to in-phase image (b). Source: Semelka 2010. Reproduced with permission of Wiley.

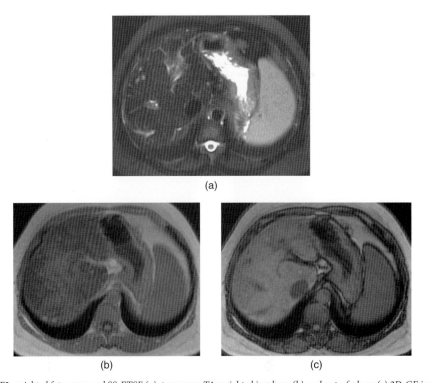

Figure 12.19 *Transverse T2-weighted fat-suppressed SS-ETSE (a), transverse T1-weighted in-phase (b) and out-of-phase (c) 2D-GE images show heterogeneous iron deposition in the liver.* The liver is cirrhotic secondary to primary sclerosing cholangitis and cirrhosis may be associated with iron deposition which is characterized by low T2 and T1 in-phase signal. No iron deposition is seen in the spleen and bone marrow.

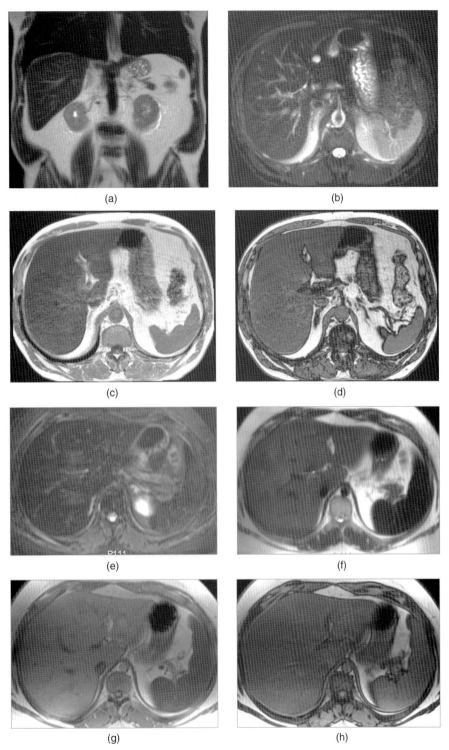

Figure 12.20 *Coronal T2-weighted SS-ETSE (a), transverse T2-weighted SS-ETSE (b), T1-weighted in-phase (c) and out-of-phase (d) 2D-GE images show combined iron and fat deposition in the liver.* The liver shows low T2 signal and T1 signal due to iron deposition. Additionally, the liver shows low signal on T1-weighted out-of-phase image (d), which is suggestive of combined fat deposition in the liver. Note the low signal of the spleen on in-phase image (c) due to iron deposition. Transverse T2-weighted STIR (e), T1-weighted fat-only DIXON 3D-GE (f), T1-weighted in-phase (g) and out-of-phase (h) 2D-GE images show combined iron and fat deposition in another patient. The liver and spleen show low T2 signal on T2-weighted image due to iron deposition. The spleen also shows low T1 signal on in-phase image (g) compared to out-of-phase image (h). The fat-only image (f) shows high liver signal and the out-of-phase image shows low liver signal due to fat deposition. Source: Semelka 2010. Reproduced with permission of Wiley.

uptake by the RES in the spleen (or RES in liver and bone marrow as well). The presence of iron deposition in the pancreas correlates with irreversible changes of cirrhosis in the liver.

- HCC cells do not contain excess iron; therefore, they are seen as higher signal intensity masses relative to iron-overloaded liver on T2-weighted images (Figure 12.17).
- Iron quantification can be performed with multi-TE T2*-weighted sequences.

- *Secondary Hemochromatosis*
- Secondary hemochromatosis can develop secondary to transfusions (Figure 12.18), cirrhosis (Figure 12.19), anemias related to ineffective erythropoiesis and myelodysplastic syndrome (many of these anemic conditions reflect the effects of blood transfusions).
- Transfusional iron overload is the most common form of secondary hemochromatosis.
- Iron deposition predominantly occurs in the RES, resulting in low signal intensity of the spleen, liver, and bone marrow on MR images, best shown on T1-weighted gradient echo images and T2-weighted images (Figure 12.18).
- Histologically, iron overload from multiple transfusions may be distinguished from HH in that iron accumulates primarily within the RES of the liver (Kupffer cells) and spleen (monocytes/macrophages) in transfusional overload, with relative sparing of functional cells (hepatocytes).
- Signal intensity of the spleen is usually normal with HH, whereas signal intensity of the pancreas is normal with secondary hemochromatosis. In massive iron overload (e.g., >100 units) direct tissue deposition may occur in tissues, including the pancreas.
- **MR features and grading**
  - In mild forms of transfusional overload, signal loss is appreciated only on T2-weighted images, and signal intensity on T1-weighted images appears relatively normal.
  - In moderate to severe forms of iron deposition, signal intensity loss on T1-weighted images is also seen in addition to the signal loss seen on T2-weighted images.
  - A variety of methods to quantify iron have been implemented/attempted. Many of these are based on multi-TE T2* decay.

- *Coexistent Fat and Iron Deposition*
- Fat and iron deposition may occur concurrently within the liver.
- Coexisting fat and iron deposition causes signal decrease on T2-weighted images (due to iron deposition) and signal decrease on T1-weighted out-of-phase images compared to in-phase images (due to fat deposition) (Figure 12.20).
- The presence of iron in the liver may obscure the detection of fat.

References

1 Heredia, V., Ramalho, M., de Campos, R.O. *et al.* (2012) Liver – vessel cancellation artifact on in-phase and out-of-phase MRI imaging: a sign of ultra-high liver fat content. J Magn Reson Imaging, 35, 1112–1118.

2 Elias, J. Jr., Altun, E., Zacks, S. *et al.* (2009) MRI findings in non-alcoholic steaotohepatitis: correlation with histopathology and clinical staging. Magn Reson Imaging, 27, 976–987.

3 Venkataraman, S., Braga, L., and Semelka, R.C. (2002) Imaging the fatty liver. Magn Reson Imaging Clin N Am, 10, 93–103.

4 Reeder, S.B. and Sirlin, C. (2010) Quantification of liver fat with magnetic resonance imaging. Magn Reson Imaging Clin N Am, 18, 337–357.

5 Qayyum, A., Chen, D.M., Breiman, R.S. *et al.* (2009) Evaluation of diffuse liver steatosis by ultrasound, computed tomography, and magnetic resonance imaging: which modality is best? Clin Imaging, 33, 110–115.

6 Hamer, O.W., Aguirre, D.A., Casola, G. *et al.* (2006) Fatty liver: imaging patterns and pitfalls. Radiographics, 26, 1637–1653.

7 Decarie, P.-O., Lepanto, L., Billiard, J.-S. *et al.* (2011) Fatty liver deposition and sparing: a pictorial review. Insights Imaging, 2, 533–538.

8 Basaran, C., Karcaaltincaba, M., Akata, D. *et al.* (2005) Fat-containing lesions of the liver: cross-sectional imaging findings with emphasis on MRI. AJR Am J Roentgenol, 184, 1103–1110.

9 Lall, C.G., Aisen, A.M., Bansal, N., and Sandrasegaran, K. (2008) Nonalcoholic fatty liver disease. AJR Am J Roentgenol, 190, 993–1002.

10 Costa, D.N., Pedrosa, I., McKenzie, C. *et al.* (2008) Body MRI using IDEAL. AJR Am J Roentgenol, 190, 1076–1084.

CHAPTER 13
Inflammatory liver diseases

Ersan Altun[1], Mohamed El-Azzazi[1,2,3,4], and Richard C. Semelka[1]

[1] The University of North Carolina at Chapel Hill, Department of Radiology, Chapel Hill, NC, USA
[2] University of Dammam, Department of Radiology, Dammam, Saudi Arabia
[3] King Fahd Hospital of the University, Department of Radiology, Khobar, Saudi Arabia
[4] University of Al Azhar, Department of Radiology, Cairo, Egypt

- Autoimmune liver disorders are inflammatory liver diseases characterized by:
  ○ Inflammatory cell infiltrate in the portal tracts.
  ○ Presence of autoantibodies and increased levels of transaminases, Ig G.
- Entities Include:
  ○ Primary sclerosing cholangitis (PSC).
  ○ Autoimmune hepatitis (AIH).
  ○ Primary biliary cirrhosis (PBC).
  ○ Overlap Syndrome.
  ○ Sarcoidosis.

Primary sclerosing cholangitis (PSC)

- Chronic cholestatic liver disease of presumed autoimmune origin.
- Characterized by diffuse cholangitis and progressive fibrosis of intrahepatic and extrahepatic bile ducts.
- PSC is more common in males. 60–80% of patients have associated inflammatory bowel disease, particularly ulcerative colitis.
- Patients with PSC have a higher risk of developing cholangiocarcinoma. The absolute increase of cholangiocarcinoma has been reported as high as in 10% of patients with PSC. In clinical practice the incidence appears much lower. Additionally, there has been increased risk of developing hepatocellular carcinoma, which is significantly lower compared to chronic hepatitis B and C.
- **Morphologic changes:**
  ○ Lymphocytic infiltrate with fibrosing cholangitis of intra and extrahepatic bile ducts and progressive obliteration of their lumens.

○ Between areas of scarring and progressive stricture, bile ducts become ectatic, presumably the result of downstream obstruction. This creates the "string of pearls" or "beaded" bile duct appearance. Multifocal strictures and dilatations.
  ○ The disease culminates in cirrhosis.
- **MR findings of PSC:**
  ○ Early Findings: Biliary ductal findings are seen without associated parenchymal findings. Mild wall thickening (<2 mm) and mildly increased enhancement of biliary ducts. Focal strictures and dilatations are apparent, but may be subtle. Best looked for on source images of a 3D MRCP image. The lateral segment of the left lobe tends to experience slightly greater disease (Figures 13.1 and 13.2).
  ○ Late Findings: Parenchymal findings are seen in addition to biliary ductal findings. Macronodular regeneration pattern, which is characteristically central regeneration in pattern, is distinctive. Central regeneration and hypertrophy of the segments 1–2–3–4 associated with peripheral atrophy is seen commonly (Figures 13.3–13.5). Central regeneration also contributes the biliary obstruction, as the regenerative liver compresses/occludes peripheral ducts (Figure 13.5). Wedge-shaped, segmental or peribiliary transient increased enhancement of the hepatic parenchyma, which becomes isointense with the remaining liver parenchyma on the later phases, may be seen, reflecting the inflammatory nature of the condition (Figure 13.5). Peripheral wedge-shaped atrophy may show mildly high signal on T2-WI, low signal on T1-WI and mildly increased enhancement, which is more prominent on the interstitial phase. Occasionally, wedge-shaped regions of mildly high T1 signal is apparently presumed to represent inspissated bile in partially obstructed bile ducts/ductules (Figure 13.4).

Liver Imaging: MRI with CT Correlation, First Edition. Edited by Ersan Altun, Mohamed El-Azzazi and Richard C. Semelka.
© 2015 John Wiley & Sons, Inc. Published 2015 by John Wiley & Sons, Inc.

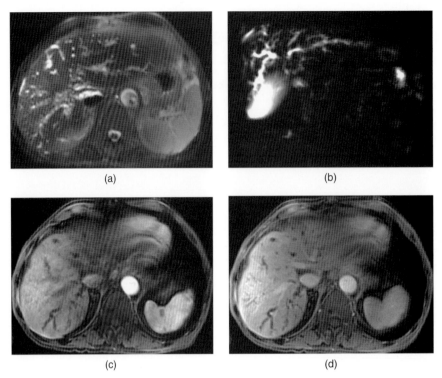

Figure 13.1 *Transverse fat-suppressed T2-weighted SS-ETSE (a), coronal thick slab MRCP (b), T1-weighted postgadolinium fat-suppressed hepatic arterial phase (c) and hepatic venous phase (d) 3D-GE images show bile duct involvement without the evidence of parenchymal changes secondary to PSC. The bile ducts show irregular focal strictures – beading with resultant dilatation.*

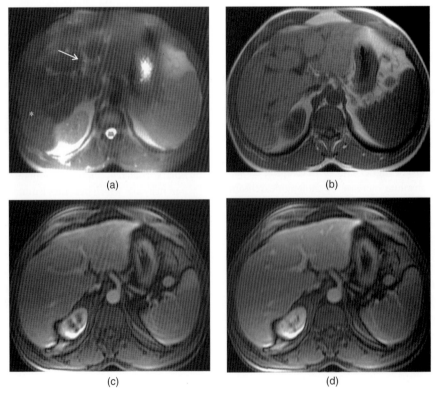

Figure 13.2 *Transverse fat-suppressed T2-weighted SS-ETSE (a), T1-weighted 2D-GE (b), T1-weighted postgadolinium fat-suppressed hepatic arterial phase (c) and hepatic venous phase (d) 3D-GE images show biliary ductal involvement with early parenchymal changes secondary to PSC. The bile ducts show mild dilatation in the left lobe of the liver (arrow, a). The segments II and III appear hypertrophic due to central regeneration. Peripheral atrophy of the posterior segment of the right lobe (asteriks, a) is noted. The atrophic segment demonstrates mildly high T2 signal (asteriks, a).*

○ MR and MRCP are superior to CT because they can visualize the bile ducts with greater contrast resolution, and higher soft tissue contrast to examine for neoplasms.

- **Differential Diagnosis**
  Chronic Budd–Chiari.
  ○ May possess similar morphologic findings:

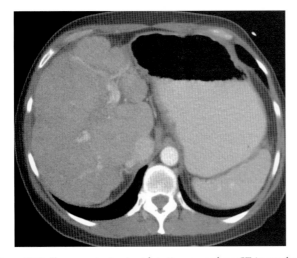

Figure 13.3 *Transverse postcontrast hepatic venous phase CT image shows advanced form of PSC with resultant cirrhosis.* The liver has nodular contours with macronodular regenerative pattern. The caudate lobe appears prominently hypertrophic.

- Hypertrophy of the caudate lobe.
- Presence of regenerative nodules and fibrosis are present in both entities. The regenerative nodules are small.
  ○ In contrast, chronic Budd–Chiari shows hepatic vein absence or thrombosis, and shows distinctive intrahepatic venous collaterals.
  ○ In PSC:
    - Central regenerative nodules involve more of the entire central region of the liver, so segment II is also involved, whereas Chronic Budd–Chiari tends to show massive segment I dilation in isolation.
    - Sarcoidosis
      Sarcoidosis may possess the identical imaging features of PSC with central regeneration. Clinical picture and lab test may allow the distinction. To date, no other hepatic condition has been identified that routinely shows this appearance.

Autoimmune hepatitis (AIH)

- The incidence of AIH is 1.9/100.000.
- The great majority of patients are middle-aged women.
- Associated with increased levels of antinuclear antibody and antismooth muscle antibody.

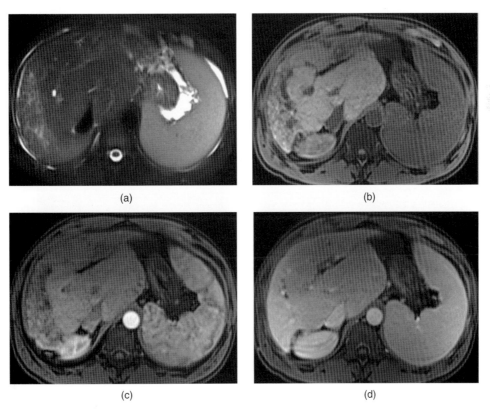

(a)   (b)

(c)   (d)

Figure 13.4 *Transverse fat-suppressed T2-weighted SS-ETSE (a), T1-weighted fat-suppressed 3D-GE (b), T1-weighted postgadolinium fat-suppressed hepatic arterial phase (c) and hepatic venous phase (d) 3D-GE images demonstrate advanced form of PSC with cirrhosis.* Central regeneration including the hypertrophy of the caudate lobe is detected. The peripheral atrophy is very prominent in both lobes. The atrophic peripheral right lobe shows increased T2 signal. Additionally, increased T1 signal is noted in the peripheral atrophic liver due to inspissated bile.

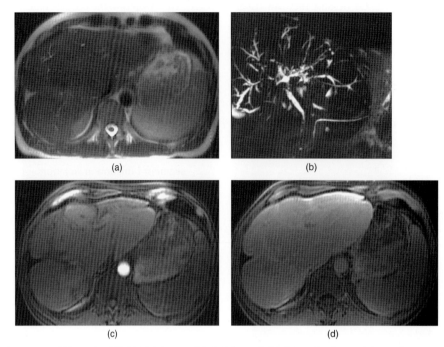

(a)　　　　　　　　　　　　(b)

(c)　　　　　　　　　　　　(d)

Figure 13.5 *Transverse fat-suppressed T2-weighted SS-ETSE (a), coronal thick slab MRCP (b), T1-weighted postgadolinium fat-suppressed hepatic arterial phase (c) and hepatic venous phase (d) 3D-GE images show prominent central regeneration of the segments I, II, III and IV with associated peripheral atrophy, which is more prominent at the right lobe.* In addition to the parenchymal changes of PSC, intrahepatic bile ducts demonstrate peripheral dilatation secondary to strictures and compression due to central regeneration.

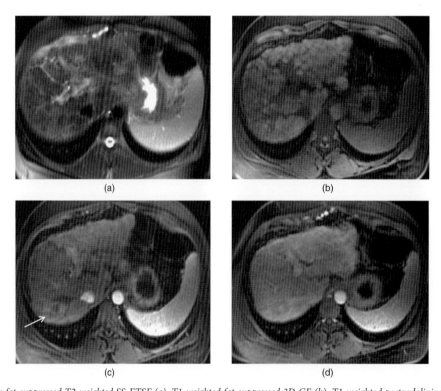

(a)　　　　　　　　　　　　(b)

(c)　　　　　　　　　　　　(d)

Figure 13.6 *Transverse fat-suppressed T2-weighted SS-ETSE (a), T1-weighted fat-suppressed 3D-GE (b), T1-weighted postgadolinium fat-suppressed hepatic arterial dominant phase (c) and hepatic venous phase (d) 3D-GE images show cirrhosis secondary to autoimmune hepatitis.* The liver shows global atrophy, which is associated with severe fibrosis. The fibrotic network shows high signal on T2-weighted image (a). The regenerative nodules demonstrate low T2 signal (a) and isointense/hyperintense signal on T1-weighted image (b). Focal early enhancing area (arrow, c), which becomes isointense with the remaining liver parenchyma, is seen in the segment VII. The fibrotic network shows enhancement on the late phase image (d).

- AIH is characterized by the presence of piecemeal necrosis with a predominant lymphoplasmacytic cell infiltrate and fibrosis which my lead to cirrhosis.
- The risk of developing HCC is low.
- On CT and MRI:
- AIH usually presents with a prominent pattern of liver fibrosis/cirrhosis with global prominent atrophy of the liver (Figure 13.6). The cirrhosis may also have bizarre shape (Figure 13.7).
- At initial presentation there may be substantial inflammatory enhancement. Patchy transient heterogeneous enhancement on the hepatic arterial dominant phase images, which fade to isointensity with the background liver parenchyma on the later phases may be seen (Figure 13.6).

Primary biliary cirrhosis (PBC)

- Chronic cholestatic progressive autoimmune liver disorder that causes obliteration of the intrahepatic bile ducts, portal inflammation, fibrosis and cirrhosis.
- A progressive necrotizing inflammatory process involving the portal triads with destruction of bile ducts, inflammatory infiltrate and fibrosis leading to cirrhosis.
- The disease occurs primarily in females (90%). Its incidence is 2.7/100.000.
- PBC is associated with elevated IgG antimitochondrial antibodies.
- Symptoms include pruritis, fatigue, jaundice, melanosis, malabsorbtion of lipids – vitamins, hepatocellular failure, portal hypertension.

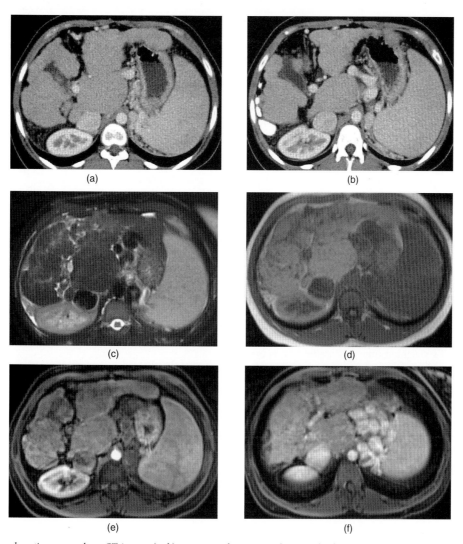

(a) (b)

(c) (d)

(e) (f)

Figure 13.7 *Transverse hepatic venous phase CT images (a, b), transverse fat-suppressed T2-weighted SS-ETSE (c), T1-weighted 2D-GE (d), T1-weighted postgadolinium fat-suppressed hepatic arterial phase (e) and hepatic venous phase (f) 3D-GE images show bizarre shaped cirrhosis secondary to autoimmune hepatitis.* The hypertrophy of the caudate lobe and atrophy of the right and left lobe are very prominent. Note the absence of bile duct changes. Extensive varices are also seen in the lesser sac.

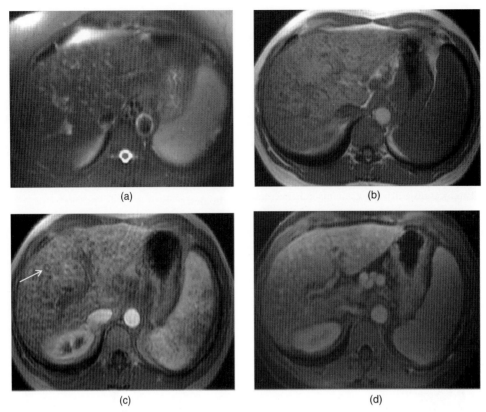

Figure 13.8 *Transverse fat-suppressed T2-weighted SS-ETSE (a), T1-weighted 2D-GE (b), T1-weighted postgadolinium hepatic arterial dominant phase 2D-GE (c) and hepatic venous phase fat-suppressed (d) 3D-GE images show cirrhosis secondary to primary biliary cirrhosis.* Fibrotic network shows reticular network with mildly high T2 signal associated with low signal intensity regenerative nodules (a). This reticular network shows increased enhancement on the hepatic venous phase. Periportal halo sign, which is characterized by low signal intensity halo, is also noted around the enhancing portal tracts (arrow, c).

- Enlarged portal lymph nodes are commonly seen.
- The risk of developing HCC is low.
- **CT and MR Imaging:** In addition to classical findings of liver fibrosis and cirrhosis, "periportal halo sign" may be seen in patients with PBC. Periportal halo sign is characterized by a hypointense round area surrounding the portal vein branches on both T2- and T1-weighted images. This finding is better appreciated on postcontrast portal venous and interstitial phase images (Figures 13.8 and 13.9). However, this sign is not specific and may be seen in patients with autoimmune hepatitis, PSC, or overlap syndrome.

Overlap syndrome

- Overlap syndrome is characterized by clinical and laboratory findings of a combination of autoimmune diseases involving the liver. These include PSC, AIH, and PBC.
- Based on imaging features, the overlap syndrome can be divided into two groups, including PSC type and non-PSC type.

- PSC-type overlap syndrome shows imaging findings similar to PSC (Figure 13.10).
- Non-PSC type overlap syndrome show imaging findings of AIH and/or PBC without bile duct findings or central regeneration/peripheral atrophy.

Sarcoidosis

- Sarcoidosis, a systemic inflammatory granulomatous disease of unknown etiology, is one of the most common causes of hepatic non-caseating granulomas. The other causes of non-caseating granulomas include tuberculosis, histoplasmosis, toxoplasmosis, and primary biliary cirrhosis.
- The liver and spleen involvement follow lymph node and lung in the frequency of involvement. The liver and spleen are involved histologically in 40–70% of patients.
- The majority of patients show minimal evidence of clinical or biochemical hepatic dysfunction.
- Hepatosplenomegaly is the most common manifestation of hepatic and splenic involvement without nodule formation.

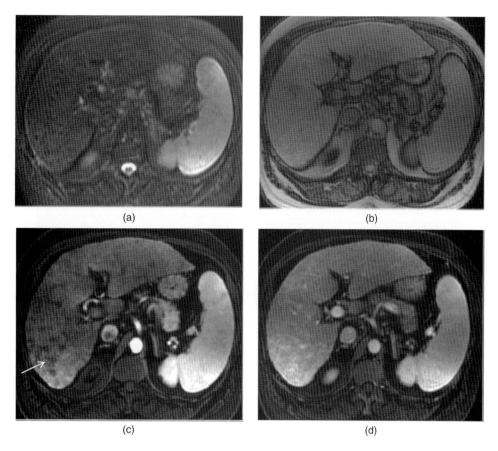

Figure 13.9 *Transverse fat-suppressed T2-weighted SS-ETSE (a), T1-weighted out-of-phase 2D-GE (b), T1-weighted postgadolinium fat-suppressed hepatic arterial phase (c) and hepatic venous phase (d) 3D-GE images show an enlarged cirrhotic liver with nodular contours secondary to primary biliary cirrhosis.* The left lobe of the liver appears enlarged and the right lobe appears atrophic. Multifocal small hypointense areas are seen in the right lobe of the liver on the arterial phase (arrow, c). Due to the arterial phase of enhancement, the portal vein branches are not opacified. Therefore, these small hypoechoic areas represent periportal halo sign without the visualization of the portal tracts.

- Secondary finding is the presence of nodules in the spleen and liver.
- Macronodular regeneration and central regeneration with peripheral atrophy mimicking PSC may be seen in the advanced forms of hepatic sarcoidosis (Figure 13.11).
  Pathological features:
- Granulomas are characterized by compact aggregates of plump epithelioid cells, sometimes with multinucleated giant cells, surrounded by a cuff of lymphocytes and macrophages.
  CT imaging features:
- Small (~0.5–2 cm in diameter) rounded hypoattenuating or isoattenuating lesions on non-contrast enhanced CT, which become more prominent and hypodense compared to the enhancing parenchyma on the later phases. Retroperitoneal lymph nodes are commonly seen.
  MRI imaging features:
- Small (~0.5–2 cm in diameter) rounded nodular lesions low in signal intensity on T2- and T1-weighted images.

- Nodules enhance in a diminished, delayed fashion on gadolinium-enhanced gradient echo images. The diminished enhancement reflects the hypovascular nature of the granulomas.
- Concomitant retroperitoneal lymph nodes are often present, exhibiting moderately high signal on T2-weighted images.

Acute toxic hepatitis

- Drugs, toxins, and alcohol can cause acute hepatitis.
- Imaging features are not different from acute viral hepatitis (Chapter 10) (Figure 13.12)

Wilson's Disease

- Inherited, rare, autosomal recessive disorder caused by impaired biliary excretion of copper, resulting in deposition of toxic levels of copper in the liver, brain, and cornea.

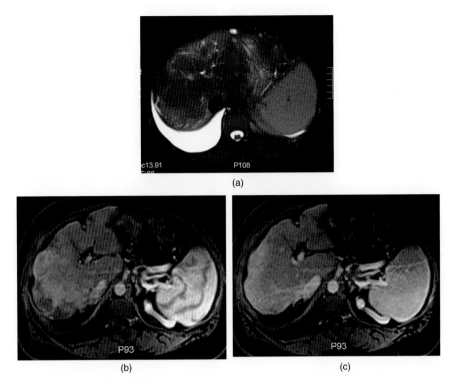

Figure 13.10 *Transverse fat-suppressed T2-weighted SS-ETSE (a), T1-weighted postgadolinium fat-suppressed hepatic arterial dominant phase (b) and hepatic venous phase (c) 3D-GE images show a PSC type overlap syndrome.* The cirrhotic liver demonstrates central regeneration with caudate lob hypertrophy and mild peripheral atrophy. Note the mild dilatation of bile ducts on T2-weighted image (a). Peripheral heterogeneous enhancement of the liver is seen in the early phase (b), which fades in the later phase (c). The presence of perisplenic varices, splenomegaly, and pleural effusion are suggestive of portal hypertension.

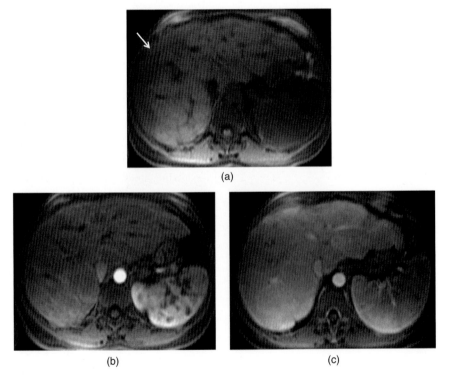

Figure 13.11 *Transverse T1-weighted fat-suppressed 3D-GE (a), T1-weighted postgadolinium fat-suppressed hepatic arterial dominant phase (b) and hepatic venous phase (c) 3D-GE images show a cirrhotic liver secondary to sarcoidosis.* The liver has macronodular regenerative nodules and demonstrates mild to moderate central regeneration with more prominent enlargement of central parts of lateral segment of the left lobe. The peripheral atrophy shows mildly low T1 signal on precontrast image (a).

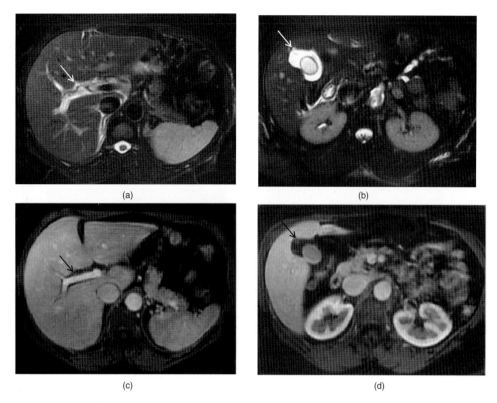

Figure 13.12 *Transverse T2-weighted fat-suppressed SS-ETSE (a, b), T1-weighted postgadolinium hepatic venous phase (c, d) images illustrate acute toxic hepatitis.* Periportal edema (arrows; a, c) is noted around the portal vein. Periportal edema is characterized by high T2 signal of the portal tracts (a) and does not show enhancement (c). Additionally, gallbladder edema (arrows; b, d) is also noted. The gallbladder edema shows homogeneously high signal on T2-weighted image (b) and no enhancement (d). Small volume of free fluid is also found around the liver. The periportal edema, ascites, and gallbladder edema may be signs of acute hepatitis in the appropriate clinical setting as they are not specific and may be seen in patients with chronic liver disease and cirrhosis.

- Copper deposition occurs in the periportal regions and along the hepatic sinusoids early in the course of disease progression. The copper deposition later leads to episodes of acute hepatitis and fatty changes, which are followed by chronic active hepatitis induced by the presence of periportal inflammation and fibrosis. Cirrhosis develops after several years.
- CT imaging findings are nonspecific and include the development of classical signs of cirrhosis and regenerative nodules. Caudate lobe hypertrophy is not common.
- MR imaging findings are nonspecific. Occasionally, multiple hypointense nodules on T2-weighted images and hyperintense/isointense nodules on T1-weighted images may develop (Figure 13.13). The low signal on T2- and high signal on T1-weighted images have been reported to develop due to deposition of copper, but likely reflect the presence of associated proteins. The development of these nodules in a young patient may be suggestive of Wilson's disease. Additionally, typical features of cirrhosis are seen except caudate lobe hypertrophy, which is an uncommon finding in Wilson's disease.

Alpha-1-antitripsin deficiency

- Autosomal recessive inherited disorder characterized by abnormally low serum levels of a major protease inhibitor.
- Hepatic involvement varies and ranges from neonatal hepatitis to childhood cirrhosis or cirrhosis late in life (Figure 13.14).

Radiation injury

- Clinical radiation injury of the liver has been reported to occur in 6–66% of patients who receive radiation, where the field includes the right upper quadrant of the abdomen. Factors that are more likely to result in hepatic toxicity include whole-liver radiation and doses greater than 30 Gy. Radiation therapy targeting the pleura, such as mesothelioma, or neoplastic diseases involving the thoracic wall, may result in radiation injury.
- Acute radiation hepatitis usually occurs within 2–6 weeks after completion of radiation therapy. However, it may be seen up to 1 year after the treatment.
- Acute radiation hepatitis and sequela, that include ascites and hepatomegaly, are currently quite rare, reflecting

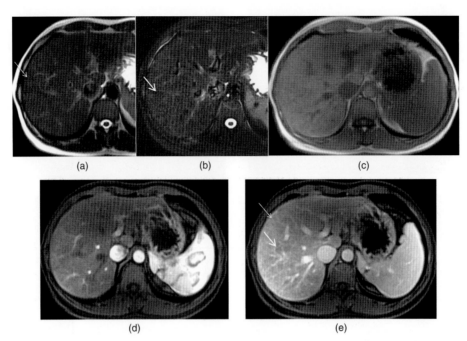

(a)   (b)   (c)

(d)   (e)

Figure 13.13 *Transverse T2-weighted SS-ETSE (a), T2-weighted fat-suppressed SS-ETSE (b), T1-weighted 2D-GE (c), T1-weighted fat-suppressed postgadolinium hepatic arterial dominant phase (d) and hepatic venous phase (e) 3D-GE images demonstrate multiple regenerative nodules (thick arrows) with reticular fibrosis (thin arrows) which develop secondary to cirrhosis in this young female patient due to Wilson's disease. The liver has a normal morphology but multiple T2-hypointense small nodules with intervening mildly high signal intensity reticular network are noted. These nodules are isointense on T1-weighted image (c). The nodules and reticular network are better seen on the hepatic venous phase image (e). The nodules appear as hypointense nodular structures on the hepatic venous phase image and the intervening reticular fibrotic network shows enhancement.*

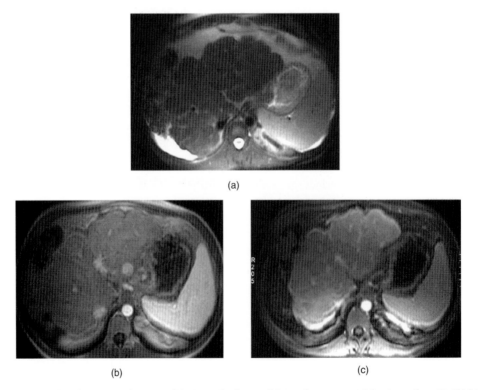

(a)

(b)   (c)

Figure 13.14 *Transverse T2-weighted fat-suppressed SS-ETSE (a), T1-weighted postgadolinium hepatic arterial dominant phase 2D-GE (b) and fat-suppressed hepatic venous phase 3D-GE (c) images demonstrate advanced cirrhosis secondary to alpha-1 antitrypsin deficiency. The liver contour is nodular due to macronodular regeneration. The omentum is also hypertrophic.*

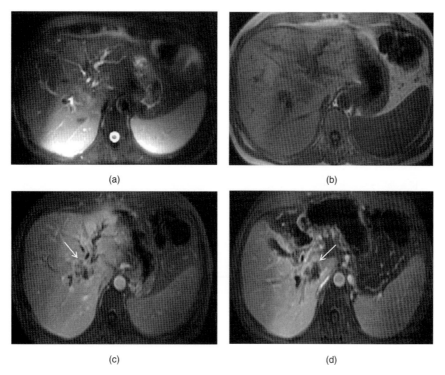

Figure 13.15 *Transverse fat-suppressed T2-weighted SS-ETSE (a), T1-weighted 2D-GE (b), T1-weighted postgadolinium fat-suppressed hepatic venous phase 2D-GE (c, d) images show subacute radiation induced injury/changes in the liver.* The radiation treatment was applied for the treatment of heterogeneous enhancing mass adjacent to the porta hepatis. A large area of liver parenchyma, which has well-defined boundaries consistent with radiation port, shows high T2 signal, low T1 signal and increased enhancement. The high T2 and low T1 signal represents edema and increased enhancement is seen due to inflammation and increased arterial flow secondary to portal vein injury.

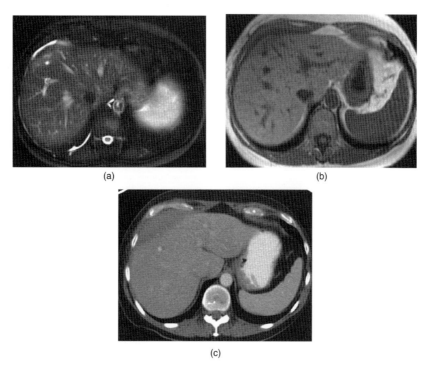

Figure 13.16 *Transverse T2-weighted fat-suppressed SS-ETSE (a), T1-weighted 2D-GE (b) MRI and postcontrast hepatic venous phase CT (a) images demonstrate chronic radiation injury in the liver.* An area of mildly high T2 signal and mildly low T1 signal is seen in the anterior part of the liver. This area has well defined borders and shows decreased enhancement on postcontrast image due to the radiation injury of the hepatic arterial branches and liver parenchyma.

improvements in radiation therapy. In the acute phase, radiation injury causes hepatocyte loss, edema, and obliterative fibrosis of small veins. In the chronic phase, fatty change, fibrosis, and atrophy of affected segments develop.

- Acute radiation hepatitis including edema usually resolves in 4 months with mild scarring. Edema may develop within 2–6 weeks after the radiation therapy and corresponds to the radiation ports, which have usually anteroposterior or oblique orientations.
- Chronic effects of radiation including perfusion changes, fatty infiltration, and fibrosis usually develop at 1 year after the initial insult, but may appear several years later.
- *Acute Radiation Injury* appears as:
  ° Decreased density on pre-contrast CT.
  ° Increased signal intensity on T2-WIs.
  ° Decreased signal intensity on T1-WIs.
  ° On the hepatic arterial dominant and hepatic venous phase of enhancement, the area of radiation injury enhances more or less than the normal parenchyma, depending on the predominant involvement of the arterial or venous system.
  ° On the interstitial phase of enhancement, increased enhancement compared to the background is seen due to injury to the small veins.
  ° Radiation changes have geographic margins corresponding to radiation ports.
  ° Figure 13.15.
- *Chronic Radiation Injury* appears as:
  ° Decreased signal intensity on both T1- and T2-weighted images and decreased early enhancement, reflecting the development of chronic fibrosis (Figure 13.16). Fat may also occur, appearing as high signal on T1.

- Fat is usually decreased within the radiation site in patients with fatty liver.

References

1 Hyslop, W.B., Kierans, A.S., Leonardou, P. *et al.* (2010) Overlap syndrome of autoimmune chronic liver diseases: MRI findings. J Magn Reson Imaging, 31, 383–389.

2 Ferreira, A., Ramalho, M., de Campos, R. *et al.* (2013) Hepatic sarcoidosis: MR appearances in patients with chronic liver disease. Magn Reson Imaging, 31, 432–438.

3 Bilaj, F., Hyslop, W.B., Rivero, H. *et al.* (2005) MR imaging findings in autoimmune hepatitis: correlation with clinical staging. Radiology, 236, 896–902.

4 Bader, T.R., Beavers, K.L., and Semelka, R.C. (2003) MR imaging features of primary sclerosing cholangitis: patterns of cirrhosis in relationship to clinical severity of disease. Radiology, 226, 675–685.

5 Tokala, A., Khalili, K., Menzes, R. *et al.* (2014) Comparative MRI analysis of morphologic patterns of bile duct disease in IgG4-related systemic disease versus primary sclerosing cholangitis. AJR Am J Roentgenol, 202, 536–543.

6 Sahni, V.A., Raghunathan, G., Mearadji, B. *et al.* (2010) Autoimmune hepatitis: CT and MR imaging features with histopathological correlation. Abdom Imaging, 35, 75–84.

7 Akhan, O., Akpinar, E., Karcaaltincaba, M. *et al.* (2009) Imaging findings of liver involvement of Wilson's disease. Eur J Radiol, 69, 147–155.

8 Meyer, C.A., White, C.S., and Sherman, K.E. (2000) Diseases of the hepatopulmonary axis. Radiographics, 20, 687–698.

9 Willemart, S., Nicaise, N., Struyven, J., and Van Gansbeke, D. (2000) Acute radiation-induced hepatic injury: evaluation by triphasic contrast enhanced helical CT. BJR, 73, 544–546.

10 Unger, E.C., Lee, J.K., and Weyman, P.J. (1987) CT and MR imaging of radiation hepatitis. J Comput Assist Tomogr, 11, 264–268.

CHAPTER 14

Vascular disorders of the liver

Ersan Altun[1], Mohamed El-Azzazi[1,2,3,4], and Richard C. Semelka[1]

[1] The University of North Carolina at Chapel Hill, Department of Radiology, Chapel Hill, NC, USA
[2] University of Dammam, Department of Radiology, Dammam, Saudi Arabia
[3] King Fahd Hospital of the University, Department of Radiology, Khobar, Saudi Arabia
[4] University of Al Azhar, Department of Radiology, Cairo, Egypt

Transient hepatic enhancement differences

- Transient increased hepatic enhancement is seen in the hepatic arterial dominant phase on CT and MRI, which characteristically should fade to background attenuation/signal with liver on more delayed acquisitions. These areas often have sharp and usually triangular borders although they may be nodular (Figure 14.1), wedge shaped (Figure 14.2), patchy (Figure 14.3) and segmental (Figure 14.3). These areas sometimes are associated with fatty infiltration, or sparing, or intrahepatic, biliary dilatation. On MR images, care should be taken to distinguish enhancement differences from differing fat content of hepatic parenchyma.
- Transient increased hepatic enhancement may be seen due to arterioportal shunts related to focal hepatic lesions; examples include hemangiomas (Figure 14.4), metastases (Figure 14.5), hepatocellular carcinoma, and focal nodular hyperplasia.
- Transient increased hepatic enhancement may be seen due to associated inflammation as in hepatic abscesses (Figure 14.6), acute cholecystitis (Figure 14.7), or acute-on-chronica hepatitis.
- Transient increased hepatic enhancement may be seen secondary to portal vein thrombosis or compression, which may be due to bland tumor thrombosis, tumor thrombosis, or tumor compression (Figures 14.8 and 14.9).
- Transient increased hepatic enhancement may also be seen due to cirrhosis (Figure 14.3) and aberrant venous drainage although it may also be idiopathic.

Portal venous thrombosis

- Portal vein thrombosis is the major cause of presinusoidal hypertension in the United States.
- Acute or Chronic.

- Causes:
  1 Extrahepatic:
     - Massive hilar lymphadenopathy.
     - Phlebitis (e.g. secondary acute appendicitis).
     - Propagation of splenic vein or superior mesenteric vein thrombosis secondary to pancreatitis.
     - Postsurgical thrombosis.
     - Hypercoagulable states.
  2 Intrahepatic:
     - Cirrhosis.
     - Cholangitis.
     - Intravascular invasion/tumor thrombosis by HCC or metastases.
- **Forms of occlusion:**
  (A) Bland thrombus.
     - Do not cause enlargement of the portal vein.
     - Bland thrombus may also show mildly high attenuation on precontrast CT images.
     - Bland thrombus may show mild high T2-signal and intermediate T1-signal on precontrast sequences if it is very prominent.
     - Bland thrombus does not show enhancement.
     - Figures 14.10–14.13
  (B) Tumor thrombus.
     - Causes enlargement of the portal vein.
     - Tumor thrombus may show mildly high attenuation on precontrast CT images.
     - Tumor thrombus may show mild-moderate high T2-signal and intermediate T1-signal on precontrast sequences.
     - Tumor thrombus usually shows heterogeneous enhancement on the hepatic arterial dominant phase and may demonstrate wash-out in later phases on postcontrast CT

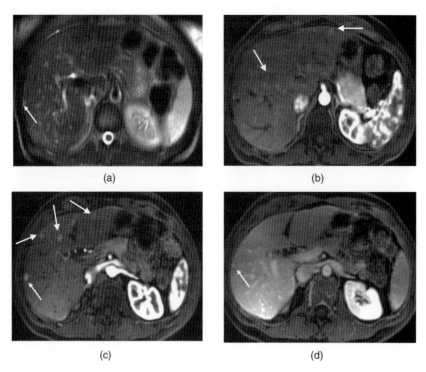

Figure 14.1 *Transverse T2-weighted fat-suppressed SS-ETSE (a), T1-weighted fat-suppressed postgadolinium hepatic arterial dominant phase (b, c), hepatic venous phase (d) 3D-GE images show multiple small wedge-shaped and nodular areas of transient perfusion abnormalities (thick arrows, b, c).* These areas do not demonstrate any signal change on precontrast sequences. These areas show early transient increased enhancement in the hepatic arterial dominant phase and become isointense on the hepatic venous phase. Note the presence of a tiny lesion with moderately high T2 signal (thin arrow, a) and prominent early enhancement (thin arrow, c) which persists in the hepatic venous phase (thin arrow, d).

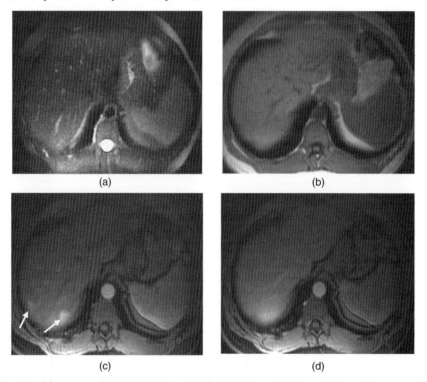

Figure 14.2 *Transverse T2-weighted fat-suppressed SS-ETSE (a), T1-weighted 2D-GE, T1-weighted postgadolinium fat-suppressed hepatic arterial dominant phase (c) and hepatic venous phase 3D-GE (d) images demonstrate MR features of focal wedge-shaped areas of transient increased perfusional abnormality/vascular shunting (arrows).* These wedge-shaped areas of perfusional abnormalities do not demonstrate any signal change on postgadolinium images and are only visible on the hepatic arterial dominant phase (c) becoming isointense on the hepatic venous phase (d).

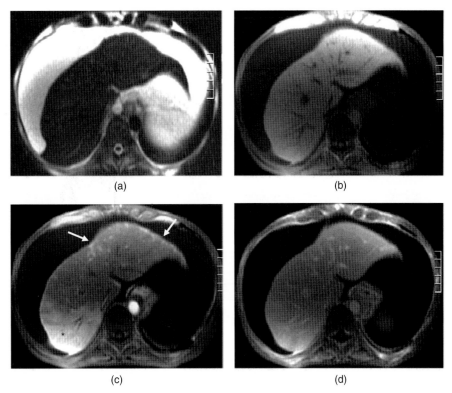

Figure 14.3 *Transverse T2-weighted fat-suppressed SS-ETSE (a), T1-weighted fat-suppressed 3D-GE (b), T1-weighted postgadolinium fat-suppressed late hepatic arterial phase (c) and hepatic venous phase (d) 3D-GE images demonstrate MR features of segmental transient perfusional abnormality in the right lobe of the liver (asterisk, c) and patchy transient perfusional abnormality in the left lobe of the liver (arrows, c) in a cirrhotic liver.* These areas of transient increased enhancement on the late hepatic arterial phase (c) do not show any signal change on precontrast images (a, b) and become isointense to the background liver on the hepatic venous phase (d). Note the large volume of ascites.

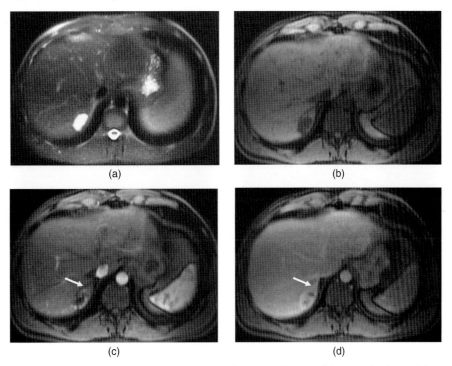

Figure 14.4 *Transverse T2-weighted fat-suppressed SS-ETSE (a), T1-weighted fat-suppressed 3D-GE (b), T1-weighted postgadolinium fat-suppressed hepatic arterial dominant phase (c) and hepatic venous phase (d) 3D-GE images show a hemangioma associated with peripheral arterioportal shunting.* The arterioportal shunt is characterized by the presence of adjacent early increased enhancement (arrow, c) which tends to fade on the later phase (arrow, d).

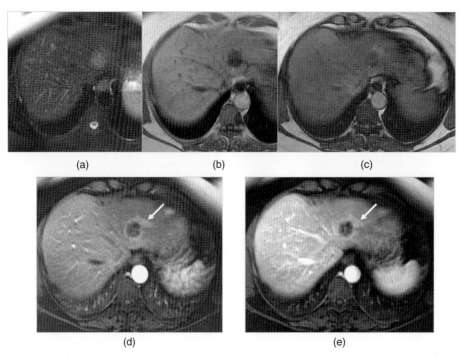

Figure 14.5   *Transverse T2-weighted fat-suppressed SS-ETSE (a), T1-weighted in-phase (b) and out-of-phase (c) 2D-GE, T1-weighted postgadolinium fat-suppressed hepatic arterial dominant phase (d) and hepatic venous phase (e) 3D-GE images show a single colorectal cancer metastasis associated with peripheral arterioportal shunting.* The arterioportal shunt is characterized by the presence of adjacent early increased enhancement (arrow, d) which tends to fade on the later phase (arrow, e). This area also shows fatty sparing on out-of-phase imaging.

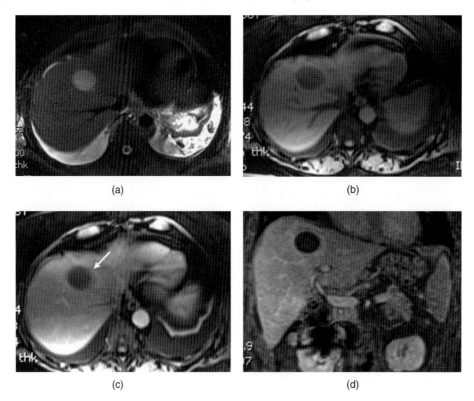

Figure 14.6   *Transverse T2-weighted fat-suppressed SS-ETSE (a), T1-weighted fat-suppressed 3D-GE (b), T1-weighted postgadolinium fat-suppressed hepatic arterial dominant phase (c) and coronal hepatic venous phase (d) 3D-GE images show a liver abscess associated with transient peripheral increased enhancement (arrow, c) on the hepatic arterial dominant phase secondary to associated inflammation, hyperemia.* The liver abscess shows high fluid content and enhancing thick wall. Note bilateral pleural effusions.

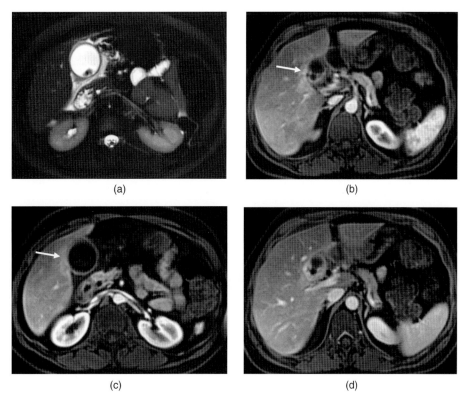

Figure 14.7 *Transverse T2-weighted fat-suppressed SS-ETSE (a), T1-weighted postgadolinium fat-suppressed hepatic arterial dominant phase (b, c) and hepatic venous phase (d) 3D-GE images show acute calcolous cholecystitis associated with adjacent transient increased enhancement of the liver parenchyma (arrows; b, c) secondary to inflammation/hyperemia.* Note the hydropic gallbladder with thick enhancing walls, pericholecystic fluid/edema and intraluminal stones.

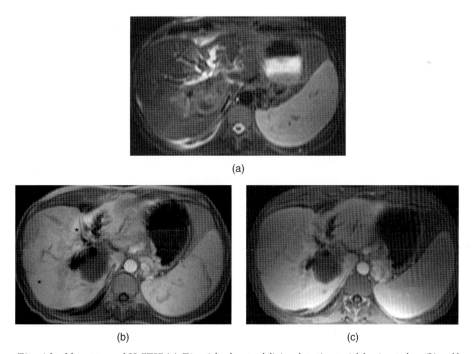

Figure 14.8 *Transverse T2-weighted fat-suppressed SS-ETSE (a), T1-weighted postgadolinium hepatic arterial dominant phase (b) and hepatic venous phase (c) 2D-GE image shows an intrahepatic cholangicocarcinoma invading the portal hilum causing intrahepatic biliary dilatation and portal vein compression.* Due to the portal vein compression, increased transient enhancement is seen in the liver (asterisk, b) in the hepatic arterial dominant phase with mildly increased enhancement in the later phase (c).

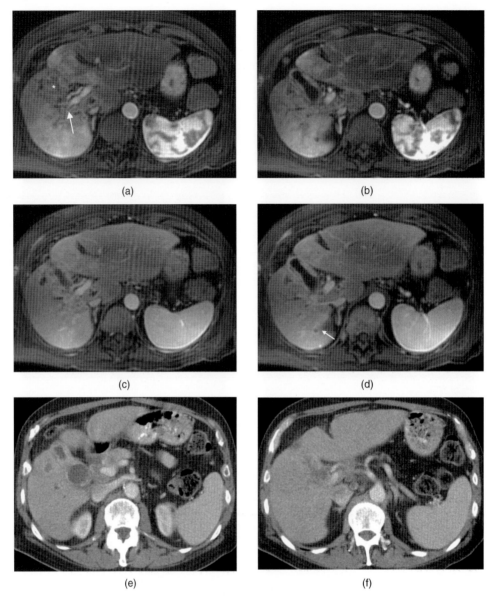

Figure 14.9 *Transverse T1-weighted postgadolinium hepatic arterial dominant phase (a, b), hepatic venous phase (c, d) and postcontrast hepatic venous phase CT (e, f) images show the right portal vein compression (arrow, a) due to the infiltrative lesion secondary to the gallbladder cancer. The gallbladder wall is diffuse* thickened and shows increased enhancement. Heterogeneously enhancing mass (asteriks, a) is seen in the right lobe. Due to the portal vein compression, early transient increased enhancement is seen in the right lobe of the liver (a, b). Note peripherally enhancing small metastases (arrow, d) in the right lobe of the liver. Postcontrast CT images (e, f) show enhancing thick walls of the gallbladder with small liver metastases.

and MRI. These features are more consistently and better observed on MRI.

- Figures 14.14–14.17.

(C) Extrinsic compression. Most commonly caused by malignant tumors, and characteristic of intrahepatic cholangiocarcinoma (Figure 14.8) and gallbladder carcinoma (Figure 14.9).

Acute portal vein thrombosis

1 Direct signs:

- Bland thrombosis is seen in the portal vein on postcontrast images as hypodense or hypointense material in the lumen (Figures 14.10–14.12).
- Involvement may be partial or complete and segmental or lobar.

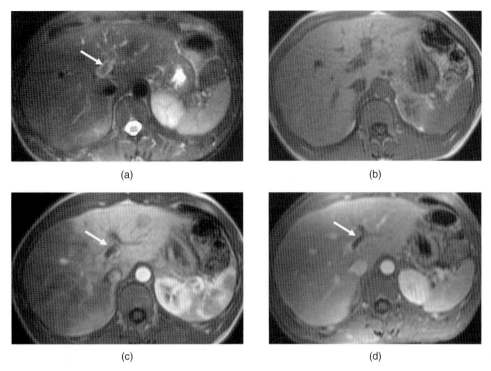

(a)

(b)

(c)

(d)

Figure 14.10 *Transverse T2-weighted fat-suppressed SS-ETSE (a), T1-weighted 2D-GE (b), T1-weighted hepatic arterial dominant phase 2D-GE (c), hepatic venous phase fat-suppressed 3D-GE (d) images show bland thrombus (arrows) in the left portal vein.* The thrombus shows mildly low signal on T2-weighted image (a) and fills the lumen of left portal vein without any enhancement on postgadolinium images (c, d). Increased transient enhancement is seen in the left lobe of the liver in the hepatic arterial dominant phase due to compensatory increase in the hepatic arterial flow and this transient increased enhancement fades in the hepatic venous phase. Note the presence of mild wall enhancement of the left portal vein on postgadolinium images secondary to inflammation.

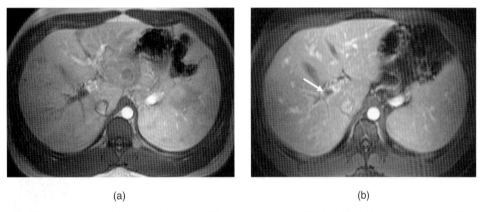

(a)

(b)

Figure 14.11 *Transverse T1-weighted postgadolinium hepatic arterial dominant phase 2D-GE (a) and hepatic venous phase 3D-GE (b) images show bland thrombus (arrow, b) in the right portal vein.* Note the presence of prominent wall enhancement of the right portal vein due to inflammation. The thrombus does not show enhancement.

° Portal vein expansion may rarely be seen, and this is a finding typical of tumor thrombosis. The most common explanation with bland thrombus is that the involved vessel is intrinsically aneurysmal, rather than the thrombus causing expansion.

° Bland thrombus is differentiated from tumor thrombus by the lack of enhancement on postgadolinium images. The wall of the portal veins may show enhancement.

° Acute bland thrombosis may appear as high attenuation in the portal vein on precontrast CT images.

° Acute bland portal vein thrombosis may show variable signal intensities on precontrast MRI sequences. In general, substantial volume acute thrombus shows moderately high signal on T2-weighted (in distinction from chronic bland thrombus which appears more dark in signal) and intermediate signal on T1-weighted precontrast images.

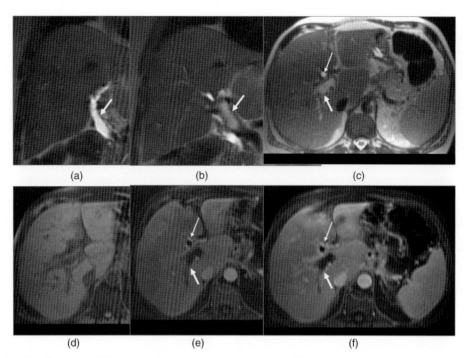

Figure 14.12 *Coronal (a, b) and transverse (c) T2-weighted SS-ETSE, transverse T1-weighted fat-suppressed 3D-GE (d), T1-weighted postgadolinium hepatic venous phase 3D-GE (e, f) images demonstrate findings of ascending cholangitis and right portal vein thrombosis.* The common bile duct is mildly dilated (arrow, a). The main portal vein and right portal vein show mildly increased T2 signal (short arrows; b, c) and the right hepatic duct appears mildly dilated (long arrow, c). The wall of the right hepatic duct is mildly thickened and shows increased enhancement (long arrows; e, f) which is suggestive of ascending cholangitis. The portal vein appears thrombosed (short arrows; e, f), which may be seen in association with ascending cholangitis.

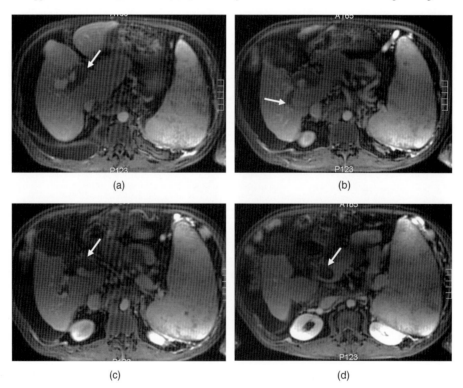

Figure 14.13 *Transverse T1-weighted fat-suppressed hepatic venous phase 3D-GE images (a–d) show large bland thrombus involving the main portal vein and portal vein branches.* The thrombus does not show any enhancement and extends into the splenic vein at the midline. Note the presence of dilated vessels at the porta hepatis representing cavernous transformation. Right-sided pleural effusion and findings of cirrhosis and portal hypertension including ascites, perisplenic/perigastric/peritoneal varices and splenomegaly are detected.

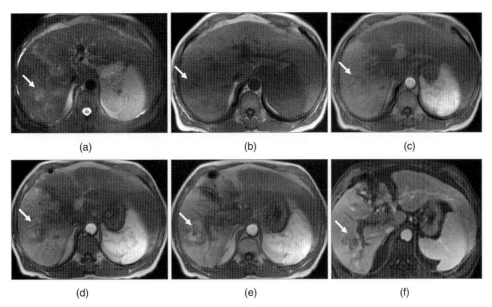

Figure 14.14 *Transverse T2-weighted fat-suppressed SS-ETSE (a), T1-weighted 2D-GE (b), T1-weighted postgadolinium hepatic arterial dominant phase 2D-GE (c–e), hepatic venous phase fat-suppressed 3D-GE (f) images demonstrate a hepatocelluar carcinoma (arrows) associated with tumor and bland thrombus. The* tumor is located in the right lobe of the liver and has mildly increased T2 signal. The tumor shows early increased heterogeneous enhancement on the hepatic arterial dominant phase (c–e) with wash-out on the hepatic venous phase (f). The right portal vein is completely thrombosed. Mild heterogeneous enhancement is seen in the superior part of the right portal vein, suggestive of tumor thrombus. Note the presence of early transient increased enhancement in the right lobe of the liver, which fades on the hepatic venous phase, secondary to compensatory increase in the hepatic arterial flow.

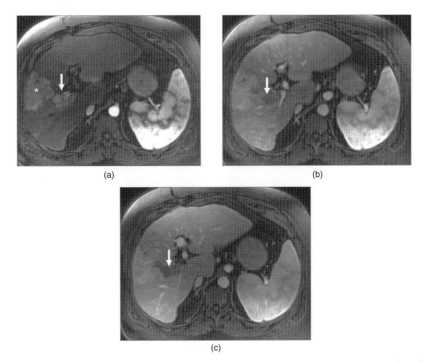

Figure 14.15 *Transverse T1-weighted postgadolinium fat-suppressed hepatic arterial dominant phase (a), hepatic venous phase (b, c) 3D-GE images show a segmental diffuse HCC associated with portal vein tumor thrombus. The wedge-shaped tumor located in the segments VIII and V shows early prominent* enhancement (asterisk, a) with small areas of wash-out in the later phases (b, c). The right portal vein (arrows; a–c) shows early increased enhancement (a) and wash-out (b, c) in the later phases.

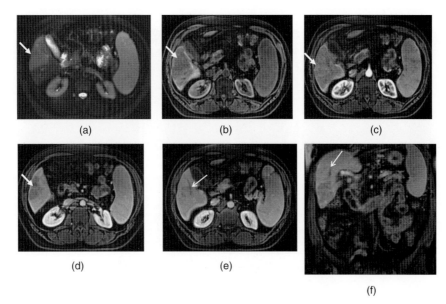

Figure 14.16 *Transverse T2-weighted fat-suppressed SS-ETSE (a), T1-weighted fat-suppressed 3D-GE (b), T1-weighted postgadolinium hepatic arterial dominant phase (c), hepatic venous phase fat-suppressed 3D-GE (d, e) and coronal postgadolinium interstitial phase fat-suppressed 3D-GE (f) images show a diffuse HCC (arrows, a–d) associated with thrombus involving a branch of the right hepatic vein (arrows; e, f). The tumor shows wedge-shaped high T2 (a) and low T1 (b) signal. The tumor shows early mildly increased enhancement (c) with later wash-out (d). An adjacent branch of the right hepatic vein does not enhance in the later phases (e, f) due to the presence of thrombus.*

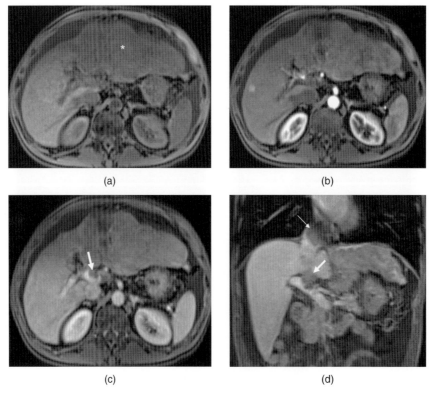

Figure 14.17 *Transverse T1-weighted fat-suppressed 3D-GE (a), T1-weighted fat-suppressed postgadolinium late hepatic arterial phase (b) and hepatic venous phase (c) 3D-GE, and coronal T1-weighted fat-suppressed postgadolinium interstitial phase 3D-GE images show a diffuse HCC (asterisk, a) involving the left lobe of the liver, which is also associated with nonocclusive tumor thrombus (thick arrows; c, d) in the portal vein. The left lobe of the liver is diffusely enlarged with lobulated contours and shows decreased T1 signal (a) due to the involvement of tumor. The tumor shows heterogeneous mild early enhancement (b) with later wash-out (d). Note that nonocclusive but prominent thrombus (thin arrow, d) is also present in the dilated inferior vena cava. Additionally, an early enhancing dysplastic nodule (b) is seen in the right lobe.*

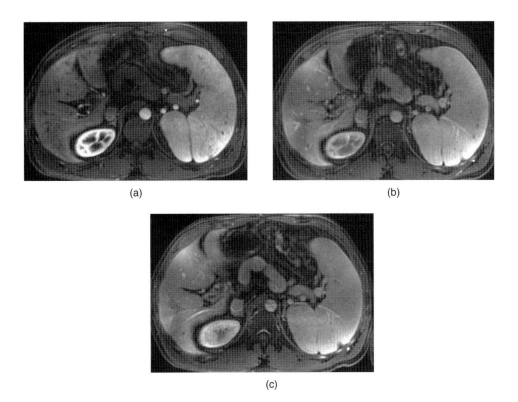

Figure 14.18 *Transverse postgadolinium T1-weighted hepatic arterial dominant phase (a), hepatic venous phase (b) and interstitial phase (c) fat-suppressed 3D-GE images demonstrate the presence of a tangle of vessels at the porta hepatis, which represents cavernous transformation.* The portal vein and its branches are not visualized since as they were chronically thrombosed.

- **Indirect signs**: Confined to liver parenchyma.
  - A flow-related phenomenon is observed in the parenchymal territory with absent or diminished portal venous supply on dynamic postcontrast images.
    1 Transient hepatic increased enhancement
    - Increased parenchymal enhancement during the hepatic arterial dominant phase is noted in the area supplied by the portal vein as this area receives increased hepatic arterial supply due to an autoregulatory mechanism (Figure 14.10). Gadolinium in the hepatic arteries is delivered faster than portal venous and in higher concentration, explaining the transient hepatic arterial dominant increased enhancement.
    2 Redistribution.
    - The area shows increased enhancement on the hepatic arterial dominant phase and on the hepatic venous phase.
  - Intrahepatic portal vein thrombosis may be associated with focal steatosis, fatty-sparing or iron deposition.

Chronic portal vein thrombosis
- Cavernous transformation may eventually develop with the formation of collateral vessels in the porta hepatis (Figure 14.18).

- Portal veins may be seen as diminutive atrophic vessels or may not be visualized.

Hepatic veno-occlusive disease

- Known as Budd–Chiari syndrome.
- Defined as lobar or segmental hepatic venous outflow obstruction at the level of hepatic veins or IVC.
- Results in the elevation of sinusoidal pressure and diminished portal venous flow, which lead to hepatocellular necrosis.
- In the acute form, hepatocellular necrosis commonly develops, since there is no collateral flow to relieve the intrahepatic pressure.
- In the subacute and chronic forms, hepatic venous outflow is less severe, reflecting conversion to partial occlusion, commonly due to presence of accessory veins.
- Because of accessory venous drainage and portal venous supply to the caudate lobe, hypertrophy of caudate lobe is noted. Central hepatic parenchymal hypertrophy and peripheral atrophy is also noted.
- Hepatic venous outflow obstruction may be primary or secondary.
- Primary causes are congenital, including webs or diaphragms.

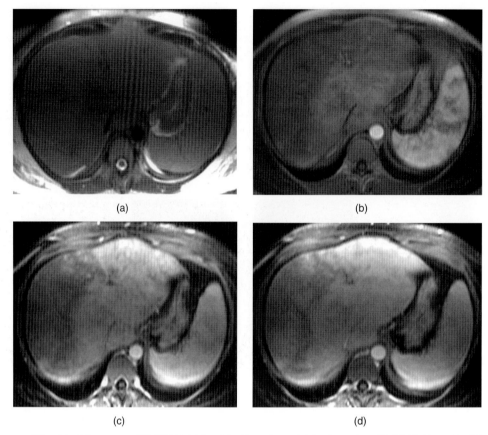

(a)

(b)

(c)

(d)

Figure 14.19 *Transverse T2-weighted fat-suppressed SS-ETSE (a), T1-weighted hepatic arterial dominant phase 2D-GE (b), T1-weighted fat-suppressed hepatic venous phase (c) and interstitial phase (d) fat-suppressed 2D-GE images demonstrate findings of Budd–Chiari syndrome.* The liver is enlarged with caudate and left lobe lateral segment hypertrophy. The liver shows heterogeneous enhancement on postgadolinium images with increased central enhancement particularly involving the caudate lobe in the hepatic arterial dominant phase. The hepatic veins could not be visualized due to veno-occlusive disease.

- Secondary causes are thrombosis, trauma, infection, or neoplasms, including HCC.
- Thrombosis may be seen due to hypercoagulability, chemotherapy, and radiation therapy.
- Is more common in women, and an underlying thrombotic tendency is present in up to one-half of patients.
- Clinical presentation may be fulminant, acute, subacute, or chronic. Fulminant form results in acute hepatic encephalopathy. Acute form results in sudden onset of ascites and jaundice. Subacute and chronic forms result in portal hypertension.
- **Imaging Findings on CT and MRI**
- *Acute changes*
- Enlarged and edematous/engorged normal-shaped liver showing low attenuation on precontrast CT, and high signal on T2-weighted images with low signal on T1-weighted images, features which are more prominent peripherally.
- On postcontrast images, increased central enhancement compared to decreased enhancement of peripheral liver is seen on the hepatic arterial dominant phase. On later phases, central increased enhancement decreases and peripheral

enhancement increases, with persistence of the enhancement differential (Figures 14.19 and 14.20).
- Hepatic veins may not be visualized or narrowed. Narrowing of IVC may be seen. Thrombosis of hepatic veins (Figure 14.21) or IVC may be seen.
- *Subacute changes*
- Mild to moderate, caudate lobe/central hypertrophy.
- Development of small, commonly capsule-based collaterals.
- Mildly edematous liver.
- Mildly increased central enhancement on the hepatic arterial dominant phase and mildly increased enhancement in the periphery on later phases relative to central liver.
- Hepatic veins may not be visualized or narrowed. Narrowing of IVC may be seen. Thrombosis of hepatic veins or IVC may be seen.
- *Chronic changes*
- Atrophy of peripheral liver with central hypertrophy.
- Subtle enhancement differences between peripheral and central liver.
- Curvilinear intrahepatic collaterals and capsule-based collaterals (Figure 14.22).
- Development of varices.

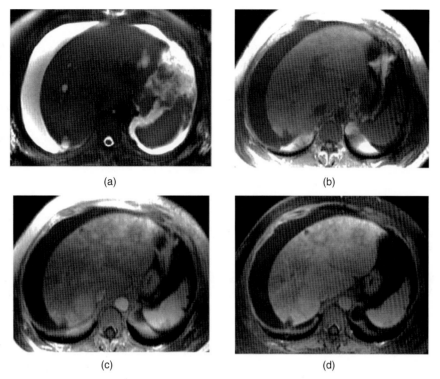

(a)   (b)

(c)   (d)

Figure 14.20 *Transverse T2-weighted fat-suppressed SS-ETSE (a), T1-weighted 2D-GE (b), T1-weighted hepatic arterial dominant phase (c), fat-suppressed hepatic venous phase (d) 2D-GE images demonstrate findings of Budd–Chiari syndrome.* The liver is enlarged with caudate and left lobe lateral segment hypertrophy. The liver shows heterogeneous enhancement on postgadolinium images with increased central enhancement particularly involving the caudate lobe. The hepatic veins could not be visualized due to veno-occlusive disease. Note the presence of a large volume of ascites and a few small cysts in the liver.

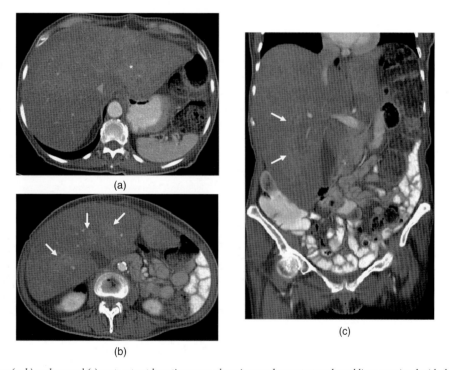

(a)

(b)

(c)

Figure 14.21 *Transverse (a, b) and coronal (c) postcontrast hepatic venous phase images demonstrate enlarged liver associated with thrombosis of the hepatic veins. The portal vein and its branches are patent.* The hepatic veins could not be visualized. The hepatic vein branches appear thrombosed with associated increased perivenular enhancement (arrows; b, c). The inferior vena cava appears compressed. Note the presence of mild heterogeneous enhancement at the left lobe of the liver (asteriks, a). The patient has amyloid infiltration in the liver.

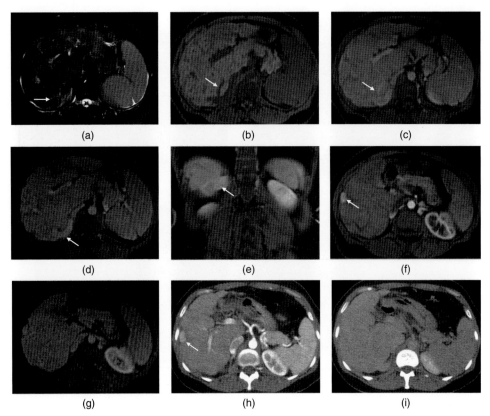

Figure 14.22 *Transverse T2-weighted SS-ETSE (a), T1-weighted fat-suppressed 3D-GE (b), T1-weighted postgadolinium transverse (c, d) and coronal hepatic venous phase (e) images demonstrate regenerative nodules, caudate lobe hypertrophy, and cirrhosis secondary to chronic Budd–Chiari syndrome.* Intrahepatic venous collaterals (arrows; a–c), which develop due to the thrombosis of hepatic veins, drain into a collateral extrahepatic large vein (arrows; d, e) which also drains into the inferior vena cava. Transverse T1-weighted fat-suppressed hepatic arterial dominant phase (f) and hepatic venous phase (g) 3D-GE images, and transverse hepatic arterial dominant phase (h) and hepatic venous phase (i) CT images demonstrate the development of early enhancing nodules in the same patient with chronic Budd Chiari syndrome. Early enhancing nodules (arrows; f, h), which tend to become isointense with the remaining liver in the later phases, can also be seen in patients with Budd–Chiari syndrome.

- Regenerative nodules and early enhancing nodules may be seen (Figure 14.22).
- Patients with HCC may develop acute or subacute Budd–Chiari syndrome because of tumor invasion of major hepatic veins.
- Patients with chronic Budd–Chiari syndrome may be at minimally increased risk for the development of HCC.

Hepatic arterial thrombosis/hepatic ischemia – infarction

Hepatic ischemia

- Most commonly seen in the setting of liver transplantation. Other common settings are severe small vessel disease (such as severe system lupus erythematosis or eclampsia in pregnancy).
- Unlike portal venous or hepatic venous thrombosis, the distribution of abnormal enhancement is not a regular pattern (segmental/lobar in portal vein abnormality, central/peripheral with hepatic venous), but appears more patchy throughout the liver (Figure 14.23)
- In the setting of more severe hepatic arterial disease, the enhanced portion of the liver, which is generally central, has a serrated margin with the less vascularized peripheral ischemic portion.

Hepatic infarction

- Hepatic infarction is rare due to dual blood supply of the liver including hepatic arterial and portal venous flows. The presence of collateral vessels is another protective factor against infarction. Hepatic arterial disease must be present to result in infarction, but often, additional portal venous compromise occurs.
- Commonly caused by iatrogenic events including liver transplantation, hepatobiliary surgery, chemoembolization, TIPS procedures.
- May also be caused by hypercoagulability, vasculitis, infection, or trauma.
- The most common cause is liver transplantation.

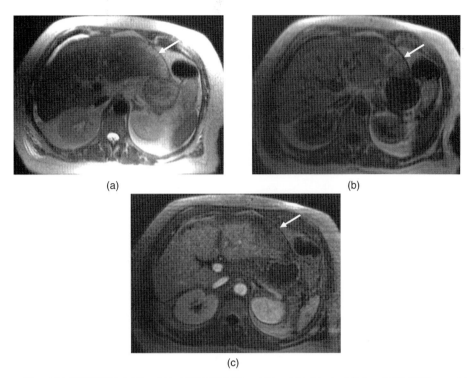

Figure 14.23 *Transverse T2-weighted SS-ETSE (a), T1-weighted MP-RAGE (b) and T1-weighted postgadolinium MP-RAGE images (c) show mild to moderately increased T2 signal at the periphery of the liver, particularly at the left hepatic lobe (a) with corresponding T1 bright signal (b) and relatively decreased enhancement (c).* These findings are suggestive of hemorrhagic changes and decreased perfusion (arrows) secondary to hepatic arterial ischemia.

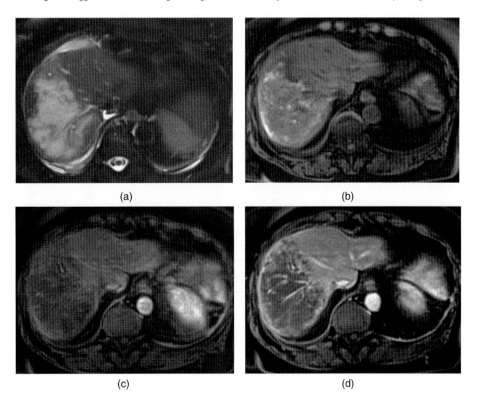

Figure 14.24 *Transverse T2-weighted fat-suppressed SS-ETSE (a), T1-weighted fat-suppressed 3D-GE (b), T1-weighted postgadolinium fat-suppressed hepatic arterial dominant phase (c) and hepatic venous phase (d) 3D-GE images show a large hemorrhagic infarct involving the right lobe of the liver.* The infarct shows mild to moderate high T2 signal (a), heterogeneous T1 signal with high signal hemorrhage on T1-weighted image (b) and decreased enhancement on postgadolinium images (c, d).

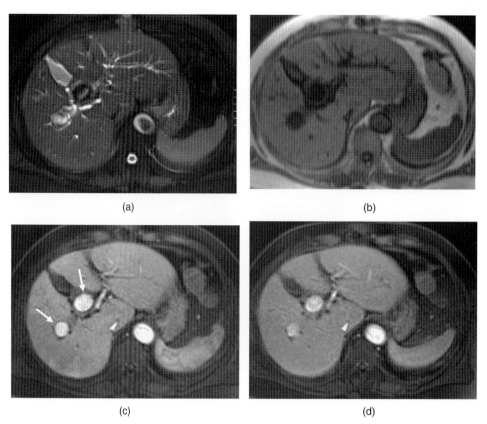

(a)   (b)

(c)   (d)

Figure 14.25 *Transverse T2-weighted fat-suppressed SS-ETSE (a), T1-weighted 2D-GE (b), T1-weighted postgadolinium fat-suppressed hepatic arterial dominant phase (c) and hepatic venous phase (d) MPRAGE images show two mycotic aneurysms of the right hepatic artery (arrows).*

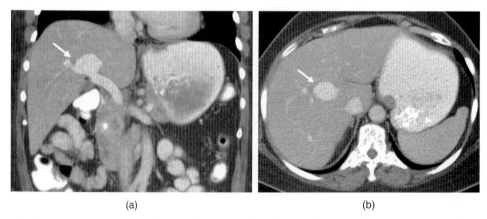

(a)   (b)

Figure 14.26 *Coronal and transverse postcontrast hepatic venous phase images show a large exophytic portal vein aneurysm (arrows).*

- **Imaging Features on CT and MRI:**
- Peripheral wedge-shaped areas or rounded/irregular shaped areas paralleling bile ducts which show low attenuation on precontrast CT and mildly high signal on T2-weighted and mildly low and/or high signal on T1-weighted precontrast images. Infarcts may also show low T2 signal uncommonly.
- Diminished enhancement of involved hepatic parenchyma is apparent, particularly on the hepatic arterial dominant

phase and on later phases (Figure 14.24). However, some heterogeneous enhancement may also be seen on later phases although nonenhancing areas reflecting necrosis, hemorrhage, or fibrosis are usually seen. Delayed enhancement of focal areas of parenchyma, which show initial diminished enhancement, generally reflects ischemic rather than necrotic hepatic parenchyma, but may at times reflect the presence of vascularized fibrotic tissue (which would be observed > 1 month after the start of the ischemic process).

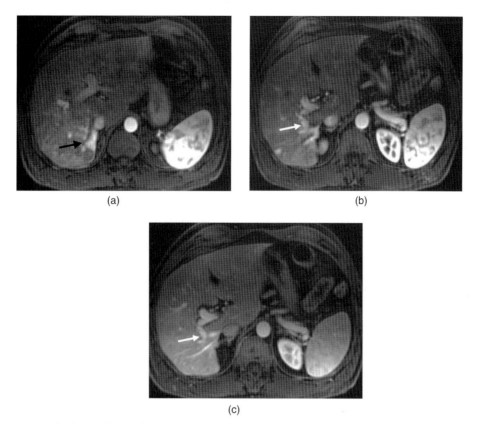

Figure 14.27 *Transverse T1-weighted postgadolinium fat-suppressed hepatic arterial dominant phase (a, b) and hepatic venous phase (c) show a vascular fistula (white arrows; b, c) located between the right portal vein and right hepatic vein. The vascular fistula between the right portal vein and right hepatic vein is seen and causes the early filling of the right hepatic vein on the hepatic arterial dominant phase. Additionally, early enhancing wedge-shaped (black arrow, a) and nodular areas are seen on the hepatic arterial dominant phase due to vascular shunting/perfusion abnormalities.*

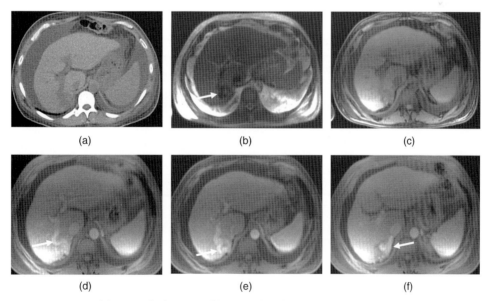

Figure 14.28 *Transverse precontrast CT (a), T2-weighted SS-ETSE (b), T1-weighted fat-suppressed 3D-GE (c), T1-weighted postgadolinium fat-suppressed 3D-GE (d–f) images show a large vascular malformation composed of a tangle of blood vessels including the dilated branches of the right portal vein and right hepatic vein, which drain into the IVC. Note that the patient has cirrhosis and ascites.*

- Bile leaks and gas formation (in sterile or infected infarcts) may be seen.

Vascular malformations/fistula/aneurysms

- Primary: Congenital
- Secondary: Occur secondary to:
  - Trauma. Percutaneous liver biopsy or surgery may cause vascular fistula.
  - Tumors.
  - Infection
  - Congenital disease such as Rendu-Osler-Weber syndrome.
- *On CT and MRI:*
  - Large fistulas/malformations/aneurysms may be seen as communicating vascular structures on precontrast CT images or T1- and T2-weighted images.
  - Fistulas/malformations/aneurysms are well depicted on postcontrast images on CT and MR, and CTA and MRA images. Fistulas and vascular malformations show enlarged feeding/draining vessels, which may be associated with transient hepatic arterial dominant phase focal parenchymal blush.
  - Large fistulas/malformations/aneurysms are seen as communicating enhancing vascular structures.
  - Figures 14.25–14.28.
  - Small fistulas/malformations are seen as enhancing oval structures, which show communication with vascular structures and enhancement parallel to the vessels.

References

1 Brancatelli, G., Vilgrain, V., Federle, M. *et al.* (2007) Budd–Chiari syndrome: spectrum of imaging findings. AJR Am J Roentgenol, 188, W168–W176.

2 Torabi, M., Hosseinzadeh, K., and Federle, M.P. (2008) CT of non-neoplastic hepatic vascular and perfusion disorders. Radiographics, 28, 1967–1982.

3 Angthong, W. and Semelka, R.C. (2014) Dealing with vascular conundrums with MR imaging. Radiol Clin North Am, 52, 861–882.

4 Sousa, M.S., Ramalho, M., Heredia, V. *et al.* (2014) Perilesional enhancement of liver cavernous hemangiomas in magnetic resonance imaging. Abdom Imaging; 39, 722–730.

5 Semelka, R.C., Lessa, T., Shaikh, F. *et al.* (2009) MRI findings of posttraumatic intravascular shunts. J Magn Reson Imaging, 29, 617–620.

6 Altun, E., Semelka, R.C., Elias, J. Jr., *et al.* (2007) Acute cholecystitis: MR findings and differentiation from chronic cholecystitis. Radiology, 244, 174–183.

7 Shah, T.U., Semelka, R.C., Voultsinos, V. *et al.* (2006) Accuracy of magnetic resonance imaging for preoperative detection of portal vein thrombosis in liver transplant candidates. Liver Transpl, 12, 1682–1688.

8 Kanematsu, M., Danet, M.I., Leonardou, P. *et al.* (2004) Early heterogeneous enhancement of the liver: magnetic resonance imaging findings and clinical significance. J Magn Reson Imaging, 20, 242–249.

9 Kanematsu, M., Kondo, H., Semelka, R.C. *et al.* (2003) Early-enhancing non-neoplastic lesions on gadolinium-enhanced MRI of the liver. Clin Radiol, 58, 778–786.

10 Bader, T.R., Braga, L., Beavers, K.L., and Semelka, R.C. (2001) MR imaging findings of infectious cholangitis. Magn Reson Imaging, 19, 781–788.

11 Semelka, R.C., Chung, J.J., Hussain, S.M. *et al.* (2001) Chronic hepatitis: correlation of early patchy and late linear enhancement patterns on gadolinium-enhanced MR images with histopathology initial experience. J Magn Reson Imaging, 13, 385–391.

12 Semelka, R.C., Hussain, S.M., Marcos, H.B., and Woosley, J.T. (2000) Perilesional enhancement of hepatic metastases: correlation between MR imaging and histopathologic findings-initial observations. Radiology, 215, 89–94.

13 Noone, T.C., Semelka, R.C., Siegelman, E.S. *et al.* (2000) Budd–Chiari syndrome: spectrum of appearances of acute, subacute, and chronic disease with magnetic resonance imaging. J Magn Reson Imaging, 11, 44–50.

14 Balci, N.C., Semelka, R.C., and Sandhu, J.S. (1999) Intrahepatic arterioportal fistula: gadolinium-enhanced 3D magnetic resonance angiography findings and angiographic embolization with steel coils. Magn Reson Imaging, 17, 475–478.

CHAPTER 15
Post-treatment changes in the liver

Ersan Altun[1], Mohamed El-Azzazi[1,2,3,4], and Richard C. Semelka[1]

[1] The University of North Carolina at Chapel Hill, Department of Radiology, Chapel Hill, NC, USA
[2] University of Dammam, Department of Radiology, Dammam, Saudi Arabia
[3] King Fahd Hospital of the University, Department of Radiology, Khobar, Saudi Arabia
[4] University of Al Azhar, Department of Radiology, Cairo, Egypt

- **Malignant liver lesions may be treated by**
  - Surgical resection
  - Liver transplantation
  - Radiation therapy
  - Systemic chemotherapy
  - Transcatheter arterial chemoembolization
  - Ablative therapies

Surgical resection

- Surgical removal with resection negative margins remains the optimal therapy for primary and secondary malignant liver tumors.
- Wedge resection, segmentectomy, and hepatectomy are the surgical resection techniques (Figures 15.1 and 15.2).
- Wedge resections and resection margins may show low attenuation on precontrast CT images and mildly high signal on T2-weighted and low signal intensity on T1-weighted precontrast MR sequences. A thin rim of enhancement may be seen along the resection margins in the hepatic arterial dominant phase, which fades to isointensity in later phases. In successful complete resection, by 6 months postprocedure negligible enhancement is seen in these resection areas on postcontrast images.
- Resection margin enhancement reflects leaky capillaries (early on), edema, and granulation tissue (>1 month) in the liver parenchyma. These changes are most prominent in the first 3 months after surgery and gradually decrease over the following 6 months.

- Hyperplasia/hypertrophy of the remaining liver may be appreciated as early as 3 months after surgery. Within 1 year, general enlargement of the remaining liver occurs. After right hepatectomy, hypertrophy of the medial segment may create the appearance of a pseudo right lobe.
- Tumor recurrence has a similar appearance to untreated malignant lesions and may arise along the resection margin. The recurrence appears as a thick rim of mildly high T2 signal/low T1 signal which shows prominent enhancement, or as a nodular lesion with mildly high T2 signal/low T1 signal that shows prominent enhancement (Figure 15.3).
- Bilomas, hematomas, and fluid collections may be seen along the resection margins (Figure 15.4).

Hepatic transplantation

- Donors and recipients may undergo a liver MR protocol with MRCP and MRA or CT with CTA for the evaluation of IVC, hepatic veins, portal vein, hepatic artery, and common bile duct.
- Recipients may receive living-related partial livers (lateral segment for small pediatric patients, right lobe for adult-to-adult recipients) or cadaveric whole or partial livers.
- In living-related hemiliver transplantation, the usual surgical procedure involves resecting the right lobe for donation and retaining the left lobe in the donor.
- In the donor liver, the resection plane is approximately 1 cm into the right lobe from the middle hepatic vein and extends inferiorly to the bifurcation between the right and left portal

Liver Imaging: MRI with CT Correlation, First Edition. Edited by Ersan Altun, Mohamed El-Azzazi and Richard C. Semelka.
© 2015 John Wiley & Sons, Inc. Published 2015 by John Wiley & Sons, Inc.

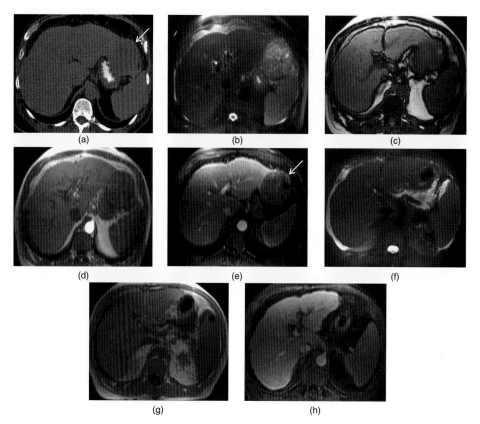

Figure 15.1 Transverse precontrast CT image (a), transverse T2-weighted fat-suppressed SS-ETSE (b), T1-weighted out-of-phase 2D-GE (c), T1-weighted postgadolinium arterial phase 2D-GE (d), fat-suppressed hepatic venous phase 3D-GE (e) images show a large heterogeneously enhancing exophytic HCC (arrows) arising from the left lobe of the liver in a patient with cirrhotic liver. The mass is surgically resected and no residual lesion is seen on postoperative MR images (f–h).

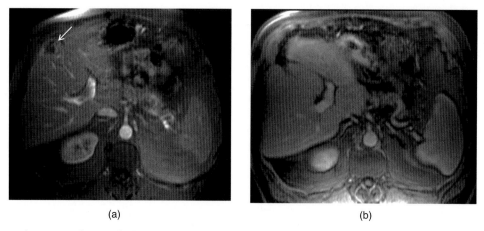

Figure 15.2 Transverse fat-suppressed T1-weighted postgadolinium 3D-GE images (a, b) show the successful interval resection of a colon carcinoma metastasis (arrow, a) located at the periphery of the liver. The lesion is not seen on the postoperative image (b).

veins, so that the donor retains the middle hepatic vein.

• Living related transplants have decreased in frequency because of the risks to the donor due to the failure of the remaining liver tissue.

• The presence of malignant disease in the recipient individual's native liver is an important determination for eligibility

for transplant. Currently, the most common indication for transplantation is the presence of limited HCC disease as determined by UNOS (The United Network for Organ Sharing)/OPTN (The Organ Procurement and Transplantation Network) criteria. The patients having a single HCC < 5 cm or not more than three HCCs, with none > 3 cm, in the

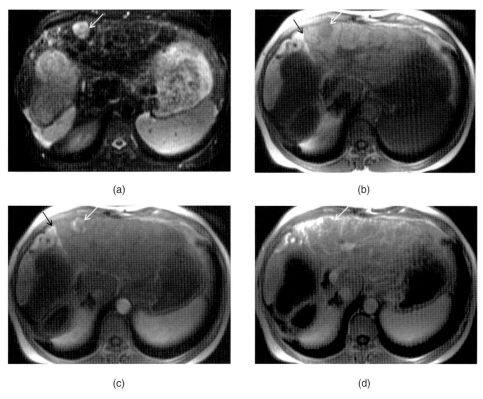

(a)   (b)

(c)   (d)

Figure 15.3 Transverse T2-weighted STIR (a), T1-weighted in-phase 2D-GE (b), T1-weighted postgadolinium hepatic arterial dominant phase 2D-GE (c), hepatic venous phase 3D-GE (d) images demonstrate the development of a recurrent enhancing HCC (white arrows, a–d) in a patient with right hepatectomy. Note that the liver is cirrhotic and the recurrent HCC is close to the resection margin (black arrows; b, c).

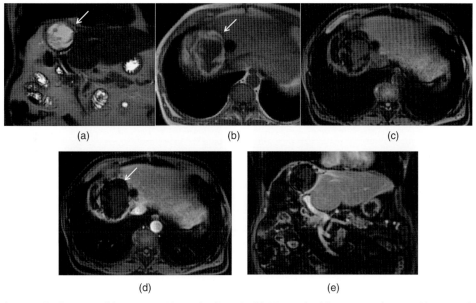

(a)   (b)   (c)

(d)   (e)

Figure 15.4 Coronal T2-weighted SS-ETSE (a), transverse T1-weighted 2D-GE (b), T1-weighted fat-suppressed 3D-GE (c), T1-weighted postgadolinium fat-suppressed hepatic venous phase (d) and coronal T1-weighted postgadolinium fat-suppressed hepatic venous phase (e) 3D-GE images show a large fluid collection (arrows) in a patient with right hepatectomy. A complex fluid collection with high T2 signal is seen along the resection margin, which represents a biloma. The fluid collection has irregular fat-containing borders, which represent the omentum. Mild stable wall enhancement is seen along the walls of the collection, which represents mild inflammation. The presence of significant wall enhancement, which is not seen in this case, may be a sign of infection and abscess. No residual disease is seen in the liver parenchyma. An oval susceptibility artifact secondary to surgical clips at the dome of the liver is seen.

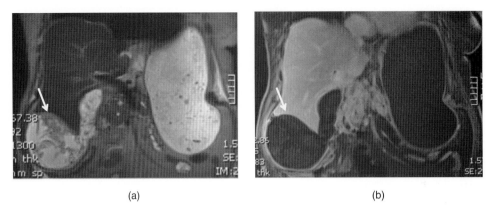

Figure 15.5 Coronal T2-weighted SS-ETSE, T1-weighted fat-suppressed hepatic venous phase 3D-GE images show a subhepatic complex fluid collection (arrow; a, b) in a patient following liver transplantation. The collection shows moderate wall enhancement, which is suggestive of infection – abscess.

absence of vascular invasion and metastases, represent the patients having limited disease and are candidates for liver transplantation.

- Complications of liver transplant surgery include fluid collections including biloma, seroma, or abscess (Figure 15.5), hematoma, vascular complications such as hepatic artery, portal vein, hepatic vein thrombosis and anastomotic strictures (Figure 15.6); biliary complications such as infection (Figure 15.7), and biliary anastomotic strictures (Figure 15.8).
- Bile leaks may develop at the anastomosis for technical reasons or may be secondary to bile duct necrosis in those patients with hepatic artery thrombosis.

- Strictures of the biliary tree are often a late complication of liver transplantation and usually occur at the anastomosis secondary to scar formation.
- Bile duct dilatation may be seen due to rejection. The differential diagnosis of rejection includes biliary obstruction, cholangitis, ischemic injury, viral infection, and drug toxicity.
- Periportal signal showing low signal intensity on T1-weighted images and high signal intensity on T2-weighted images may also be seen after transplantation and the differential includes lymphatic leak (due to failure of development of lymphatic channel continuity), lymphocytic infiltration due

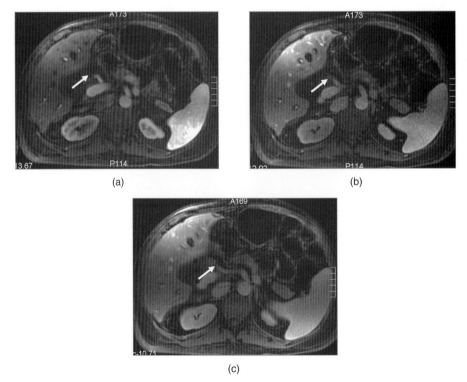

Figure 15.6 Transverse T1-weighted fat-suppressed postgadolinium hepatic arterial dominant phase (a), hepatic venous phase (b, c) 3D-GE images show significant hepatic arterial stenosis (arrows) in a patient with liver transplantation. The common hepatic artery shows significant narrowing at its midportion and its distal part cannot be visualized. Note the presence of periportal edema in the liver around the portal tracts.

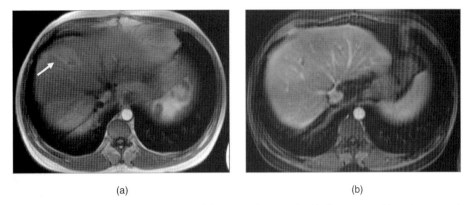

(a)   (b)

Figure 15.7 Transverse postgadolinium T1-weighted hepatic arterial dominant phase 2D-GE (a), fat-suppressed hepatic venous phase 3D-GE (b) images show mild focal segmental bile duct dilatation with transient early increased enhancement (arrow) at segment VIII in a patient with liver transplantation. These findings may develop secondary to mild ascending cholangitis and clinical correlation is required as focal bile duct dilatation with mild inflammation (without infection) secondary to postsurgical changes/bile duct ischemia may also be associated with early transient increased enhancement. The presence of bile duct wall enhancement in the later phases is suggestive of more prominent inflammation/infection.

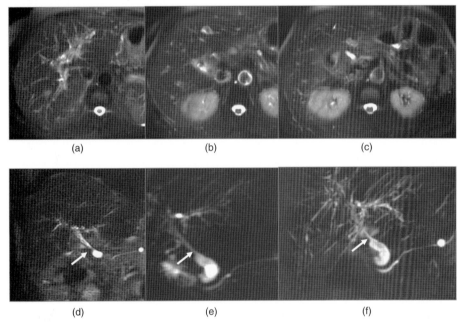

(a)   (b)   (c)

(d)   (e)   (f)

Figure 15.8 Transverse T2-weighted fat-suppressed SS-ETSE (a–c), coronal T2-weighted fat-suppressed SS-ETSE, single shot coronal thick slab heavily T2-weighted MRCP and reconstructed 3D MIP image of thin slab heavily T2-weighted MRCP images show prominent ischemic changes of the intrahepatic biliary ducts. The intrahepatic biliary ducts demonstrate multiple diffuse strictures and dilatations on the 3D reconstructed image (f). Mild edema is seen along the central intrahepatic bile ducts. The common bile duct also appears diffusely thin, which again may develop secondary to ischemic changes and a moderate stricture is also seen at the anastomosis line (arrows; d–f). Note that a small cyst is also seen at the pancreatic tail.

to rejection, and posttransplant lymphoproliferative disease (PTLD).

Radiation therapy

- Rarely used for liver lesions.
- More commonly used after the development of targeted radiotherapy such as cyberknife.
- Usually reserved for settings where surgery or ablative therapy is not considered reasonable therapy for a patient.

- Following radiation therapy, partial or complete response is initially characterized by lack of malignant lesion growth. The lesion shows progressively decreasing enhancement with the development of necrosis. After 3–6 months, responsive lesions become much smaller and the enhancement decreases prominently. Unresponsive or partially responsive lesions demonstrate further growth over this period of time with enhancement.
- In the first 3 months, edema may be seen around the lesion in the liver parenchyma, which is characterized by low attenuation on CT and moderately high T2 signal and low

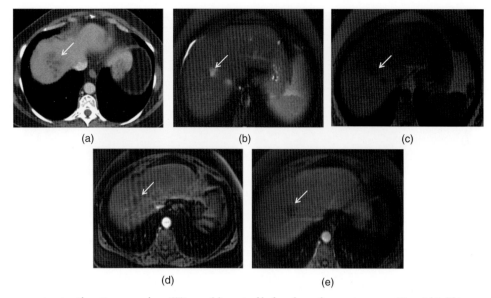

Figure 15.9 Transverse postcontrast hepatic venous phase CT image (a) acquired before chemotherapy, transverse T2-weighted fat-suppressed SS-ETSE (b), T1-weighted in-phase 2D-GE (c), T1-weighted postgadolinium fat-suppressed hepatic arterial dominant phase 2D-GE (d) and hepatic venous phase 3D-GE (e) images acquired after chemotherapy demonstrate interval prominent decrease in the size of metastasis (arrows) located at the dome of the liver. Note that the enhancement of the lesion has also decreased prominently compared to CT image.

T1 signal on precontrast sequences. This area is usually consistent with radiation port. Increased early enhancement of this area, which fades to isointensity/isodensity in later phases, may be seen due to the presence of inflammation secondary to radiation. Fibrosis and atrophy of the affected area may develop, commencing at 3 months.

- Targeted radiation therapies, such as cyberknife, are being increasingly used, due to the tighter collimation of the radiation port, and hence less surrounding hepatic damage, including in solitary smaller tumors (<3 cm). In successfully treated lesions, mildly increased thin rim-like enhancement may be seen in the hepatic arterial dominant phase, which tends to become isointense/isodense in later phases, due to the presence of peripheral inflammation.

- Recurrent disease is characterized by the presence of a thick rim of tissue or nodular tissue showing mildly high signal on T2/low T1 MRI signal or low attenuation on precontrast CT. Recurrent tumors usually show early increased enhancement or progressively increasing enhancement. Depending on the specific tumor type, wash-out may be seen in the later phases. However, some recurrent metastases may show fading in the later phases after treatment.

Systemic chemotherapy

- Responsive lesions show size decrease beginning 1 month after the start of treatment.
- In the first 3 months following treatment-start, in addition to decrease in size, responsive lesions initially become more well-defined and demonstrate progressive decrease in the

enhancement on postcontrast images (Figures 15.9–15.11). Treated small metastases may show early peripheral enhancement with progressive centripetal enhancement in later phases, with retention of contrast, at approximately 1 year following treatment. This can simulate the appearance of a hemangioma. Good response of metastases is often reflected by mild early intensity of ring enhancement on the hepatic arterial dominant phase, with progressively intense enhancement of the ring on delayed phases. This presumably reflects the enhancement pattern of fibrosis.

- With continued responsive treatment, the lesions show decreasing T2 signal and increasing T1 signal on precontrast images and tend to become isodense/isointense compared to the background liver.

- Fibrosis develops in chronically treated lesions and chronically treated lesions show irregular, angular, and polygonal margins. Treated subcapsular and peripheral lesions may be associated with capsular retraction. Fibrotic chronically treated lesions show progressive enhancement, which is more prominent in the interstitial phase.

- Unresponsive lesions demonstrate increase in size (Figure 15.12).

Transcatheter arterial chemoembolization

- Chemoembolic therapy is based on the pathophysiologic premise that hypervascular malignant tumors receive greater blood supply from hepatic arteries than surrounding intact liver and thus cytotoxic agents are preferentially delivered to malignant cells. Therefore, chemoembolization is used

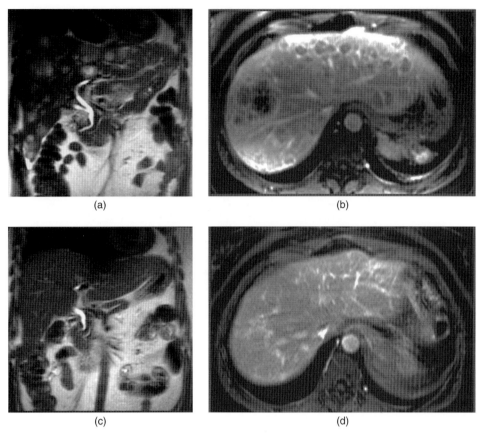

Figure 15.10 Coronal T2-weighted SS-ETSE (a), transverse T1-weighted fat-suppressed postgadolinium 3D-GE (b) images show multiple peripherally enhancing nodular metastatic lesions in the liver. After the completion of chemotherapy, the lesions decreased in number and size significantly, as seen on the corresponding MR images (c, d).

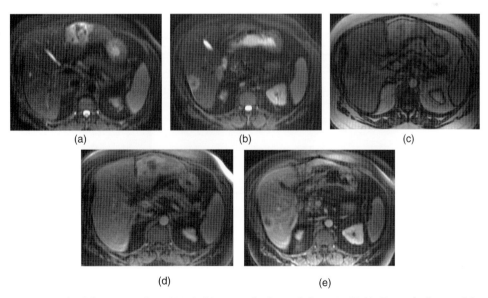

Figure 15.11 Transverse T2-weighted fat-suppressed SS-ETSE (a, b), T1-weighted out-of-phase 2D-GE (c), T1-weighted postgadolinium fat-suppressed hepatic venous phase 2D-GE (d, e) images show peripherally enhancing metastases in both lobes of the liver. After the completion of chemotherapy, the lesions demonstrated significant decrease in size and enhancement on the corresponding T2-weighted images (f, g) and postgadolinium T1-weighed images (h, i).

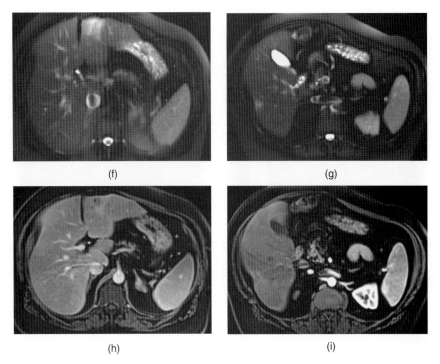

(f)

(g)

(h)

(i)

Figure 15.11 *(Continued)*

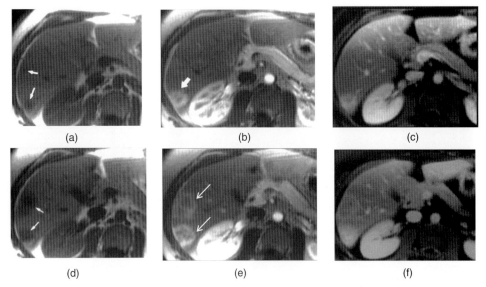

(a)

(b)

(c)

(d)

(e)

(f)

Figure 15.12 Transverse T1-weighted 2D-GE (a), T1-weighted postgadolinium hepatic arterial dominant phase (b), T1-weighted fat-suppressed post-gadolinium 3D-GE (c) images show two enhancing metastases in the right lobe of the liver. After the completion of chemotherapy, the metastases show interval prominent increase in size compared to prior examination, as seen on the corresponding images (d–f), as the metastases are unresponsive to the chemotherapy.

for hypervascular tumors such as HCC, carcinoid, and neuroendocrine tumors.

- Following chemoembolization, within the first month, partial or complete response of hypervascular lesions is seen.

- Complete response is characterized by low signal on T2-weighted images and lack of enhancing tumor tissue on postcontrast images associated with decreasing tumor size (Figures 15.13 and 15.14). This low T2-signal is characteristic

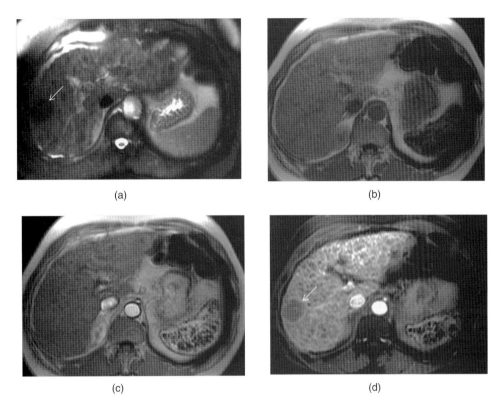

Figure 15.13 Transverse T2-weighted fat-suppressed SS-ETSE (a), T1-weighted in-phase 2D-GE (b), T1-weighted postgadolinium hepatic arterial dominant phase 2D-GE (c) and hepatic venous phase fat-suppressed 3D-GE (d) images show an effectively treated HCC with TACE (arrows; a, d) in a patient with cirrhotic liver. The oval lesion shows low signal intensity on T2-weighted image (a), isointense to mildly hyperintense signal on T1-weighted image (b) and no enhancement on postgadolinium images except a mild peripheral rim type of enhancement on the hepatic venous phase image (d). The absence of enhancement in the lesion is a sign of effective treatment (c, d). The peripheral rim type of enhancement may be a sign of posttreatment inflammatory response; however, it should be followed up.

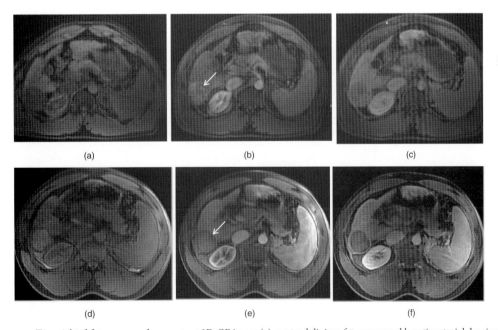

Figure 15.14 Transverse T1-weighted fat-suppressed precontrast 3D-GE image (a), postgadolinium fat-suppressed hepatic arterial dominant phase (b) and hepatic venous phase (c) 3D-GE images demonstrate a HCC with early enhancement and later wash-out in segment VI. After the TACE, the lesion shows no enhancement on the corresponding images (d, e) except a peripheral rim type of enhancement on the hepatic venous image (f), which may be suggestive of posttreatment inflammatory response. These findings indicate that the TACE is effective.

of chemo-embolization, as most other therapies are associated with capillary leakage/damage and increased T2 signal.

- Partial response is characterized by decreasing tumor size with the presence of persistent arterial enhancement on postcontrast images (Figure 15.15).
- Liver infarction, liver abscess, gallbladder injury, tumor rupture, and liver failure are complications of chemoembolization.
- Sterile gas may be rarely seen in lesions postchemo-embolization therapy, reflecting necrosis and nitrogen release. Care must be taken to distinguish this from abscess, with the latter often being associated with intense hepatic arterial dominant perilesional enhancement and later peripheral rim type of enhancement.
- Perfusion abnormalities related to the treatment, with increased and heterogeneous enhancement present in hepatic arterial dominant phase images, should fade in later phases. No wash-out is seen in later phases.

Ablative therapies

- Radiofrequency (RF) ablation, microwave ablation, cryoablation, ethanol ablation, and laser ablation are various ablative methods to treat focal liver malignancies.
- These may be performed in combination with surgical resection, or when curative resection is considered not optimal.

- The ablated area must exceed the tumor margins by approximately 1.0 cm to achieve complete treatment.
- A useful prediction of successful ablation is the size of the devascularized tissue after intervention.
- A successful ablation site demonstrates progressive decrease in size with time.
- Small necrotic areas may disappear completely with the development of fibrosis.
- Enlargement of the ablated area on follow-up examinations is suggestive of unsuccessful intervention.
- On CT, ablation sites usually demonstrate mild to moderately high density for the first 3 months and tend to become isodense with the remaining liver parenchyma later on.
- Up to 1 week after ablation, the signal intensity on T2-weighted and T1-weighted images is determined by the stage of hemorrhage and the presence of either liquefactive or coagulative necrosis. After the first week, the ablation site shows mildly low signal on T2-weighted image and high signal on T1-weighted precontrast images. Mildly low signal on T2 is a helpful feature to suggest a lesion is a posttreated region, as HCCs should be either isointense or mildly hyperintense.
- A thin rim of enhancement, with a peripheral ill-defined margin with surrounding liver, is usually seen encompassing the ablation site on the hepatic arterial dominant phase for the first 3 months, due to inflammatory reaction. No internal enhancement or thick rim of enhancement is seen in successfully ablated lesions (Figures 15.16–15.21).

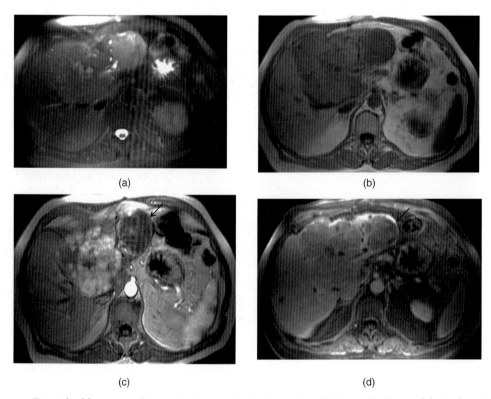

(a) (b)

(c) (d)

Figure 15.15 Transverse T2-weighted fat-suppressed SS-ETSE (a), T1-weighted in-phase 2D-GE (b), T1-weighted postgadolinium hepatic arterial dominant phase 2D-GE (c) and hepatic venous phase fat-suppressed 3D-GE (d) images show the result of an ineffective TACE treatment. This large HCC still shows heterogeneous enhancement except a small lateral part (arrows; c, d) showing decreased enhancement due to the treatment.

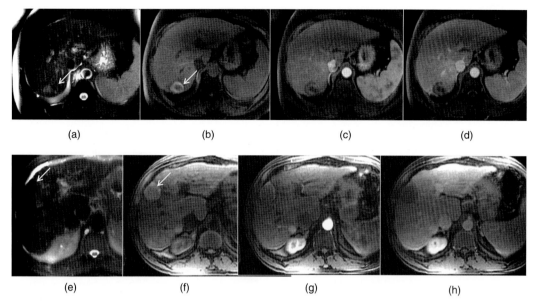

(a)   (b)   (c)   (d)

(e)   (f)   (g)   (h)

Figure 15.16 Transverse T2-weighted fat-suppressed SS-ETSE (a, e), T1-weighted fat-suppressed 3D-GE (b, f), T1-weighted postgadolinium fat-suppressed hepatic arterial dominant phase (c, g) and hepatic venous phase 3D-GE (d, h) images show two successfully ablated HCCs without residual disease. Both ablation sites show high T1 signal (b, f) due to their high protein content on T1-weighted precontrast images. The first lesion shows liquefactive necrosis with high T2 signal (a) and the second lesion shows coagulative necrosis with low T2 signal (e). No enhancement is seen on postgadolinium images, suggestive of successful ablation without residual disease.

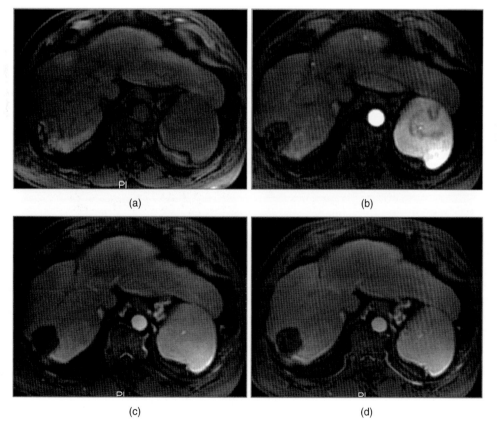

(a)   (b)

(c)   (d)

Figure 15.17 Transverse T1-weighted fat-suppressed 3D-GE (a), T1-weighted fat-suppressed postgadolinium hepatic arterial dominant phase (b), hepatic venous phase (c), interstitial phase (d) 3D-GE images show a successfully ablated HCC without residual disease. The ablation site does not demonstrate any enhancement, which indicates successful ablation.

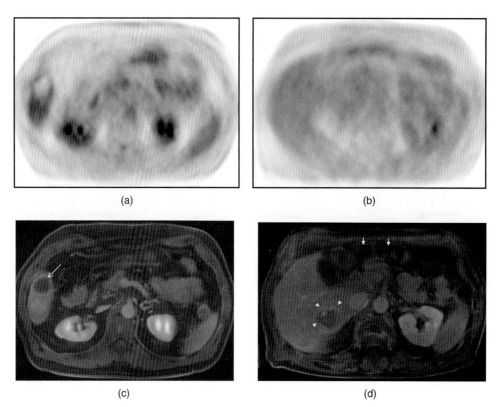

(a)

(b)

(c)

(d)

Figure 15.18 Transverse PET images (a, b) and fused MR-PET (c, d) postgadolinium T1-weighted hepatic venous phase images demonstrate successfully ablated HCCs (arrow, c; arrowheads, d) without any uptake or enhancement in two different patients. The omentum is also indicated in the second patient, indicating good registration with PET images.

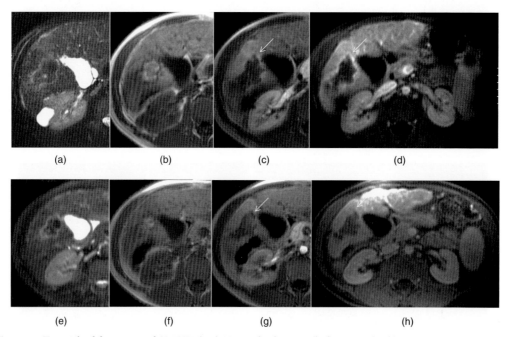

(a)   (b)   (c)   (d)

(e)   (f)   (g)   (h)

Figure 15.19 Transverse T2-weighted fat-suppressed SS-ETSE (a, e), T1-weighted 2D-GE (b, f), T1-weighted hepatic arterial dominant phase 2D-GE (c, g), T1-weighted hepatic venous phase fat-suppressed 3D-GE (d, h) images show an ablated HCC with no residual disease. The first set of images (a–d) were acquired 3 weeks after the ablation and show an ablation cavity with low T2 (a)/high T1 (b) signal, demonstrating mild thin peripheral rim type of enhancement (arrows; c, d) in the hepatic arterial dominant and hepatic venous phase. The second set of images were acquired 3 months after the ablation and show interval decrease in cavity size with no peripheral enhancement. Typically, after a successful ablation, a thin rim of peripheral enhancement is usually seen in 1 month, representing early inflammation and granulation tissue. This thin peripheral rim type of enhancement resolves in 2 months after the ablation and is no longer seen. The ablation cavity should also decrease in size and shrink with time.

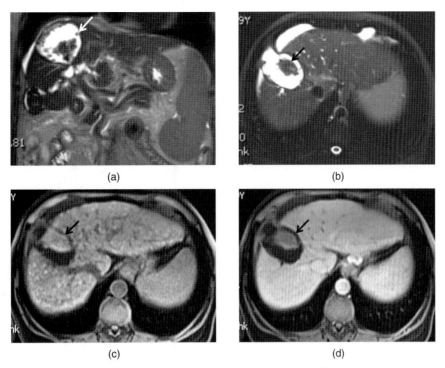

Figure 15.20 Coronal T2-weighted SS-ETSE (a), transverse T2-weighted fat-suppressed SS-ETSE (b), T1-weighted fat-suppressed 3D-GE (c) and post-gadolinium hepatic venous phase fat-suppressed 3D-GE (d) images demonstrate a complex fluid collection (white arrow, a) at the site of ablation. The fluid collection contains bile and a focal hematoma (black arrows; b–d) as well. The focal hematoma shows low signal on T2 weighted images (a, b), high signal on T1-weighted precontrast image (c) and no enhancement on the postgadolinium image (d). The complex fluid collection does not show any abnormal enhancement and no findings suggestive of infection, residual/recurrent disease is seen. Please note the presence of perihepatic free fluid. Additionally, focal central bile duct dilatation is detected adjacent to the complex fluid collection secondary to bile duct injury.

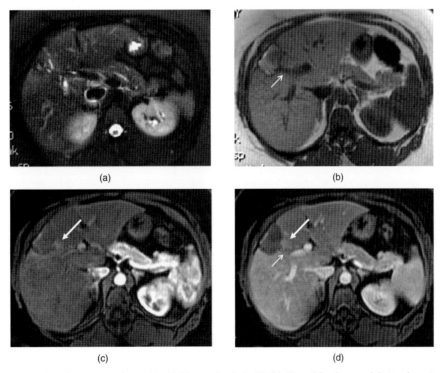

Figure 15.21 Transverse T2-weighted fat-suppressed SS-ETSE (a), T1-weighted 2D-GE (b), T1-weighted postgadolinium hepatic arterial dominant phase (c) and hepatic venous phase (d) 3D-GE images show an ablation site without evidence of residual or recurrent disease. However, a focal early enhancing area is noted posterior to the ablation site (long arrow, c) and tends to fade in the hepatic venous phase (long arrow, d). No precontrast T1 or T2 signal correlation is seen at this location. This focal early enhancement mimics residual/recurrent disease; however, it develops secondary to the compensatory increase in the arterial flow due to the thrombosis of the segmental branch of the portal vein (short arrows; b, d). This segmental portal vein branch located posterior to the lesion was thrombosed during the ablation procedure and these findings were stable for more than a year. Note that mild focal intrahepatic bile duct dilatation is also seen at the apex of the ablation site on T2-weighted image (a) secondary to focal mild bile duct injury.

- Recurrent disease is characterized by the presence of a thick rim of tissue, or nodular tissue, that shows mildly high signal on T2, mildly low T1 signal, or low attenuation on precontrast CT, and early enhancement on postcontrast images. Recurrent tumors usually show early increased enhancement or progressively increasing enhancement. Depending on the specific tumor type, wash-out may be seen in the later phases (Figures 15.22–15.24). However, some recurrent metastases may show fading in the later phases after treatment.

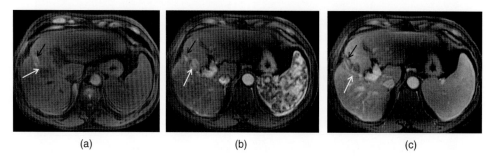

(a)　　　　(b)　　　　(c)

Figure 15.22 Transverse T1-weighted fat-suppressed 3D-GE (a), T1-weighted fat-suppressed postgadolinium hepatic arterial dominant (b) and hepatic venous phase (c) images show a recurrent HCC (white arrows; a–c) at the posteromedial portion of the ablation site. The ablation site (black arrows; a–c) shows high T1 signal on pre and postgadolinium images without any enhancement. The recurrent tumor (white arrows; a–c) shows early increased enhancement (b) and later washout with capsular enhancement (c).

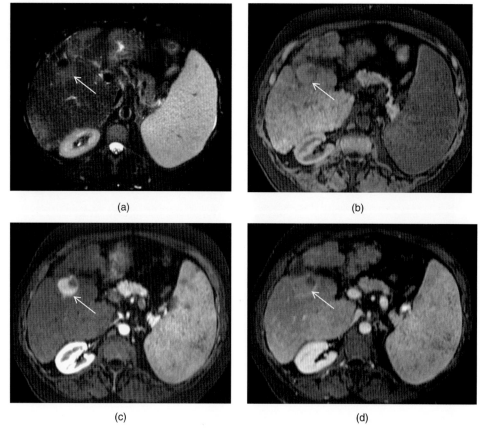

(a)　　　　(b)

(c)　　　　(d)

Figure 15.23 Transverse T2-weighted fat-suppressed SS-ETSE (a), T1-weighted fat-suppressed 3D-GE (b), T1-weighted postgadolinium fat-suppressed hepatic arterial dominant phase (c) and hepatic venous phase 3D-GE (d) images show a recurrent HCC (arrows; a–d) at the ablation site. The ablation site is replaced by a soft tissue showing high T2 signal (a), isointense T1 signal (b), early increased enhancement (c) and later wash-out (d).

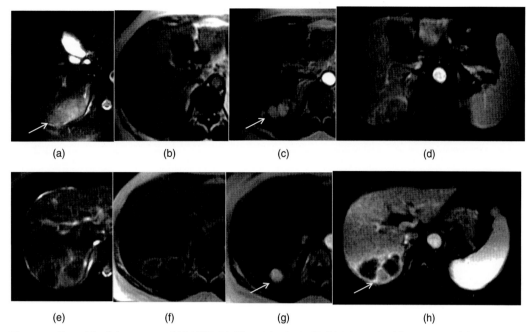

(a)   (b)   (c)   (d)

(e)   (f)   (g)   (h)

Figure 15.24 Transverse T2-weighted fat-suppressed SS-ETSE (a), T1-weighted 2D-GE (b), T1-weighted hepatic arterial dominant phase 2D-GE (c), T1-weighted hepatic venous phase fat-suppressed 3D-GE (d) images show a typical HCC (arrows; a, c) located in the right lobe of the liver, showing high T2 signal (a), early enhancement (c) and later wash-out with capsular enhancement (d). Transverse T2-weighted fat-suppressed SS-ETSE (e), T1-weighted 2D-GE (f), T1-weighted hepatic arterial dominant phase 2D-GE (g), T1-weighted hepatic venous phase fat-suppressed 3D-GE (h) images demonstrate interval ablation of this lesion. However, residual disease showing early enhancement and later wash-out is seen in the posterior part of the lesion.

- Rarely, tiny locules of sterile gas may be present in the ablated lesions for the first month.

References

1 Sainani, N.I., Gervais, D.A., Mueller, P.R., and Arellano, R.S. (2013) Imaging after percutaneous ablation of hepatic tumors. Part 1, Normal findings. AJR Am J Roentgenol, 200, 184–193.

2 Sainani, N.I., Gervais, D.A., Mueller, P.R., and Arellano, R.S. (2013) Imaging after percutaneous ablation of hepatic tumors. Part 2, Abnormal findings. AJR Am J Roentgenol, 200, 194–204.

3 Lim, S.H., Jeong, Y.Y., Kang, H.K. *et al.* (2006) Imaging features of hepatocellular carcinoma after transcatheter arterial chemoembolization and radiofrequency ablation. AJR Am J Roentgenol, 187, W341–W349.

4 Braga, L. and Semelka, R.C. (2005) Magnetic resonance imaging features of focal liver lesions after intervention. Top Magn Reson Imaging, 16, 99–106.

5 Khandani, A.H. and Semelka, R.C. (2005) Can the relation between gadopentetate dimeglumine and FDG uptake in colorectal liver metastases be used clinically? Radiology, 237, 1–2.

6 Braga, L., Semelka, R.C., Pietroborn, R. *et al.* (2004) Does hypervascularity of liver metastases as detected on MRI predict disease progression in breast cancer patients? AJR Am J Roentgenol, 182, 1207–1213.

7 Lee, C.H., Braga, L., de Campos, R.O., and Semelka, R.C. (2011) Hepatic tumor response evaluation by MRI. NMR Biomed, 24, 721–733.

8 Kierans, A.S., Elazzazi, M., Braga, L. *et al.* (2010) Thermoablative treatments for malignant liver lesions: 10-year experience of MRI appearances of treatment response. AJR Am J Roentgenol, 194, 523–529.

9 Braga, L., Guller, U., and Semelka, R.C. (2005) Pre-, peri-, posttreatment imaging of liver lesions. Radiol Clin North Am, 43, 915–927.

10 Braga, L., Semelka, R.C., Pedro, M.S., and de Barros, N. (2002) Post-treatment malignant liver lesions. MR imaging. Magn Reson Imaging Clin N Am, 10, 53–73.

CHAPTER 16

Liver trauma

Ersan Altun[1], Mohamed El-Azzazi[1,2,3,4], and Richard C. Semelka[1]

[1] The University of North Carolina at Chapel Hill, Department of Radiology, Chapel Hill, NC, USA
[2] University of Dammam, Department of Radiology, Dammam, Saudi Arabia
[3] King Fahd Hospital of the University, Department of Radiology, Khobar, Saudi Arabia
[4] University of Al Azhar, Department of Radiology, Cairo, Egypt

- Blunt and penetrating trauma.
- Blunt trauma is more common.
- Blunt trauma most commonly involves the right hepatic lobe as it constitutes the greatest volume of the liver. The posterior segment is the most commonly involved segment as it is susceptible to blunt impact (occasionally penetrating) from the ribs and spine and relative fixation of the liver by the coronary ligaments.
- **CT and MRI findings of hepatic injury:**
  1. **Laceration or fracture through the hepatic parenchyma:**
     - Contrast enhanced examinations are essential for the evaluation both on CT and MRI.
     - Appear as irregular linear, branching, or rounded areas of low attenuation within the normally enhancing liver on contrast enhanced CT images. These areas may not be detected on unenhanced CT images. They demonstrate mild to moderately high signal on precontrast T2-WI and low signal on T1-WI on MRI.
     - High-attenuation foci of freshly clotted blood may be seen in the areas of laceration on unenhanced and contrast enhanced CT images. These areas demonstrate variable MRI signal according to the age of blood products; however, they usually demonstrate high signal on precontrast T1-weighted images.
     - Lacerations commonly parallel the hepatic or portal venous vasculature and often extend to the periphery of the liver. They may have a configuration that has been termed the bear claw pattern due to its radiating, parallel, and jagged appearance.
     - On occasion, hepatic lacerations may demonstrate a branching pattern that superficially simulates the appearance of dilated bile ducts.
     - Lacerations extending into the perihilar region of the liver have an increased incidence of bile duct injury.
  2. **Intraparenchymal hematoma:**
     - They tend to be rounded or oval in configuration, and often display a central high-attenuation area of clotted blood surrounded by a larger low-attenuation region of lysed clot and contused liver parenchyma on unenhanced and contrast enhanced CT.
     - Hematomas demonstrate variable MRI signal on precontrast T1- and T2-WI according to the age of blood products. They commonly show heterogeneously increased T2 signal containing low signal intensity areas and heterogeneously low T1 signal containing high signal intensity areas (Figures 16.1 and 16.2). Layering blood products may be seen.
  3. **Subcapsular hematoma:**
     - Subcapsular hematomas usually appear as peripheral, well-marginated, lenticular, or crescent-shaped fluid collections that characteristically flatten or indent the underlying liver parenchyma (Figure 4.19).
     - On CT, the attenuation of the collection depends on the age of the hematoma, generally being of higher attenuation early when clotted blood is present and then decreasing in attenuation over time as clot lysis takes place.

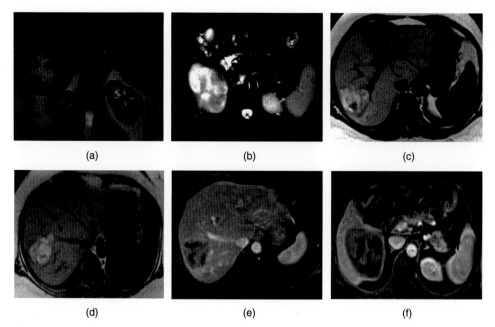

Figure 16.1 *Coronal T2-weighted SS-ETSE (a), transverse T2-weighted fat-suppressed SS-ETSE (b), T1-weighted out-of-phase (c) and in-phase (d) 2D-GE, T1-weighted postgadolinium fat-suppressed hepatic venous phase 3D-GE (e, f) images demonstrate posttraumatic hematoma in the right lobe of the liver. The* hematoma shows heterogeneously increased T2 signal (a, b) and prominently increased T1 signal (c, d) which represents blood products. The hematoma does not show enhancement. Compressed liver parenchyma shows mildly increased enhancement around the hematoma.

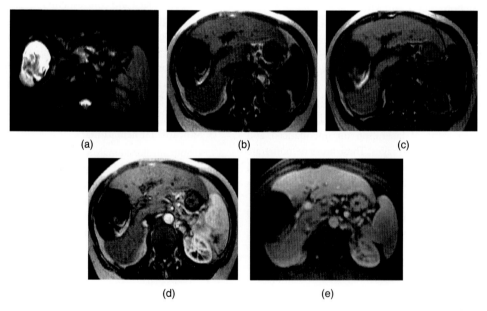

Figure 16.2 *Transverse fat-suppressed SS-ETSE (a), T1-weighted in-phase (b) and out-of-phase (c) 2D-GE, T1-weighted postgadolinium hepatic arterial dominant phase (d) and fat-suppressed hepatic venous phase 2D-GE (e) images show another posttraumatic fluid collection composed of hematoma–biloma complex in the right lobe of the liver. The blood products show low T2 signal (a) and high T1 (b, c) signal on precontrast images. This complex fluid collection does* not show any enhancement.

- MRI signal intensity features depend on the age of blood products and are similar to the characteristics of intra-parenchymal hematoma.
- **Five stages that reflect the age of hemorrhage on MRI have been described on the basis of the signal features of break-down products:**

  (a) Hyperacute; oxyhemoglobin is present, which does not have paramagnetic properties and appears as simple fluid (high signal on T2-and low signal on T1-weighted images.)

  (b) Acute, deoxyhemoglobin produces a strong effect on T2-weighted images (near signal void on T2 and low signal on T1-weighted images.)

  (c) Early subacute, intracellular methemoglobin still has a strong effect on T2-weighted images creating near signal void signal, and also has an effect on T1-weighted images, creating high signal intensity.

  (d) Late subacute extracellular methemoglobin causes high signal intensity on T1, and high signal on T2-weighted images.

  (e) Chronic hemorrhage is low signal intensity on T2-weighted and T1-weighted images due to hemosiderin and ferritin effects.
- Active bleeding can be shown as progressive accumulation of high signal or density resulting from the extravasation of gadolinium or iodine on serial post-gadolinium images or contrast enhanced CT.
- Subcapsular liver hematomas usually resolve in 6 to 8 weeks.
- Rarely, gas may be seen in areas of hepatic laceration or hematoma within 2 to 3 days following blunt abdominal trauma, which could be secondary to the trauma itself or due to underlying infection, ischemia, or necrosis.
- Periportal edema surrounding portal venous branches is frequently seen.
- Hemoperitoneum, which usually appears as high-density fluid on CT and high signal intensity fluid on T1-WI, may be seen.
- Bile duct injury may lead to collections of bile adjacent to the liver, termed *bilomas*, or free intraperitoneal leak of bile. Increasing amount of free fluid in the abdomen following liver trauma may represent intraperitoneal hemorrhage or bile leak.
- Grading of the liver trauma may be performed on CT and MRI findings.
- Associated findings of trauma, including the solid, vascular, and visceral organ injuries and bone injuries in the body should also be examined on CT and/or MRI.
- **Grading of liver trauma according to the American Association for the Surgery of Trauma:**
  1 **Grade I**
     - Hematoma: Subcapsular, <10% surface area
     - Laceration: Capsular tear, <1 cm parenchymal depth

2 **Grade II**
   - Hematoma: Subcapsular, 10–50% surface area
   - Hematoma: Intraparenchymal < 10 cm diameter
   - Laceration: Capsular tear, 1–3 cm parenchymal depth, <10 cm length

3 **Grade III**
   - Hematoma: Subcapsular, >50% surface area, or ruptured with active bleeding
   - Hematoma: Intraparenchymal > 10 cm diameter
   - Laceration: Capsular tear, >3 cm depth

4 **Grade IV**
   - Laceration: Parenchymal disruption involving 25–75% hepatic lobes or involving 1–3 Couinaud's segments

5 **Grade V**
   - Laceration: Parenchymal disruption involving >75% hepatic lobe or involving > 3 Couinaud's segments (within one lobe)
   - Vascular: Juxtahepatic venous injuries (IVC, major hepatic vein)

6 **Grade VI**
   - Vascular: Hepatic avulsion

- **Mimics of lacerations**
  ° Beam-hardening artifact from adjacent ribs can usually be recognized by their typical location, deep to an overlying rib, and by their tendency to fade centrally.
  ° Streak artifacts from air–contrast interfaces are more regular and linear in appearance than true lacerations.

References

1 Poletti, P.A., Mirvis, S.E., Shanmuganathan, K. *et al.* (2000) Ct criteria for management of blunt liver trauma: correlation with angiographic and surgical findings. Radiology, 216, 418–427.

2 McGehee, M., Kier, R., Cohn, S.M. *et al.* (1993) Comparison of MRI with postcontrast CT for the evaluation of acute abdominal trauma. J Comput Assist Tomogr, 17, 410–413.

3 Terk, M.R. and Rozenberg, D. (1998) Gadolinium-enhanced MR imaging of traumatic hepatic injury. AJR Am J Roentgenol, 171, 665–669.

4 Willmann, J.K., Ross, J.E., Platz, A. *et al.* (2002) Multidetector CT: detection of active hemorrhage in patients with blunt abdominal trauma. AJR Am J Roentgenol, 179, 437–444.

5 Patten, R.M., Gunberg, S.R., Bradenburger, D.K., and Richardson, M.L. (2000) CT detection of hepatic and splenic injuries: usefulness of liver window settings. AJR Am J Roentgenol, 175, 1107–1110.

6 Lubner, M., Menias, C., Rucker, C. *et al.* (2007) Blood in the belly: CT findings of hemoperitoneum. Radiographics, 27, 109–125.

7 Yoon, W., Jeong, J.J., Kim, J.K. *et al.* (2005) CT in blunt liver trauma. Radiographics, 25, 87–104.

Index